EMERGENCY MEDICINE CLINICS OF NORTH AMERICA

Bioterrorism

ROBERT G. DARLING, MD, FACEP,
JERRY L. MOTHERSHEAD, MD, FACEP,
JOSEPH F. WAECKERLE, MD, FACEP, and
EDWARD M. EITZEN, Jr., MD, MPH, FACEP, GUEST EDITORS

VOLUME 20 • NUMBER 2 • MAY 2002

W.B. SAUNDERS COMPANY
A Division of Elsevier Science
PHILADELPHIA LONDON TORONTO MONTREAL SYDNEY TOKYO

W.B. SAUNDERS COMPANY
A Division of Elsevier Science

The Curtis Center • Independence Square West • Philadelphia, Pennsylvania 19106

http://www.wbsaunders.com

EMERGENCY MEDICINE CLINICS	Volume 20, Number 2
OF NORTH AMERICA	ISSN 0733-8627
May 2002	ISBN 0-7216-0119-7
Editor: Karen Sorensen	

The ideas and opinions expressed in *Emergency Medicine Clinics of North America* do not necessarily reflect those of the Publisher. The Publisher does not assume any responsibility for any injury and/or damage to persons or property arising out of or related to any use of the material contained in this periodical. The reader is advised to check the appropriate medical literature and the product information currently provided by the manufacturer of each drug to be administered to verify the dosage, the method and duration of administration, or contraindications. It is the responsibility of the treating physician or other health care professional, relying on independent experience and knowledge of the patient, to determine drug dosages and the best treatment for the patient. Mention of any product in this issue should not be construed as endorsement by the contributors, editors, or the Publisher of the product or manufacturers' claims.

Emergency Medicine Clinics of North America (ISSN 0733-8627) is published quarterly by W.B. Saunders Company. Corporate and Editorial Offices: The Curtis Center, Independence Square West, Philadelphia, PA 19106-3399. Accounting and Circulation Offices: 6277 Sea Harbor Drive, Orlando, FL 32887-4800. Periodicals postage paid at Orlando, FL 32862, and additional mailing offices. Subscription prices are $149.00 per year (US individuals), $208.00 per year (US institutions), $198.00 per year (international individuals), $252.00 per year (international institutions), $179.00 per year (Canadian individuals), and $252.00 per year (Canadian institutions). International air speed delivery is included in all *Clinics*' subscription prices. All prices are subject to change without notice. POSTMASTER: Send address changes to *Emergency Medicine Clinics of North America*, W.B. Saunders Company, Periodicals Fulfillment, Orlando, FL 32887-4800. **Customer Service: 1-800-654-2452 (US). From outside of the US, call 1-407-345-4000.** E-mail: hhspcs@harcourt.com.

Emergency Medicine Clinics of North America is covered in *Index Medicus, Current Contents/Clinical Medicine, EMBASE/Excerpta Medica, BIOSIS, SciSearch, CINAHL, ISI/BIOMED,* and *Research Alert.*

Printed in the United States of America.

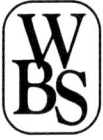

Emerg Med Clin N Am
20 (2002) iii

EMERGENCY
MEDICINE
CLINICS OF
NORTH AMERICA

Dedication

This book is dedicated to the innocent victims of terrorism who lost their lives during and after the events of September 11, 2001.

GUEST EDITORS

ROBERT G. DARLING, MD, FACEP, Captain, Medical Corps, Flight Surgeon, United States Navy; Medical Director, Aeromedical Isolation Team and Containment Care, Operational Medicine Division, US Army Medical Research Institute of Infectious Diseases (USAMRIID), Fort Detrick, Maryland; Adjunct Clinical Assistant Professor, Military and Emergency Medicine, Uniformed Services University of the Health Sciences (USUHS), Bethesda, Maryland

JERRY L. MOTHERSHEAD, MD, FACEP, Commander, Medical Corps, United States Navy; Senior Medical Consultant, Navy Medicine Office of Homeland Security; Specialty Leader, Emergency Medical Services and Prehospital Care, Navy Bureau of Medicine and Surgery; Chemical, Biological, Radiological, and Environmental Defense Officer, Navy Environmental Health Center, Norfolk, Virginia

JOSEPH F. WAECKERLE, MD, FACEP, Editor in Chief, *Annals of Emergency Medicine*; Chair, Department of Emergency Medicine, Baptist Medical Center, Menorah Medical Center and Research Medical Center; Clinical Professor, University of Missouri at Kansas City School of Medicine, Leawood, Kansas

EDWARD M. EITZEN, Jr., MD, MPH, FACEP, Colonel, Medical Corps, United States Army; Commander, US Army Medical Research Institute of Infectious Diseases (USAMRIID), Fort Detrick, Maryland; Adjunct Associate Professor of Pediatrics and Emergency Medicine, Uniformed Services University of the Health Sciences (USUHS), Bethesda, Maryland

CONTRIBUTORS

STEVEN M. BECKER, PhD, Director, Social/Behavioral and Public Policy Unit, Center for Disaster Preparedness; Assistant Professor of Public Health and Medicine, and Lister Hill Scholar in Health Policy, The University of Alabama at Birmingham, Birmingham, Alabama

DAVID M. BENEDEK, MD, Major, Medical Corps, United States Army; Chief, Forensic Psychiatry Service, Walter Reed Army Medical Center, Washington, DC

THOMAS H. BLACKWELL, MD, FACEP, Medical Director, The Center for Prehospital Medicine, Department of Emergency Medicine, Carolinas Medical Center, Charlotte, North Carolina

FREDERICK M. BURKLE, Jr., MD, MPH, FAAP, FACEP, Senior Scholar, Scientist and Visiting Professor, The Center for International Emergency, Disaster and Refugee Studies; Departments of Emergency Medicine and International Health, Schools of Medicine and Public Health, The Johns Hopkins University Medical Institutions, Baltimore, Maryland; Senior Medical and Public Health Advisor, Advanced

Systems Concept Office, Defense Threat Reduction Agency, Fort Belvior, Virginia; Captain, Medical Corps, United States Naval Reserve (Ret)

CHRISTINA L. CATLETT, MD, FACEP, Assistant Professor of Emergency Medicine, The Johns Hopkins School of Medicine; Deputy Director, The Johns Hopkins University Office of Critical Event Preparedness and Response, The Johns Hopkins University Medical Institutions, Baltimore, Maryland

THEODORE J. CIESLAK, MD, FAAP, Colonel, Medical Corps, Flight Surgeon, United States Army; Chairman, Department of Pediatrics, Brooke Army Medical Center, Fort San Houston, Texas; Adjunct Clinical Associate Professor of Pediatrics, Uniformed Services University of the Health Sciences (USUHS), Bethesda, Maryland

ROBERT G. DARLING, MD, FACEP, Captain, Medical Corps, Flight Surgeon, United States Navy; Medical Director, Aeromedical Isolation Team and Containment Care, Operational Medicine Division, US Army Medical Research Institute of Infectious Diseases (USAMRIID), Fort Detrick, Maryland; Adjunct Clinical Assistant Professor, Military and Emergency Medicine, Uniformed Services University of the Health Sciences (USUHS), Bethesda, Maryland

RICHARD G. DUKES, MD, Department of Emergency Medicine, Wayne State University School of Medicine and Detroit Medical Center, Detroit, Michigan

EDWARD M. EITZEN, Jr., MD, MPH, FACEP, Colonel, Medical Corps, United States Army; Commander, US Army Medical Research Institute of Infectious Diseases (USAMRIID), Fort Detrick, Maryland, Adjunct Associate Professor of Pediatrics and Emergency Medicine, Uniformed Services University of the Health Sciences (USUHS), Bethesda, Maryland

MORRIS FIELD, DO, Visiting Clinician, US Army Medical Research Institute of Infectious Diseases (USAMRIID), Operational Medicine Division, Fort Detrick, Maryland

GARY R. FLEISHER, MD, Chief, Division of Emergency Medicine; Interim Physician in Chief, Children's Hospital; Professor of Pediatrics, Harvard Medical School, Boston, Massachusetts

LYNN K. FLOWERS, MD, MHA, FACEP, Lieutenant Commander, Medical Corps, United States Navy; EMS Fellow, The Center for Prehospital Medicine, Department of Emergency Medicine, Carolinas Medical Center, Charlotte, North Carolina

DAVID R. FRANZ, DVM, PhD, Vice President, Chemical and Biological Defense Division, Southern Research Institute; Research Professor, Department of Emergency Medicine, University of Alabama at Birmingham, Birmingham, Alabama

MARY J. R. GILCHRIST, PhD, Director, University Hygienic Laboratory, University of Iowa, Iowa City, Iowa

FRED M. HENRETIG, MD, FACEP, Professor of Pediatrics and Emergency Medicine, Division of Emergency Medicine, Children's Hospital of Philadelphia; Director, Section of Clinical Toxicology, Children's Hospital of Philadelphia; Medical Director, Philadelphia Poison Control Center, Philadelphia, Pennsylvania

HARRY C. HOLLOWAY, MD, Professor of Psychiatry and Neuroscience, Department of Psychiatry, Uniformed Services University of the Health Sciences (USUHS), Bethesda, Maryland

KERMIT D. HUEBNER, MD, Captain, Medical Corps, United States Army; Chief Resident, Emergency Medicine Residency Program, Darnall Army Community Hospital, Fort Hood, Texas

DAVID G. JARRETT, MD, FACEP, Colonel, Medical Corps, Flight Surgeon, United States Army; Doctrine Development, Operational Medicine Division, US Army Medical Research Institute of Infectious Diseases (USAMRIID), Fort Detrick, Maryland

JESSICA JONES, MD, Associate Fellow, Department of Medicine, University of Alabama at Birmingham; VA National Quality Scholars Program, Birmingham VA Medical Center, Birmingham, Alabama

KRISTI L. KOENIG, MD, FACEP, National Director, Emergency Management Strategic Healthcare Group, Veterans Health Administration, Department of Veterans Affairs; Clinical Professor of Emergency Medicine, George Washington University School of Medicine and Health Sciences, Washington, DC

MARK G. KORTEPETER, MD, MPH, FACP, Lieutenant Colonel, Medical Corps, United States Army; Chief, Medical Division, US Army Medical Research Institute of Infectious Diseases (USAMRIID), Fort Detrick, Maryland

GREGORY J. MORAN, MD, FACEP, Associate Professor of Medicine, UCLA School of Medicine, Department of Emergency Medicine and Division of Infectious Diseases, Olive View-UCLA Medical Center, Sylmar, California

JERRY L. MOTHERSHEAD, MD, FACEP, Commander, United States Navy; Senior Medical Consultant, Navy Medicine Office of Homeland Security; Specialty Leader, Emergency Medical Services and Prehospital Care, Navy Bureau of Medicine and Surgery; Chemical, Biological, Radiological, and Environmental Defense Officer, Navy Environmental Health Center, Norfolk, Virginia

DONALD L. NOAH, DVM, MPH, DACVPM, Lieutenant Colonel, United States Air Force; Chief, Epidemiology and Public Health, Operational Medicine Division, US Army Medical Research Institute of Infectious Diseases (USAMRIID), Fort Detrick, Maryland

GARY D. OSWEILER, DVM, PhD, MS, Professor and Director, Veterinary Diagnostic and Production Animal Medicine, Iowa State University Veterinary Diagnostic Laboratory, Ames, Iowa

JULIE A. PAVLIN, MD, MPH, Lieutenant Colonel, Medical Corps, United States Army; Chief, Strategic Surveillance, Department of Defense Global Emerging Infections Surveillance and Response System, Silver Spring, Maryland

CARL H. SCHULTZ, MD, FACEP, Director, EMS and Disaster Medicine Fellowship, Department of Emergency Medicine, University of California – Irvine Medical Center; Professor of Emergency Medicine, UCI College of Medicine, Irvine, California

THOMAS E. TERNDRUP, MD, FACEP, Professor and Chair, Department of Emergency Medicine; Director, Center for Disaster Preparedness, University of Alabama at Birmingham, Birmingham, Alabama

KEVIN TONAT, DrPH, MPH, Captain, United States Public Health Service; Director, Division of Program Development, Office of Emergency Preparedness, Department of Health and Human Services, Washington, DC

JOSEPH F. WAECKERLE, MD, FACEP, Editor in Chief, *Annals of Emergency Medicine*; Chair, Department of Emergency Medicine, Baptist Medical Center, Menorah Medical Center and Research Medical Center; Clinical Professor, University of Missouri at Kansas City School of Medicine, Leawood, Kansas

SUZANNE R. WHITE, MD, FACEP, Associate Professor of Emergency Medicine and Pediatrics, Wayne State University School of Medicine; Medical Director, Children's Hospital of Michigan Regional Poison Control Center, Detroit, Michigan

NEAL E. WOOLLEN, DVM, PhD, Major, Veterinary Corps, United States Army; Diagnostic Systems Division, US Army Medical Research Institute of Infectious Diseases (USAMRIID), Fort Detrick, Maryland

JAMES A. ZIMBLE, MD, Vice Admiral, United States Navy (Ret); President, Uniformed Services University of the Health Sciences (USUHS), Bethesda, Maryland

CONTENTS

efforts to find solutions to what could become a catastrophic public health disaster. Management options are becoming more robust, as are reliable detection devices and rapid access to stockpiled antibiotics and vaccines. There is much to be done, however, especially in the organizing, warehousing, and granting/exercising authority for resource allocations. The introduction of these new options should encourage one to believe that, in time, evolving standards of care will make it possible to rethink the currently unthinkable consequences.

continue to be enhanced, building on existing structures, to provide emergency mitigation and relief in the event of such an attack. This article discusses the various federal initiatives and programs targeting bioterrorism preparedness and response, and outlines the current framework for overall federal response to bioterrorism.

Bioterrorism represents one of the great challenges of our day. Fortunately, recent advances in biotechnology promise new developments in clinical and laboratory diagnostics, recombinant vaccines, antiviral drugs, and environmental detection. This article discusses some of the latest advances and future challenges in responding to bioterrorism.

FORTHCOMING ISSUES

RECENT ISSUES

VISIT OUR WEB SITE

For more information about Clinics:
http://www.wbsaunders.com

The *Emergency Medicine Clinics of North America* Continuing Medical Education program is planned and produced in accordance with the Accreditation Council for Continuing Medical Education (ACCME) essentials through joint sponsorship of the University of Virginia School of Medicine and W.B. Saunders. The University of Virginia School of Medicine is accredited by the ACCME to provide continuing medical education for physicians.

GOAL

The goal of *Emergency Medicine Clinics of North America* is to keep practicing physicians and residents up to date with current clinical practice in pediatrics by providing timely articles reviewing the state-of-the-art in patient care.

OBJECTIVES

After reading this issue of *Emergency Medicine Clinics of North America*, Physicians will be able to:

- Review agents that can be used as biological weapons.
- Define the CDC categorization system for potential biological weapons.
- Describe the clinical presentation of infections caused by biological weapons.
- Review the diagnostic methods and treatments of infections caused by biological weapons.
- Explain the role of the emergency department in bioterrorism events.

ACCREDITATION

The *Emergency Medicine Clinics of North America* is planned and implemented in accordance with the Essential Areas and Policies of the Accreditation Council for Continuing Medical Education (ACCME) through the joint sponsorship of the University of Virginia School of Medicine and WB Saunders Company. The University of Virginia School of Medicine is accredited by the ACCME to provide continuing medical education for physicians.

The University of Virginia School of Medicine designates this continuing medical education activity for up to 90 credit hour(s) per year (15 hours per issue/test) in category 1 credit toward the AMA Physician's Recognition Award. Each physician should claim only those hours of credit that he/she actually spent in the educational activity.

Category 1 credit can be earned by reading the text material, taking the CME examination, and completing the evaluation. All answers need to be recorded on the answer sheet. Credit will be awarded upon attainment of a score of 80% of higher.

FACULTY DISCLOSURE

Disclosure of faculty financial affiliations: As a provider accredited by the Accreditation Council for Continuing Medical Education, the Office of Continuing Medical Education of the University of Virginia School of Medicine must insure balance, independence, objectivity and scientific rigor in all its individually sponsored or jointly sponsored educational activities. All faculty participating in a sponsored activity are expected to disclose to the activity audience any significant financial interest or other relationship (1) with the manufacturer(s) of any commercial product(s) and/or provider(s) of commercial services discussed in an educational presentation and (2) with any commercial supporters of the activity (significant financial interest or other relationship can include such things as grants or research support, employee, consultant, major stock holder, member of speakers bureau, etc.). The intent of this disclosure is not to prevent a speaker with a significant financial or other relationship from making a presentation, but rather to provide listeners with information on which they can make their own judgements. It remains for the audience to determine whether the speaker's interests or relationships may influence the presentation with regard to exposition or conclusion.

The faculty presenters listed below have identified no professional or financial affiliations related to their presentation: Marcel J. Casavant, MD; Joseph A. Congeni, MD; Philomenia J. Dias, MBBS, MD; Amanda J. Gruber, MD; Richard B. Heyman, MD; Steven L. Jaffe, MD; Jonathan D. Klein, MD, MPH; John R. Knight, MD; Cheryl M. Kodjo, MD, MPH; Patricia K. Kokotailo, MD, MPH; Stephen C. Koesters, MD; Sharon Levy, MD; Stephen F. Miller, MD; Harrison P. Pope, Jr., MD, MPH; Peter D. Rogers, MD, MPH; Victor C. Strasburger, MD; and, Brigid L. Vaughan, MD.

Disclosure of discussion of non-FDA approved uses for pharmaceutical products and/or medical devices: The University of Virginia School of Medicine, as an ACCME provider, requires that all faculty presenters identify and disclose any "off label" uses for pharmaceutical and medical device products. The University of Virginia School of Medicine recommends that each physician fully review all the available data on new products or procedures prior to instituting them with patients.

The faculty who provided disclosures have indicated that they will not be discussing off-label uses.

The faculty presenters listed below have not provided disclosure or off-label information: Robert T. Brown, MD; Chrisitiana R. Rajasingham, MD; Deborah R. Simkin, MD, and Molissa Weddle, MD, MPH

TO ENROLL

To enroll in the *Emergency Medicine Clinics of North America* Continuing Medical Education Program, call customer service at **1-800-654-2452**. The CME program is available to subscribers for an additional annual fee of $176.00.

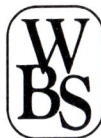

EMERGENCY
MEDICINE
CLINICS OF
NORTH AMERICA

Emerg Med Clin N Am
20 (2002) xvii–xviii

Foreword

Bioterrorism

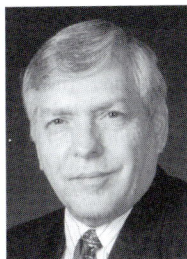

James A. Zimble, MD

The end of the Cold War and the perceived geographic protection afforded by two large oceans have engendered complacency among the American citizenry concerning the collective safety of those within our "island" nation. Until recently, the public has been relatively oblivious to the possibility of an imminent terrorist threat. Acts of terror occur somewhere else ... on the other side of the Atlantic or Pacific. There had been no act of war on continental U.S. soil since the War of 1812. Even the explosion at the World Trade Center in 1993 and the wanton destruction of the Murrah Federal Building in 1995 did little to shake that sense of well-being. This sense of protection and security was suddenly, violently, and irrevocably shattered by the multiple terrorist attacks of September 11, 2001 ..."9-1-1" events that have surely raised the public's sense of apprehension. Since then, the public has become considerably aware that it really *can* happen here.

Subsequent to the September 11th event, the delivery of letters laden with anthrax spores to media and governmental representatives by the U.S. Postal Service led to unprecedented fear and illness and death, considerable expense and significant disruption of our daily lives. These latter events further underscored our vulnerability to terrorist acts and raised public anxiety to unparalleled levels. Before those mailings, the deliberate use of a biological agent as a weapon of terror was considered by many to be so "morally repugnant" and difficult to accomplish as to be a near impossibility.

The recognition that citizens and visitors residing in the continental United States might well be exposed to terrorism, including the employment of *biowarfare*, has abruptly become all-too-real. America has received its "wake-up call." Protection from and response to weapons of mass destruction are now the highest of priorities for federal, state and local officials, and emergency planners. Readiness and capability to respond is "topic A" in the media. Communities across the country are engaged in building the expertise, obtaining the resources, and developing the plans necessary to effectively respond.

Fire fighters, police, and emergency medical technicians are considered the traditional first-responders to those abrupt acts of terror caused by fire, explosion, or dispersal of a chemical or radiological agent. The consequences of such events are immediate, readily discerned, and well defined in scope. Not so, however, with the biological weapon. In the event of a deliberate introduction of a biological agent, emergency health care professionals (EHCP) will likely be the "first responders." The initial effects of such an attack will be delayed, insidious, and difficult to distinguish from a naturally occurring event. EHCPs must therefore be astute enough to identify those patients whose signs and symptoms or whose frequency of occurrence are extraordinary presentations of such an abhorrent event. The EHCP will be confronted with conditions either never taught, or only superficially and briefly addressed in school, and only rarely, if ever are a part of the routine of emergency medical practice. He or she must be able to recognize a possible evolving bioterrorist event, discern the responsible agent, quickly initiate appropriate therapy, and rapidly mobilize resources necessary to contain the incident and manage its myriad consequences.

One cornerstone of preparedness is education and training. This volume of the *Emergency Medicine Clinics of North America* is an exceptional treatise to begin that preparation. It presents the myriad clinical and operational facets of bioterrorism. Use it as a tutorial, reference, and teaching guide. With the unfortunate possibility of another dreadful act of bioterrorism being ever present, this monograph will be invaluable in helping the emergency health care professional appropriately and effectively mitigate its consequences.

James A. Zimble, MD
President, Uniformed Services
University of the Health Sciences (USUHS)
Vice Admiral, United States Navy (Ret)
4301 Jones Bridge Road
Bethesda, MD 20814

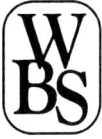

EMERGENCY
MEDICINE
CLINICS OF
NORTH AMERICA

Emerg Med Clin N Am
20 (2002) xix–xxi

Preface

Bioterrorism

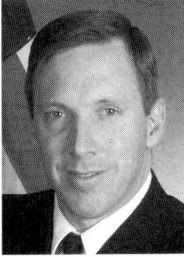

Robert G. Darling, MD, FACEP

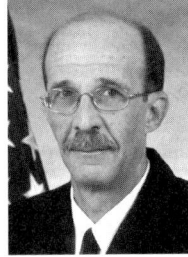

Jerry L. Mothershead, MD, FACEP

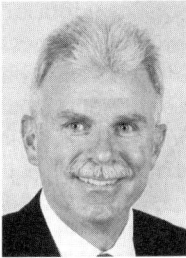

Joseph F. Waeckerle, MD, FACEP

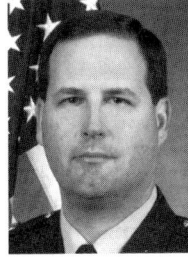

Edward M. Eitzen, Jr., MD, MPH, FACEP

Guest Editors

Few events in American history have so traumatized and galvanized a nation as the events of September 11, 2001, and the subsequent acts of bioterrorism involving weaponized anthrax spores. Those of us who have been working in the field of defense against weapons of mass destruction had been deeply concerned about these threats and our vulnerabilities, even before those horrific attacks. Since Operation Desert Storm, this unease has evolved from a battlefield focus to include terrorist use of these weapons against our homeland. Many of us maintained the hope that the use of such weapons by even the most determined enemy was highly unlikely for a number of reasons. First, despite occasional media reports to the contrary, production of biological weapons that could produce massive casualties was considered beyond the capability of most terrorists unless they were well funded or had state sponsorship. Secondly, their use was considered so heinous that only the most uncivilized adversary would even consider their deployment. Finally, any attack against the United States or its citizens would most assuredly have resulted in the most severe of retaliatory actions.

Unfortunately, the events of and since September 11th have shredded these hopes and perceptions. Our enemies appear determined to strike us in anyway that they can—regardless of the consequences. The behavior of anthrax spores released from sealed letters was also unexpected, and we realize now more than ever how much research and preparation needs to be accomplished in the areas of standoff detection, personal protection, laboratory analysis, decontamination, prophylaxis, treatment and finally education and training.

It is hoped that this collection of papers will serve as an essential resource for medical and public health professionals—including public health practitioners, epidemiologists, physicians, nurses, physician assistants, and other allied health care providers and emergency medical responders—who would seek to improve their ability to counter acts of biological terrorism. Much of what is contained herein may also be of value to governmental officials and non-medical emergency planners in understanding the complexities of bioterrorism preparedness and response. Mitigating disasters always requires an integrated horizontal and vertical approach involving diverse response elements. Unlike in most disasters, however, primary care and emergency providers will be the sentinels, and the health care community will serve as the vanguard, in the response to an attack using biological agents.

This issue of the *Emergency Medicine Clinics of North America* begins with a historical discussion of biological weapons and the evolution of the threat from the early nineteenth century to the present. Next we discuss the agents of bioterrorism. Although there are several ways to classify biological agents, we elected to review the Centers for Disease Control and Prevention's classification scheme according to their "Critical Biological Agents threat list—Categories A, B and C." Category A agents pose the greatest threat to our medical and public health systems and are therefore reviewed in some depth. Next we discuss the role of the laboratory and some of the unique medical management issues pertaining to bioterrorism. We include an interesting article that describes an algorithmic approach to managing suspected victims of bioterrorism. A separate chapter is devoted entirely to emergency mental health management. Most mental health professionals predict, and research supports, that psychological casualties will vastly outnumber those patients truly exposed to a biological weapon and may be difficult, if not impossible, to differentiate. The immediate and long-term psychological toll on the community and responders will also be severe. Deliberate planning will be necessary if we are to mount an effective response. Equally important, we must prospectively address the difficulties in the triage of thousands of patients. In his scholarly paper, Dr. Burkle argues that effective management of such an evolving disaster can only be achieved through the employment of principles and practices that are relatively alien to the health care community. A series of articles explores the many operational issues in preparing for and responding to bioterrorism events in the emergency department and hospital, and at the local, state, and federal levels. We conclude with a discussion of the profound future challenges to our efforts to stay one step ahead of those who wish us harm.

These challenges are indeed great. Fortunately, we are blessed with strong leadership at the highest levels of government. With their guidance, the determined efforts of scientists, physicians, the emergency response community, and a people united, we will overcome this threat to our way of life. We as a nation have overcome more serious threats that would have surely caused lesser societies to fall. I am confident that with our determination, ingenuity and solidarity, America will conquer this challenge as well.

I express my thanks and gratitude to the contributing authors who provided the scholarly input into each of their well-written articles. I also thank my coeditors Dr. Joseph Waeckerle and Dr. Edward Eitzen, who provided valuable insight and editorial critique. Special thanks go to my coeditor and good friend Dr. Jerry Mothershead. Without his incredible work ethic, writing, and editorial acumen and his encyclopedic knowledge of the field of disaster medicine, this project would have taken many more months to complete and would have been of far lesser quality.

Robert G. Darling, MD, FACEP
Guest Editor
Medical Director
Aeromedical Isolation Team and Containment Center
Operational Medicine Division
United States Army Medical Research
Institute of Infectious Diseases (USAMRIID)
1425 Porter Street
Fort Detrick, MD 21702-5011

Adjunct Clinical Assistant Professor of Military
and Emergency Medicine
Uniformed Services University of the Health Sciences (USUHS)
4301 Jones Bridge Road
Bethesda, MD 20814

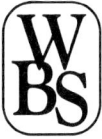

EMERGENCY
MEDICINE
CLINICS OF
NORTH AMERICA

Emerg Med Clin N Am
20 (2002) 255–271

The history and threat of biological warfare and terrorism

Donald L. Noah, DVM, MPH, DACVPM[a,*],
Kermit D. Huebner, MD[b], Robert G. Darling, MD,
FACEP[c], Joseph F. Waeckerle, MD, FACEP[d]

[a]US Air Force, Chief, Epidemiology and Public Health Department,
Operational Medicine Division, US Army Medical Research Institute of Infectious Diseases,
Fort Detrick, MD, USA
[b]US Army, Emergency Medicine Residency Program, Darnall Army Community Hospital,
36000 Darnall Loop, Fort Hood, TX 76544, USA
[c]Captain (Flight Surgeon), United States Navy, Medical Director, Aeromedical Isolation
Team and Containment Care; Operational Medicine Division, US Army Medical Research
Institute of Infectious Diseases (USAMRIID), 1425 Porter Street,
ATTN: MCMR-UIM-O, Fort Detrick, MD 21702-5011, USA
[d]University of Missouri at Kansas City, School of Medicine,
4601 West 143rd Street, Leawood, KS 66224, USA

"Until bioterrorism's true nature as an epidemic disease event is fully recognized, our nation's preparedness programs will continue to be inadequately designed: the wrong first responders will be trained and equipped; we will fail to fully build the critical infrastructure we need to detect and respond; the wrong research agendas will be developed; and we will never effectively grapple with the long-term consequence management needs that such an event would entail."

— Dr. Margaret Hamburg, in testimony to the US House Committee on Government Reform, 23 July 2001

"...more than ever we risk substantial surprise."

— Mr. George Tenet, Director of Central Intelligence, in testimony to the US Senate Select Committee on Intelligence regarding the global threat from weapons of mass destruction, 2 February 2000

* Corresponding author.
E-mail address: Noahd@mail.policy.osd.mil (D.L. Noah).

The opinions and assertions contained herein are the private views of the authors and are not to be construed as official or as necessarily reflecting the views of the Department of Defense or the US Army Medical Research Institute of Infectious Diseases.

New weapons have emerged in our modern world that demand our attention. Preeminent among them are biological warfare agents. Before the recent anthrax incidents there was very little experience with actual bioweapon use in our country. This is no longer true—Americans have suffered and died. Even with these tragic terrorists' actions, however, America's experience with bioterrorism has been with small, isolated events not indicating the true potential enormity and seriousness of bioagents.

Biological weapons are a formidable challenge. The use of a bioagent as a weapon is a multidimensional problem because of the diversity of bioagents (each with particular threat characteristics), the plethora of vulnerable targets, and the varied routes of dissemination. There are no typical presentations and no easily recognizable signatures to allow early detection or identification of a bioagent. There are limited treatment options and a disturbing array of significant consequences. Biological warfare can decimate a large population. It can destabilize a nation. As evidenced by recent events, bioterrorism can inflict enormous psychologic and economic hardship and political unrest by attacking small populations in multiple sites over a protracted period.

A biological attack on America will impose unparalleled demands on all aspects of our government and our societal infrastructure. Although the probability of such an attack is difficult to measure, America will be at great risk should a bioweapon be used. This risk must not be dismissed. To do so is to ignore man's history of warfare and, more importantly, to ignore the uncertainty of the future.

The medical and public health communities are the cornerstone of America's preparation and response to a bioweapons incident. They are essential to this effort and must be involved early in developing and implementing a comprehensive national strategy. Medical and public health professionals will benefit from understanding the history of the use of biological agents during times of war and as weapons of terror. We must learn from the past to prepare for the future. In addition, medical professionals can better appreciate the challenges of preparation if they have some understanding of the assessment and analysis of the threats and risks. This article begins with a historical summary of the use of biological agents and ends with a discussion of the current threat and the United States' vulnerability to attack.

Historical summary

Early examples

One of the first recorded uses of a biological agent in warfare occurred in 184 BC. Carthaginian soldiers lead by Hannibal were preparing for a naval battle against King Eumenes of Perganum. Hannibal ordered that earthen pots be filled with "serpents of every kind." During the battle, Carthaginians hurled these pots onto the decks of Perganum ships. Initially humored by the earthen pots launched as ammunition, the Perganum soldiers soon found themselves battling an additional enemy and Hannibal lead the Carthaginians to victory [1].

During the Middle Ages, Gabriel de Mussis, a notary, recorded the attack of the Tatars on the city of Caffa, a well-fortified, Genoese-controlled port (now Feodosiya, Ukraine). He described how Tatar soldiers surrounded the city and placed it under siege. De Mussis noted that the Tatars were fatigued by a "plague and pestiferous disease" and ordered "cadavers placed on their hurling machines" and catapulted into the city where the inhabitants "died wildly" [2]. It is unknown if the catapulted bodies led to the development of plague in Caffa or if this was a coincident event. The tactic of hurling bodies of dead plague victims over city walls occurred in other conflicts and was also reportedly used by Russian troops battling Swedish forces in 1710 [3].

Smallpox, historically one of humankind's most dreaded diseases, was used as a weapon on several occasions during the fifteenth and eighteenth centuries. In the fifteenth century, Pizarro presented indigenous peoples of South America with variola-contaminated clothing. This also occurred during the French and Indian Wars of 1754–1767 when Sir Jeffery Amherst ordered the provision of smallpox-laden blankets to indigenous Indians loyal to the French. The resulting epidemic lead to the loss of Fort Carillon to the English. In 1763 at Fort Pitt, Captain Ecuyer of the Royal Americans, fearing an attack from Native Americans, acquired two variola virus-contaminated blankets and a handkerchief from a smallpox hospital and distributed them to the Native Americans in a false gesture of goodwill. The unsuspecting Indians accepted the gifts and several outbreaks of smallpox occurred in various tribes in the Ohio Region [1]. Having knowledge of these effects on the outcome of military campaigns, General George Washington ordered the Continental Army to undergo variolation, a process of active immunization using live smallpox virus taken from the lesions of infected victims [4]. Approximately 1 in 200 vaccinates developed full-blown smallpox as a result of this procedure [5].

Pre-World War II era

World War I saw the use of chemical warfare agents to break the stalemates of trench warfare. There was also a lesser-known biological weapons campaign carried out to disrupt the supply and mobility of forces. It has been reported that Germany shipped horses and cattle inoculated with *Bacillus anthracis* and *Pseudomonas pseudomallei* to the United States and other countries. The Germans were also suspected of similarly infecting sheep in Romania that were to be shipped to Russia. Cultures confiscated from the German Legation in Romania in 1916 were identified as *B. anthracis* and *P. pseudomallei* at the Bucharest Institute of Bacteriology and Pathology. In 1917 a German saboteur was arrested in Mesopotamia after infecting 4500 mules with glanders. Germany was also accused of spreading cholera in Italy and plague in St. Petersburg, Russia in 1915. These accusations were denied and in 1924 a subcommittee of the League of Nations curiously found no evidence of the use of bacterial agents in World War I [1]. Signed in 1925, the Protocol for the Prohibition of the Use in War of Asphyxiating, Poisonous, or Other Gases and of Bacteriological Methods of Warfare, otherwise known as the Geneva Protocol, was the first multilateral agreement extending prohibition of chemical and biological agents [6]. Although a landmark event in the international process of limiting the production and use of biological weapons, its long-term effectiveness was nil because it contained no provision for verification inspections. Many countries ratified the treaty while stipulating the right of retaliation, and others, such as the United States, did not ratify the treaty until 1975 [7].

World War II

The modern era of biological weapons development began immediately before and during World War II. The Japanese began one of history's most notorious biological weapons programs in 1932, and numerous human experiments were conducted at the infamous Unit 731 throughout the war. Located near Pingfan, Manchuria, Unit 731 sprawled across 150 buildings, 5 satellite camps, and had a staff of more than 3000 scientists and technicians [7].

In October 1940, Japanese planes scattered *Yersinia pestis*-contaminated rice and fleas over the city of Shusien in Chekiang province. This was followed by an outbreak of bubonic plague in this region where it had not been previously recorded. At least 11 similar flights over other Chinese cities occurred and, although suspicion for the intentional spread of plague was high, there was a failure to associate disease outbreaks with the materials dropped by the Japanese planes. Unit 731 allegedly used at least 3000 prisoners of war (including Chinese, Koreans, Mongolians, Soviets, Americans, British, and Australians) for experimentation with biological agents [8]. Of these, more than 1000 were estimated to have died following experiments using anthrax, botulism, brucellosis, cholera, dysentery, gas gangrene, meningococcal infection, and plague. These allegations were supported during a military tribunal held in the former Soviet Union in December 1949. Twelve Japanese soldiers, including the Commander in Chief of the Japanese Kwantang Army, testified that no fewer than 600 prisoners were killed annually at Unit 731 [9].

The German Minister of Propaganda, Dr. Joseph Goebbels, accused the British of attempting to introduce yellow fever into India by transporting infected mosquitoes from West Africa. Although this specific accusation was unfounded, the British in fact had been performing trials with *Bacillus anthracis* on Gruinard Island off the coast of Scotland. These trials, consisting of the detonation of numerous bomblets containing viable anthrax spores, left the island heavily contaminated until successful decontamination was accomplished in 1986 using formaldehyde and seawater [10]. Consistent with US doctrine at the time, it has been reported that Winston Churchill seriously considered using anthrax in retaliation had Nazi Germany used biological agents against Britain [1].

The US offensive biological weapons program

The US offensive biological weapons program began in 1942 with the establishment of the War Research Service, a civilian agency that conducted research and development at Camp Detrick, Maryland. Drawing on information gleaned from Japanese scientists from Unit 731, who were controversially granted full immunity from war crimes tribunals, testing sites were created in Mississippi and Utah and a production facility was started at Terre Haute, Indiana. Pre-production testing at this facility, using *Bacillus subtilis* as a simulant, however, revealed shortfalls in safety procedures that precluded mass production. Although approximately 5000 anthrax bombs were prepared at Camp Detrick, none were used during the war [1]. Although research and development efforts continued, this facility was later converted to a civilian commercial pharmaceutical plant.

During the Korean War, the American program was expanded and another production facility was constructed at Pine Bluff, Arkansas. Research continued on proper production and storage techniques, methods of deployment, the effects of climate and ultraviolet radiation, and the behavior of aerosols dispersed over large areas that included the use of simulant agents in and around US cities during 1949–1968 [7]. During this war, the United States was accused by the Soviet Union, China, and North Korea of using biological warfare agents against North Korea and China [11]. Although it was later revealed as a propaganda event, a group of international scientists met in 1952 and concluded that tests of biological weapons were being conducted by the United States against the two countries. As a further illustration of the fallacy of these allegations, a letter was discovered in the Archives of the Polish Academy of Science that contained a request from the Korean government that Polish financial assistance be redirected to pay for clothing instead of the sera and vaccines they had been receiving [12].

In 1953 research was begun on defensive aspects of biological agents and studies were performed to evaluate the effectiveness of vaccines, chemoprophylaxes, and therapeutic regimens. Following Congressional approval in 1954, "Project Whitecoat" was initiated to further these defensive efforts. Volunteer members of the Seventh Day Adventist Church, who wished to serve the United States without taking up arms, were exposed (under informed consent) to aerosols of *Francisella tularensis* and *Coxiella burnetii*. Although some of these volunteers certainly became ill, no deaths occurred and all recovered fully [1].

In July of 1969, Great Britain submitted a recommendation to the Conference of the Committee on Disarmament prohibiting the "development, production, and stockpiling of bacteriological and toxic weapons" [13]. In September of that year, the Soviet Union recommended a disarmament convention to the United Nations General Assembly. On November 25, 1969,

President Nixon signed an Executive Order that changed the US policy on biological warfare. At Fort Detrick, Maryland he announced that the US offensive program would be terminated and that only small research quantities of agents would be retained for continued use in the defensive program to develop appropriate biological protective measures, diagnostic procedures, and therapeutics. A new laboratory was opened in 1971 and was named the US Army Medical Research Institute of Infectious Diseases (USAMRIID). Between May 1971 and May 1972 all antipersonnel biological warfare stocks were destroyed under the supervision of the Department of Agriculture, Department of Health, Education, and Welfare, and the Departments of Natural Resources of the states of Arkansas, Colorado, and Maryland. The production facility at Pine Bluff, Arkansas was converted to a civilian toxicologic research laboratory [1].

The 1972 Biological Weapons Convention

The Convention on the Prohibition of the Development, Production, and Stockpiling of Bacteriological and Toxin Weapons and their Destruction, otherwise known as the 1972 Biological Weapons Convention, was designed to stop the proliferation of biological agents as weapons and to destroy current stockpiles internationally. This agreement has been signed and ratified by at least 140 nations [14] and calls for nations to never develop, produce, stockpile, or otherwise acquire or retain microbial or other biological agents or toxins, whatever their origin or method of production, of types and in quantities that have no justification for prophylactic, protective, or other peaceful purposes, and weapons, equipment, or means of delivery designed to use such agents or toxins for hostile purposes or in armed conflict [6]. The agreement went into effect in 1975, however, there have been difficulties with verification and interpretation of "defensive" research. Under this agreement, each country was required to submit a list of all facilities, scientific conferences at these facilities, exchange of information on biological warfare agents, and disease outbreaks. There was no direct oversight by outside nations and the Security Council maintained the right to veto any request for an investigation if an alleged infraction occurred. There are on-going international efforts to address these shortcomings and to produce a lasting agreement that deters the proliferation of offensive biological weapons while protecting the pursuit of legitimate public and private biological science.

The Soviets and biological weapons

In April 1979 an outbreak of inhalational anthrax was reported near a heavily guarded facility at the Soviet Institute of Microbiology and Virology at Sverdlovsk, USSR. The 77 identified cases, including 66 deaths, comprise the largest reported epidemic of inhalational anthrax [7]. At the time, the Soviet government explained that the epidemic resulted from the improper handling of food by black marketeers, who had allowed meat contaminated with anthrax to be distributed in the region. This explanation raised concern in the United States because the type of anthrax reported results from the inhalation of anthrax spores, not from their ingestion. In 1992, after epidemiologic evidence had mounted to debunk the tainted meat theory, Russian President Boris Yeltsin finally admitted that the outbreak was the result of military developments and that there had indeed been an accidental release of anthrax spores from a secret biological warfare facility [15]. He also revealed that the country had conducted extensive research on the offensive use of biological warfare agents and had not destroyed previously existing stockpiles as directed by the 1972 Biological Weapons Convention. President Yeltsin subsequently outlawed all activities that were in disagreement with the 1972 Biological Weapons Convention and a separate "Trilateral Agreement" was eventually reached between the United States, the United Kingdom, and the Soviet Union.

The defection of Dr. Kanatjan Alibekov (later changed to Ken Alibek), second in command at the huge civilian biological warfare research organization "Biopreparat," led to further revelations of the secret yet massive Soviet biological weapons program. Dr. Alibek revealed to the United States that soon after signing the 1972 Biological Weapons Convention, the Soviets began willfully violating it. At one point, the Soviets used as many as 50,000 scientists and technicians, and had over 40 facilities devoted to the research or production of offensive biological weapons [16]. After the dissolution of the Soviet Union in 1989, many of these facilities went into disrepair and many of the previously well-paid scientists became unemployed. There are grave concerns that many of these scientists may make themselves available for hire to third world countries or sub-national groups to develop biological weapons programs and that stores of biological agents, including smallpox, may have been smuggled out of the country and into the hands of these subversive factions.

The Gulf War

During Operations Desert Shield/Desert Storm, there was speculation that the Iraqi government possessed biological weapons and would use them against Allied Coalition troops. This fear was bolstered by the fact Iraq had used chemical weapons against Iranian soldiers and its own Kurdish minority in northern Iraq some years earlier. Although there is no evidence that biological agents were used against Allied troops, speculation about Iraq's offensive biological warfare capability continued to mount. United Nations Special Commission Teams inspected Iraq for this evidence and the Iraqi government eventually admitted that it had conducted research into the offensive use of *Bacillus anthracis*, *Clostridium botulinum* toxin, and *Clostridium perfringens*. Furthermore, after the defection of Iraqi General Hussein Kamal Hussan in August 1995, the Iraqi government disclosed that it had filled warheads with biological agents, including 166 bombs (100 with botulinum toxin, 50 with anthrax, and 16 with aflatoxin); 25 Scud missiles (13 with botulinum toxin, 10 with anthrax, and 2 with aflatoxin); 122 millimeter rockets with anthrax, botulinum toxin, and aflatoxin; and spray tanks that could be fitted to aircraft to aerosolize 2000 liters of agent over a target [1].

The Aum Shinrikyo

The religious cult Aum Shinrikyo intentionally contaminated the Tokyo subway system with sarin in March 1995, resulting in more than 5500 health care facility visits, of which 20 percent resulted in hospitalizations, and 12 deaths [17]. During the subsequent criminal investigation it was revealed that the Aum was also developing biological weapons and had apparently worked with *Bacillus anthracis, Clostridium botulinum,* and *Coxiella burnetii.* Although attempts were made to release anthrax or botulinum toxin in or around Tokyo on several occasions, none were successful. In a chilling illustration of their interest in novel biological warfare agents, cult members were even sent to Africa during the 1995 Ebola outbreak to try and obtain the virus for weaponization [1].

Threat of biological warfare and terrorism

Much has been written and spoken concerning the true threat of biological warfare and terrorism. In general, an assessment of threat is a combined function of the perceived adversary's *capability* to produce and effectively disseminate biological agents, his *intent* to do so, and our own *vulnerability* to such an action. Herein lies the inherent difficulty in definitively assessing the foreign or domestic intentional biological threat. At best, we have direct knowledge and control over only our own vulnerability. Our awareness of the adversary's capabilities and doctrine likely is incomplete, if present at all. Comprehensive assessments are therefore rare; commonly, "threat assessments" boil down to being mere functions of domestic vulnerabilities.

A recent study sponsored by the National Intelligence Council offered an analysis of global trends and their effects on regional and global politics. Among the biotechnologic technologies predicted to significantly advance in the next 15 years are biomedical engineering, prevention and therapy developments, and genetic modification. Although these improvements will be made primarily in the more advanced nations and regions, the general result will be to lower the capability threshold of those countries and subnational groups in producing and disseminating effective biological weapons. Regarding those dissemination methods, this study concluded that the threat of a missile attack against US forces or interests using weapons of mass destruction (WMD) warheads is greater today than during much of the Cold War—a trend that is likely to continue [18].

Despite current trends in globalization, the United States likely will maintain a significant technologic edge over potential adversaries during the next 15 years. This disparity will force those adversaries to consider unconventional threats, necessitating an on-going process of threat assessment. Among those unconventional threats are (1) "asymmetric threats" from state and non-state actors (including small groups and individuals) who seek to level the playing field by devising strategies, tactics, and weaponry that minimize US strengths and exploit perceived weaknesses, (2) strategic WMD threats, in which such countries as Russia, China, and most likely North Korea, probably Iran, and possibly Iraq may have the capability to strike the United States, and (3) regional conventional military threats posed by large standing armies guided by a mix of Cold War and post-Cold War ideologies and tactics [18]. Glaring examples of this asymmetric threat are the heinous attacks on New York City, Washington DC, and Pennsylvania on September 11, 2001. The subsequent mailings of numerous letters containing viable anthrax spores throughout the United States and several other countries serve to remind us of the inherent uncertainties when preparing defenses against biological terrorism. Small-scale attacks on US troops or citizens at home or abroad have occurred and will continue to do so, given inherent political, social, ethical, cultural, moral, and religious differences.

Although the general motive of a biological attack, similar to that of any application of force, is to influence the thoughts and actions of other people, the actual targets may not be humans. For example, biological attacks could be directed toward animals, with either zoonotic or epizootic disease agents to influence international trade commodities, against crops to devaluate certain food supplies or foliage, or against physical material, as certain microorganisms preferentially erode materials such as rubber and plastics. This discussion will be limited to those agents targeted directly at humans.

Capabilities and intentions

Traditional agents of offensive biological warfare programs have included the causative organisms of anthrax, plague, tularemia, brucellosis, glanders, melioidosis, various food borne illnesses, cryptosporidiosis, cryptococcosis, Q fever, psittacosis, dengue fever, smallpox, viral equine encephalitides, and the arena/bunya/filo/flaviviral fevers. Toxins with historical biological warfare application include Salmonella, Staphylococcus enterotoxin B, ricin, *Clostridium botulinum* toxin, and trichothecene (T-2) mycotoxins [19–22].

Because of varying disease properties and dissemination potentials, terrorists may choose from a slightly different list of biological agents. Infectious disease organisms associated with past crimes and terrorism include *Bacillus anthracis, Ascaris suum, Coxiella burnetii, Giardia lamblia,* HIV, *Rickettsia prowazekii, Salmonella typhimurium, Salmonella typhi, Shigella spp, Schistosoma* spp, *Vibrio cholerae,* viral hemorrhagic fevers, yellow fever virus, *Yersinia enterocolitica,* and *Yersinia pestis.* Toxins associated with terrorism include *Clostridium botulinum* toxin, cholera endotoxin, diphtheria toxin, nicotine, ricin, snake toxin, and tetrodotoxin [22]. Partial listings of the agents available to terrorists are presented by organism type (Table 1) and their categorical effect (Table 2). Additionally, the Centers for Disease Control and Prevention (CDC) has developed a list of Critical Biological

Table 1
Agents of biological terrorism

Bacterial diseases	Viral diseases	Intoxications (biological toxins)
Anthrax	Smallpox	Botulinum toxin
Plague	Viral hemorrhagic fever	Staphylococcal enterotoxin B
Tularemia	Viruses (Ebola, Marburg, Lassa,	T-2 mycotoxins
Q fever	Junin, Machupo)	Ricin
Brucellosis	Alphaviruses	
Glanders	VEE, EEE, and WEE	
Melioidosis		
Typhus		
Psittacosis		
Salmonellosis		
Shigellosis		
Cryptosporidiosis		

Agents (categories A, B, and C) (Table 3). Criteria used to develop this list include (1) the severity of impact on public health and person-to-person transmissibility, (2) the potential for delivery as a weapon, (3) the need for special preparation requirements such as vaccine and medication stockpiling or special laboratory detection techniques, and (4) the ability to generate fear or terror in a population. Category A agents would cause the gravest harm to the population at risk if intentionally released by a terrorist. Category B agents could cause significant morbidity and mortality but would have less impact on the medical and public health systems than category A. Category C agents are classified as emerging pathogens or genetically engineered agents.

Finally, threats can be categorized as originating from states (e.g., Russia and China), state-sponsored groups (e.g., Osama bin-Laden's Al Qaeda network), non-state terrorist groups (e.g., Aum Shinrikyo cult and The Covenant, the Sword, and the Arm of the Lord), and "lone wolf" individuals (e.g., Larry Wayne Harris).

Table 2
Agents of biological terrorism

Lethal	Incapacitating
Anthrax	Q fever
Plague	Brucellosis
Melioidosis	Alphaviruses
Tularemia	T-2 mycotoxins
Viral hemorrhagic fevers	Typhus
Botulinum toxin	Psittacosis
Ricin toxin	Salmonellosis
Glanders	Shigellosis
Smallpox	Cryptosporidiosis

Table 3
Centers for disease control and prevention critical biological agents

Category A

Biological agent	Disease
Variola major	Smallpox
Bacillus anthracis	Anthrax
Yersinia pestis	Plague
Clostridium botulinum toxin	Botulism
Francisella tularensis	Tularemia
Filoviruses (Ebola, Marburg)	Viral hemorrhagic fever
Arenaviruses (Lassa, Junin, Machupo)	

Category B

Biological agent	Disease
Coxiella burnetti	Q fever
Brucella species	Brucellosis
Burkholderia mallei/pseudomallei	Glanders/Melioidosis
Alphaviruses (Venezuelan, eastern and western equine encephalomyelitis)	Encephalitis
Toxins (Ricin, epsilon toxin of *C. perfringens*, SEB)	Toxic syndromes
Rickettsia prowazekii	Typhus
Chlamydia psittaci	Psittacosis

Food safety threat agents
Salmonella species, *Shigella dysenteriae, Escherichia coli* 0157:H7

Water safety threat agents
Cryptosporidium parvum, Vibrio cholerae

Category C
Emerging pathogens that could be engineered for mass dissemination in the future because of availability, ease of production and dissemination, and potential for high morbidity and mortality and major health impact:
Nipah virus, hantavirus, tickborne hemorrhagic fever viruses, tickborne encephalitis virus, yellow fever, and multidrug-resistant tuberculosis

Foreign state/national programs

The following nations are judged to possess offensive biological weapons programs: Iraq, Iran, Syria, Libya, China, North Korea, Russia, Israel, Taiwan, and possibly Sudan, India, Pakistan, and Kazakstan [23]. The probability of a large-scale attack by a nation such as Russia or China is arguably less likely than it was a decade ago. Nonetheless, aging biological warfare production and dissemination equipment and personal scientific expertise may be sold to other nations or groups to generate much-needed funds for reindustrialization programs. From the mid-1980s to the mid-1990s, when the Soviet Union was dissolving, the aforementioned 50,000 biological scientists in the combined civilian-military program were left to embark on other careers or ply their trade on the international market [16]. The Soviet (then Russian) State Research Center for Virology and

Biotechnology (VECTOR) lost an estimated 3500 scientists and the State Research Center for Applied Microbiology lost 54% of its staff [24]. Examples of this scientific export phenomenon include allegations that former Soviet Union scientists provided technical assistance to Iran and South African expatriate scientists assisted Libya [25,26]. In the case of the smaller national programs such as those of North Korea and Iran, these efforts can also be used as income-generators because the production and dissemination of materials (to include ballistic missiles) can easily be exported.

Although the direct risk of mass attack from foreign states such as the former Soviet Union may be on the decline, Russia likely will continue to invest disproportionate resources into weapons of mass destruction to bolster its flagging international influence and counter perceived shortcomings in conventional weapons and strategic defenses. Additionally, the influence of regional hegemonists will remain an on-going source of destabilization. For example, in the Middle East, internal economic fluctuations, regional border clashes, and reactions to a US military presence may fan nationalistic sentiments [27]. Similarly, although the nature and extent of its WMD programs are unclear, China has stated its intention to continue its expanding scope of power "without regard to US interests." Finally, short of an unlikely reunification with the South, North Korea's mid- and long-range missile programs remain at least a regional source of destabilization [18]. That situation will change for the worse over the course of the next 15 years, according to the Director of the Central Intelligence Agency (CIA), as North Korea, Iran, and Iraq will all develop missiles capable of reaching the continental United States [28].

Terrorist groups and individuals

As the fall 2001 instances of anthrax-laden envelopes seem to confirm, independent or obscurely backed terrorist groups and individuals likely will present the most significant domestic biological terrorism threat in the present and near future. Vague, unpredictable motivations and methods render these groups difficult to identify, track, and counter. Among those motivations are religious fanaticism, economic disruption, exacting revenge, creating chaos, mimicking God, displaying an "aura of science," millenarianism, getting attention, and copying the acts of others [29]. According to the CIA and individual analysts, interest in chemical and biological weapons among non-state and terrorist organizations is increasing, as is the number of potential perpetrators [30–32]. Evidence of this increased activity is provided by the Federal Bureau of Investigation, which reportedly logged 27 bioterrorism threats in 1997, 112 in 1998, 187 in 1999, and more than 115 in 2000 [23].

Among the fastest growing domestic terrorist groups are the religiously oriented groups. Motivated by a desire to impress God and humble mankind, they are unconstrained by governmental influences and have shown a greater tendency toward violence than secular groups [29]. In 1968, the

Rand Corporation identified 11 international terrorist groups, none of which were religiously oriented. A similar Rand study in 1994, however, identified 49 international terrorist groups, of which a third were classified as religious [33]. With 751 reported illnesses, the largest example of recognized biological terrorism in the United States occurred in 1984 when members of a religious commune deliberately contaminated several community salad bars with *Salmonella typhimurium* in an effort to make patrons too ill to vote in upcoming local elections [34]. Although affecting smaller numbers of people and stemming from as yet-unknown sources, the fall 2001 domestic biological attacks occurred concurrently with a religious-based war on Western nations initiated by Osama bin-Laden's Al Qaeda organization. These attacks resulted in, as of this writing, 11 cases of inhalational anthrax, including five deaths, and 12 cases of cutaneous anthrax, all of which continue to cause widespread concern and frustration.

Lone operators may be even more unpredictable as they are far less constrained than larger interest groups because they are not dependent on any segment of the population for financing, approval, or assistance. They are also free to formulate and carry out plans of their own design—without the potentially stifling influence from a group dynamic. They are also unlikely to be proactively detected by law enforcement or intelligence nonproliferation/counterproliferation efforts. Finally, the recent explosion in communication capabilities caters almost specifically to the lone individual who no longer needs to rely on a larger group to gather the necessary information for obtaining and using biological weapons [35].

Although the likelihood of activity in the biological realm by independent or international terrorist groups and lone individuals may be greater than that by state-sponsored groups, that activity is characterized by fewer and more focused groups of target individuals [35]. In another example of domestic bioterrorism with obscure motivations, a disgruntled medical laboratory worker in 1996 deliberately contaminated coworkers' food with *Shigella dysenteriae*, resulting in 12 illnesses [36]. Fig. 1 depicts the present inverse relationship between the ease of accomplishing biological attacks and the number of casualties generated. As these groups and individuals become more sophisticated in capabilities and methods, however, the relationship may move the line in the direction indicated—resulting in greater lethality and number of attacks—to include mass casualty situations [18,21].

Vulnerabilities

Although a national-level risk assessment of potential chemical and biological terrorist incidents has not yet been performed, [32] the last few years have seen a sharp increase in the number and scope of national WMD readiness exercises designed to test our vulnerability and responsiveness. Among these were the 2000 TOPOFF and the 2001 Dark Winter exercises. The largest exercise of its kind to date, the $3 million TOPOFF scenario was

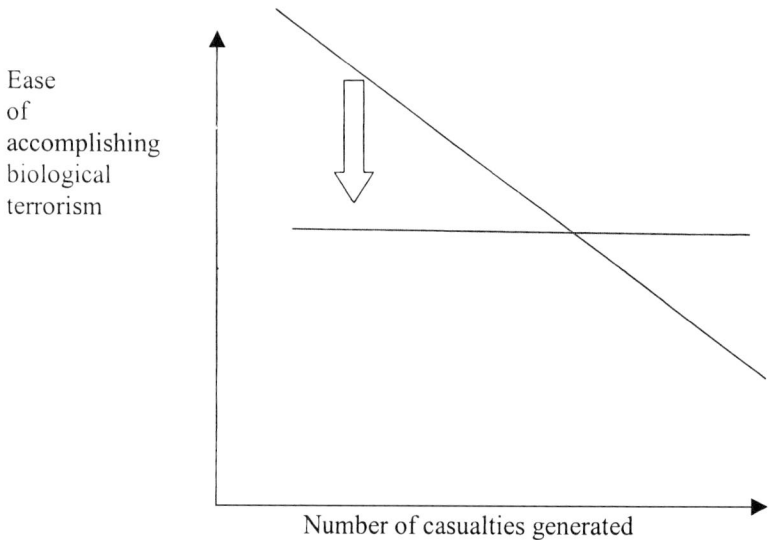

Fig. 1. Inverse relationship between Aease of accomplishment and number of casualties for biological warfare/terrorism cases. (*Adapted from* Franz DR, Zajtchuk R. Biological terrorism: understanding the threat, preparation, and medical response. Dis Mon 2000;127–90.)

designed to test the readiness of top governmental officials (hence, its name) to attacks using weapons of mass destruction. Characterized by notional attacks against Portsmouth, New Hampshire (chemical weapons), Washington, DC (radiologic contamination), and Denver, Colorado (biological [plague] weapons), TOPOFF identified key weaknesses in the public health community's ability to identify and respond to an intentional biological event in a timely and effective manner. The necessary degrees of political authority, human resources, public health communication, and prioritized decision-making templates were judged inadequate. Equally revealing was the inadequacy of the community hospitals' response capabilities. The local health care facilities were overwhelmed with the patient numbers, quickly understaffed, short of critical supplies, equipment, and medicines, not prepared for strict crowd control, and not capable of insuring the safety of their workers or patients [37].

Dark Winter was a multi-state (Pennsylvania, Georgia, and Oklahoma) exercise to simulate a smallpox outbreak during the winter of 2001–2002. Among the lessons learned from this exercise were that (1) an attack on the United States using biological weapons could threaten vital national security interests, (2) current organizational structures and capabilities are not well-suited for the management of a biological attack, (3) there is no surge capability in the US health care and public health systems or the pharmaceutical and vaccine industries, and (4) should a contagious biological agent be used, containing the spread of disease will present significant ethical, political, cultural, operational, and legal challenges [23].

In a 1997 study published by the CDC, researchers concluded that an attack on a fictionalized population of 100,000 people using an aerosolized *Bacillus anthracis* product would result in 50,000 cases of illness, with 32,875 deaths resulting. Similar attacks using *Francisella tularensis* and *Brucella melitensis* would result in 82,500 cases of illness (with 6,188 deaths resulting) and 82,500 cases of illness (with 413 deaths resulting), respectively [38]. The study also pointed out that the morbidity and mortality could be drastically reduced through a combination of surveillance and the early administration of appropriate antibiotics. Although this type of large-scale response is currently being developed, however, it likely will remain problematic, especially in a covert attack situation.

Summary

The inevitable conclusion is that the availability of biological warfare agents and supporting technologic infrastructure, coupled with the fact that there are many people motivated to do harm to the United States, means that America must be prepared to defend her homeland against biological agents. Some have argued to the contrary, that the threat and risks from a biological weapon attack are not to be considered serious, because [39]:

- They've not been used yet on a large scale so they probably won't be in the near future.
- Their use is so morally repugnant that they probably won't be used at all.
- The technologic hurdles associated with isolating, growing, purifying, weaponizing, and disseminating adequate quantities of pathologic agents are so high that only the most advanced laboratories could attempt the process.
- Similar to a 'nuclear winter,' the aftermath of a biological attack is so unthinkable that none would attempt it.

Unfortunately, the trends associated with biotechnology globalization, terrorist group dynamics, and global/regional politics render these beliefs untenable and inappropriate, as recent events have underscored.

To that end, the United States has accelerated its program of defense against biological weapons, as it must. Biological weapons are such dreadful weapons of uniqueness and complexity that a specific defense strategy is paramount. Elements of this program include pharmaceutical stockpiles, heightened surveillance systems, energized vaccine development programs, and comprehensive training initiatives. Although the depth and breadth of these efforts are unprecedented, above all these efforts is the absolute necessity for medical and public health care professionals to be educated and actively involved. These professionals are the sine qua non of future defensive readiness. This is just the start; unfortunately, there is no end yet in sight.

References

[1] Eitzen EM, Takafuji ET. Historical overview of biological warfare. In: Sidell FR, Takafuji EF, Franz DR, editors. Medical aspects of chemical and biological warfare. Washington, DC: Borden Institute; 1997. p. 415–23.

[2] Derbes VJ. De Mussi and the great plague of 1348: a forgotten episode of bacteriological war. JAMA 1966;196(1):59–62.

[3] Stockholm International Peace Research Institute (SIPRI). The rise of CB weapons, Vol 1. In: The problem of chemical and biological warfare. New York, NY: Humanities Press; 1971.

[4] Bayne-Jones S. The evolution of preventive medicine in the United States army, 1607–1939. Washington, DC: Department of the Army, Office of the Surgeon General; 1968.

[5] Baxby D. Jenner's smallpox vaccine. London, England: Heinemann Educational Books; 1981.

[6] Geissler E, editor. Biological and toxin weapons today. Oxford, England: Oxford University Press, Stockholm International Peace Research Institute; 1986.

[7] Christopher GW, Cieslak TJ, Pavlin JA, et al. Biological warfare: a historical perspective. JAMA 1997;278(5):412–7.

[8] Williams P, Wallace D. Unit 731: Japan's secret biological warfare in World War II. New York: Free Press; 1989.

[9] Harris SH. Factories of death. New York: Routledge; 1994.

[10] Manchee R, Stewart W. The decontamination of Gruinard Island. Chem Br. 1998;July: 690–1.

[11] Cowdrey AE. The medic's war. Washington, DC: Center of Military History, US Army; 1987.

[12] Rolicka M. New studies disputing allegations of bacteriological warfare during the Korean War. Milit Med 1995;160:97–100.

[13] Bernstein BJ. The birth of the US biological-warfare program. Sci Am 1987;256:116–21.

[14] Kadlec RP, Zelicoff AP, Vrtis AM. Biological weapons control: prospects and implications for the future. JAMA 1997;278:351–6.

[15] Smith JR. Yeltsin blames '79 anthrax on germ warfare efforts. Washington Post, June 16, 1992:A-1.

[16] Tucker JB. Biological weapons in the former Soviet Union: an interview with Dr. Kenneth Alibek. Nonproliferation Rev Spring–Summer (5) 1999. Available at: http://cns.mis.edu/pubs/npr/vol 06/63/alibek 63.pdf. Accessed 1 April 2002.

[17] Sidell FR, Franz DR. Overview: defense against the effects of chemical and biological warfare agents. Sidell FR, Takafuji ET, Franz DR, editors. In: Medical aspects of chemical and biological warfare. Washington, DC: Borden Institute; 1997. p. 1–7.

[18] US Government. Global trends 2015: a dialogue about the future with nongovernmental experts. Washington, DC: National Intelligence Council; 2000. p. 1–85.

[19] Burrows WD, Renner SE. Biological warfare agents as threats to potable water. Environ Health Perspect 1999;107:975–84.

[20] Eitzen EM. Use of biological weapons. In: Sidell FR, Takafuji ET, Franz DR, editors. Medical aspects of chemical and biological warfare. Washington, DC: Borden Institute; 1997. p. 437–50.

[21] Greenwood DP. A relative assessment of putative biological-warfare agents [technical report 1040]. Lexington, MA: Lincoln Laboratory, Massachusetts Institute of Technology; 1997. p. 1–79.

[22] Kortepeter MG, Parker GW. Potential biological weapons threats. Emerg Infect Dis 1999;5:523–7.

[23] House of Representatives Committee on Government Reform, Subcommittee on National Security, Veterans Affairs, and International Relations. Hearing on combating terrorism: federal response to a biological weapons attack. July 23, 2001. Available at: http://www.house.gov/reform/ns/web_resources/briefing_memo_july_23.htm. Accessed 4 Dec 2001.

[24] Tucker JB. Bioweapons from Russia: stemming the flow. Issues Sci Technol; Spring 1999 p. 34–8.

[25] Adams J. Gadaffi lures South African top germ warfare scientists. Sunday Times, February 26, 1995.

[26] Miller J, Broad WJ. Bio-weapons in mind, Iranians lure needy ex-Soviet scientists. New York Times, November 8, 1998.

[27] Caudle LC. The biological warfare threat. In: Sidell FR, Takafuji ET, Franz DR, editors. Medical aspects of chemical and biological warfare. Washington, DC: Borden Institute; 1997. p. 451–66.

[28] Tenet GJ, Statement before the Senate Select Committee on Intelligence on the worldwide threat in 2000: global realities of our national securities. February 2, 2000. Available at: http://www.cia.gov/cia/public_affairs/speeches/archives/2000/dci_speech_020200.html. Accessed 4 Dec 2001.

[29] Stern J. The prospect of domestic bioterrorism. Emerg Infect Dis 1999;5:517–22.

[30] Pilat JF. Prospects for NBC terrorism after Tokyo. In: Roberts B, editor. Terrorism with chemical and biological weapons—calibrating risks and responses. Alexandria, VA: Chemical and Biological Arms Control Institute; 1997. p. 1–21.

[31] Purver R. Understanding past non-use of CBW by terrorists. In: Roberts B, editor. Terrorism with chemical and biological weapons–calibrating risks and responses. Alexandria, VA: Chemical and Biological Arms Control Institute; 1997. p. 65–73.

[32] US General Accounting Office. Combating terrorism: need for comprehensive threat and risk assessments of chemical and biological attacks. Washington, DC: US General Accounting Office; 1999. Publication GAO/NSIAD-99-163.

[33] Hoffman B. Terrorism and WMD: some preliminary hypotheses [viewpoint]. Nonproliferation Rev Spring–Summer 1997;45–52.

[34] Torok TJ, Tauxe RV, Wise RP, et al. A large community outbreak of salmonellosis caused by intentional contamination of restaurant salad bars. JAMA 1997;278:389–95.

[35] Simon JD. Lone operators and weapons of mass destruction. In: Roberts B, editor. Hype or reality: the "new terrorism" and mass casualty attacks. Alexandria, VA: Chemical and Biological Arms Control Institute; 2000. p. 69–81.

[36] Kolavic SA, Kimura A, Simons SL, et al. An outbreak of *Shigella dysenteriae* Type 2 among laboratory workers due to intentional food contamination. JAMA 1997;278:396–8.

[37] Inglesby T, Grossman R, O'Toole T. A plague on your city: observations from TOPOFF. Biodefense Quarterly 2000;2:1–10.

[38] Kaufmann AF, Meltzer MI, Schmid GP. The economic impact of a bioterrorist attack: are prevention and postattack intervention programs justifiable? Emerg Infect Dis 1997;3: 83–94.

[39] Henderson DA. Biological terrorism. Presented at the Conference on New and Emerging Infections. Atlanta, GA, March 10, 1998.

Emerg Med Clin N Am
20 (2002) 273–309

EMERGENCY
MEDICINE
CLINICS OF
NORTH AMERICA

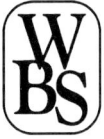

Threats in bioterrorism I:
CDC category A agents

Robert G. Darling, MD, FACEP[a,b,*],
Christina L. Catlett, MD, FACEP[c],
Kermit D. Huebner, MD[d],
David G. Jarrett, MD, FACEP[e]

[a]Captain (Flight Surgeon), United States Navy, Medical Director,
Aeromedical Isolation Team and Containment Care
[b]Operational Medicine Division, US Army Medical Research Institute of Infectious
Diseases (USAMRIID), 1425 Porter Street, ATTN: MCMR-UIM-O,
Fort Detrick, MD 21702-5011, USA
[c]The Johns Hopkins Hospital Department of Emergency Medicine,
600 North Wolfe Street, Baltimore, MD 21287-2080, USA
[d]Darnall Army Community Hospital, 26000 Darnall Loop, Fort Hood, TX 76544, USA
[e]Colonel (Flight Surgeon), United States Army, Chief, Doctrine Development

Before the anthrax attacks of 2001, the threat of bioterrorism was based primarily on the events surrounding the sarin nerve agent attacks in Japan in 1995 [1,2,9] and the biological weapons production and stockpiling programs of the former Soviet Union [3] and Iraq [4]. Now that terrorists have used the US Postal Service to disseminate anthrax spores contained in letters, the threat of lethal bioterrorism has become a reality.

Numerous strategies exist to reduce vulnerabilities to an attack with a biological weapon, of which education and training are important components [5,6]. Each physician can and should make education his or her responsibility [7]. To facilitate rapid disease recognition, the clinician must focus on syndromes and symptom complexes associated with these agents, especially those deemed to be the most credible threats [8].

In June of 1999 the Centers for Disease Control and Prevention (CDC) and a multidisciplinary panel of experts formed a strategic workgroup to outline steps to strengthen the US public health infrastructure and healthcare capacity to protect against bioterrorism [5]. This group identified a list

* Corresponding author.
E-mail address: Robert.Darling@det.amedd.army.mil (R.G. Darling).

0733-8627/02/$ - see front matter © 2002, Elsevier Science (USA). All rights reserved.
PII: S 0 7 3 3 - 8 6 2 7 (0 2) 0 0 0 0 5 - 6

of "Critical Biological Agents" that if intentionally released into a susceptible population would have the greatest impact on US health and security. Those of greatest concern were designated category A and were chosen because of their ease of dissemination or ability for person-to-person transmission, high mortality rate, potential major impact on public health, ability to incite panic and social disruption, and the requirement for additional major public health preparedness measures. Other potential agents of concern were assigned to categories B or C by using the above criteria to rate each pathogen's impact on the medical and public health systems if intentionally released as a weapon.

This article reviews the category A agents with a discussion of their history and significance, clinical presentation, diagnostic evaluation, infection control precautions, treatment, and prophylaxis. Table 1 provides a summary of the important properties and characteristics of these agents.

Bacillus anthracis (anthrax)

History and significance

It would be difficult to create a more "perfect" biological weapon than *Bacillus anthracis*, the causative agent of anthrax. Anthrax, a zoonotic disease of herbivores such as horses, cattle, sheep, and goats can occur naturally in humans handling contaminated animal products such as hair, hides, blood, and waste products of infected animals or from products such as bone meal. Infection, usually by spores, is introduced through scratches or abrasions of the skin, inhalation, eating insufficiently cooked infected meat, or by the bites of flies. Anthrax spores may remain stable for decades or can be produced, weaponized, and delivered as a wet or dry aerosol cloud. A Canadian study demonstrated the ease with which weapons-grade anthrax spores can spread throughout a building even when delivered in a contained letter [10]. In this form, the spores behave like a gas and can disperse over wide geographic areas with the potential to infect great numbers of people [11].

Anthrax spores were manufactured into biological weapons by the United States during its offensive biological weapons program [12]. Other countries have weaponized this agent or are suspected of doing so [13]. Anthrax bacteria are easy to cultivate and spore production is readily induced. Spores are moderately resistant to sunlight, heat, and disinfectants—desirable properties when choosing a bacterial weapon. Iraq admitted in August of 1991 that it had performed research on the offensive use of *B. anthracis* before the Persian Gulf War, and in 1995 admitted to weaponizing anthrax [4]. A defector from the former Soviet Union's biological weapons program revealed that the Soviets had produced anthrax in ton quantities for use as a weapon [3]. An outbreak of inhalational anthrax occurred near one of their facilities in 1979, with a resultant 77 infections and 66 deaths, with some victims becoming ill up to six weeks after the exposure [15]. The Japanese cult group

Table 1
Category A agent characteristics

Disease	Clinical presentation	Transmit human to human	Isolation precautions	Incubation period	Duration of illness	Lethality (approx. case fatality rates)	Persistence of organism	Diagnostic testing	Treatment	Prophylaxis	Vaccine
Inhalational Anthrax	Fever, malaise, fatigue, cough, and chest discomfort leading to respiratory distress and shock	No	Standard	1–6 days	Without aggressive treatment, death in 24–36 hours after onset of severe symptoms	High (45% in 2001 attack)	Very stable —spores remain viable for >40 years in soil	Blood, Gram stain, Ag-ELISA, serology: ELISA, PCR	Ciprofloxacin or doxycycline plus one or two other (Note 1)	Ciprofloxacin or doxycycline × 60 days Consider vaccination	FDA licensed vaccine 0.5 ml SQ at 0, 2, 4 weeks then 6, 12, and 18 months with annual boosters
Smallpox	Fever, malaise, headache, follow d by severe pustular rash	High	Airborne	7–17 days	4 weeks	Moderate to high	Very stable	Pharyngeal swab, scab material. ELISA, PCR, virus isolation	Possibly cidofivir (some effectiveness in vitro)	Vaccinia immune globulin 0.6 ml/kg IM (within 3 days of exposure, best within 24 hours) Also used for adverse reactions to vaccinia vaccination	Vaccinia vaccination by way of scarification —effective if positive "take" within last 3 years

(continued on next page)

Table 1 (continued)

Disease	Clinical presentation	Transmit human to human	Isolation precautions	Incubation period	Duration of illness	Lethality (approx. case fatality rates)	Persistence of organism	Diagnostic testing	Treatment	Prophylaxis	Vaccine
Pneumonic plague	Fever, chills, malaise, and cough leading to dyspnea, stridor, hemoptysis, cyanosis, and death	High	Droplet until 3 days of treatment completed	2–3 days	1–6 days usually fatal	High unless treated within 24 hours	For up to 1 year in soil; 270 days in live tissue	Blood, sputum, lymph node aspirate/ Gram stain, Ag-ELISA, culture, serology: ELISA, IFA	Streptomycin Gentamycin Doxycycline Chloramphenicol	Tetracycline × 7 days Doxycycline × 7 days	Killed vaccine for bubonic plague, not effective against aerosol exposure (no longer manufactured)
Typhoidal tularemia	Fever, malaise, prostration, headache, weight loss, and nonproductive cough	No	Standard	2–10 days (avg. 3–5)	2 weeks or more	Moderate if untreated	For months in moist soil or other media	Blood, sputum, serum, EM of tissue, culture, serology: agglutination	Streptomycin Gentamycin	Doxycycline × 14 days Tetracycline × 14 days	Investigational live attenuated vaccine
Viral hemorrhagic fevers	Fever, prostration, myalgia, conjunctival injection followed by systemic coagulopathies	Moderate	Contact; consider additional precautions if massive hemorrhage	4–21 days	7–16 days	Moderate to high	Relatively unstable —depends on agent	Serum, blood viral isolation, Ag-ELISA, RT-PCR serology: Ab-ELISA	Supportive care Ribavirin for CCHF/ arenaviruses	NA	Licensed vaccine for Yellow fever only

| Botulism | Ptosis, diplopia, dry mouth followed by descending paralysis and respiratory arrest | No | Standard | 1–5 days | Death in 24–72 hours; lasts months if not lethal | High without respiratory support | For weeks in nonmoving water and food | nasal swab, Ag-ELISA mouse neutralization | Passive antibody for AHF, BHF, Lassa fever, and CCHF | DOD heptavalent antitoxin for Serotypes A–G (IND); CDC trivalent equine antitoxin for serotypes A, B, E (licensed) | NA | Pentavalent toxoid vaccine (types A–E) available as IND |

Abbreviations: Ab, antibody; AHF, Argentine hemorrhagic fever; Ag, Antigen; BHF, Bolivian/Brazilian hemorrhagic fever; CCHF, Crimean-Congo hemorrhagic fever; CDC, Centers for Disease Control and Prevention; DOD, Department of Defense; ELISA, Enzyme-linked immunosorbent assay; HHF, Hantaan hemorrhagic fever; IFA, Immunofluorescent assay; IND, Investigational New Drug; PCR, Polymerase chain reaction; RT-PCR, reverse transcriptose PCR; SC, subcutaneous.

Standard precautions: Handwashing after contact, wear gloves when handling blood, body fluids, or secretions, wear mask and eye protection or a face shield if splashes of fluid are likely.

Droplet precautions: Standard precautions plus private room or cohort with patient with same infection, wear mask when within 3 feet of patient, limit movement of patient, and place mask on patient before moving.

Airborne precautions: Standard precautions plus negative-pressure private room, wear respiratory protection on entering room, limit movement of patient, and place mask on patient before moving.

Note 1. Rifampin, vancomycin, penicillin, ampicillin, streptomycin, chloramphenicol, imipenem, clindamycin, or clarithromycin.

Adapted from 1) Franz et al. Clinical recognition and management of patients exposed to biological warfare agents. Summary of biological warfare agents. JAMA Aug 6, 1997, p. 400–40.

2) USAMRIID's medical management of biological casualties Handbook, 4th edition. February 2001 (appendix C (www.USAMRIID.army.mil)) with permission.

Aum Shinrikyo developed an anthrax weapon, but was unable to successfully release the weapon even after several attempts [16].

On October 4, 2001, a 63-year-old man died from inhalational anthrax. This represented the first such case in the United States since 1976 [17,18]. As of January 2002, 18 cases of anthrax (11 inhalational and 7 cutaneous) have been confirmed [18–25]. All but two of the inhalational cases were traced to direct exposure to *B. anthracis* contained in envelopes sent through the US Postal Service. In two of the fatal cases, the source of exposure remains a mystery. More than 30,000 potentially exposed patients were placed on postexposure prophylaxis. To date none of these patients have subsequently developed inhalational anthrax.

Clinical presentation

Anthrax presents as three clinically distinct syndromes in humans: cutaneous, inhalational, and gastrointestinal [26,27]. The cutaneous form occurs most frequently on the hands and forearms of persons who work with infected livestock. It may also appear on the face. It begins as a papule followed by the formation of a fluid-filled vesicle. The vesicle typically dries and forms a coal-black scab (eschar), hence the term anthrax (Greek for "coal") (Fig. 1). This local infection has a mortality rate of less than 1% if treated, but can occasionally become systemic with mortality rates

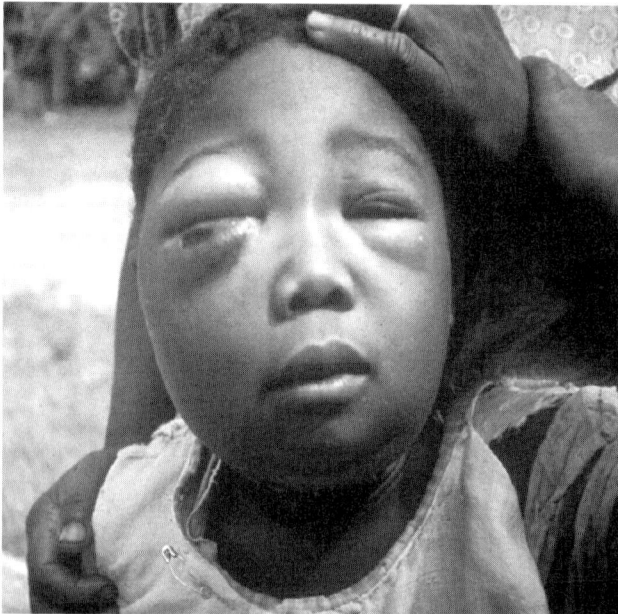

Fig. 1. Cutaneous anthrax. Young African female with cutaneous anthrax involving upper and lower eyelids. Note marked lid edema and central black eschar involving lower eyelid. The lesion is generally not painful. (*Courtesy of* Arnold Kaufman, Centers for Disease Control [public domain].)

approaching 20% [28]. Early in its course, anthrax may present in a more atypical fashion without the classic black eschar (Fig. 2). With appropriate antibiotic use, death from cutaneous anthrax is unlikely.

Gastrointestinal anthrax, rare in humans, is contracted by the ingestion of insufficiently cooked meat from infected animals which may contain vegetative organisms or spores. Spores may germinate in the upper or lower gastrointestinal tract, with the development of oropharyngeal disease or disease of the terminal ileum or cecum, respectively. Patients with upper tract disease present with an ulcer involving the mouth or esophagus that may then progress to regional lymphadenopathy and edema. As the disease progresses patients may develop systemic illness and sepsis. Patients with lower tract involvement may present with nausea, vomiting, and abdominal pain that rapidly progresses to bloody diarrhea and sepsis. The mortality rate of gastrointestinal anthrax may be high once the disease process becomes systemic [28].

Woolsorters' disease (endemic inhalational anthrax) is a rare infection contracted by the inhalation of spores. Only 18 cases have been reported in the twentieth century in the United States. It occurs mainly among industrial workers handling infected hides, wool, and furs [29]. After an incubation period of one to six days, presumably dependent on the dose and strain of inhaled spores, onset of symptoms is gradual and nonspecific. Fever, malaise, and fatigue may be present, sometimes in association with a nonproductive cough and mild chest discomfort [30]. Initial symptoms are sometimes

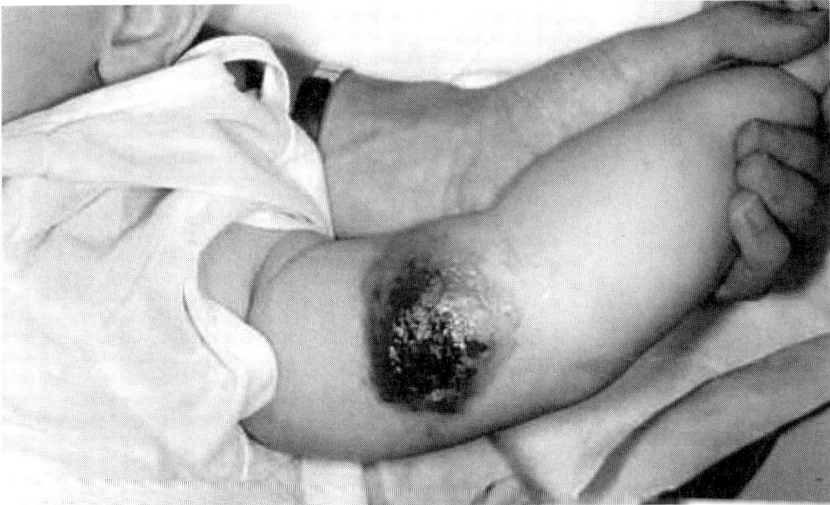

Fig. 2. Cutaneous anthrax. Seven-month-old male infant with 2-cm open sore accompanied by erythema, induration, and weeping clear yellow fluid. The entire arm is swollen but nontender. The initial diagnosis when this patient presented was *Loxosceles reclusa* spider bite with superimposed cellulites. Once anthrax was suspected the diagnosis was confirmed by way of polymerase chain reaction and immunostaining of 2 punch biopsies from the lesion. (*From* N Eng J Med 2001;345; Copyright © 2001 Massachusetts Medical Society. All rights reserved.)

followed by a short period of improvement (hours to two to three days), followed by the abrupt development of severe respiratory distress with dyspnea, diaphoresis, stridor, and cyanosis. Septicemia, shock, and death usually follow within 24–36 hours after the onset of respiratory distress [19]. Physical findings are typically non-specific, especially in the early phase of the disease.

The bioterrorism-related inhalational anthrax cases that occurred during the fall of 2001 presented in a predictable manner with a few exceptions. Nearly all patients initially developed fatigue and malaise followed by minimal or nonproductive cough. They soon developed fever, chills, nausea, vomiting, and drenching sweats. This progressed to chest pain and dyspnea. Only 1 of 11 presented with rhinorrhea and 2 of 11 with sore throat. No patients reported even a brief interval of improvement that has been noted to occur sometimes in patients with Woolsorters' disease. Ten of 11 patients revealed some abnormality on plain chest radiography or computed tomography. Seven had infiltrates, eight had pleural effusions, and seven demonstrated mediastinal widening. The large number of patients with infiltrates on chest radiographs or computed tomography was somewhat unexpected because previously it was believed that inhalational anthrax was primarily a disease of the mediastinum. It is clear from this cluster of cases that pneumonic processes may also be prominent features of inhalational anthrax [18,19,25,31,32] (Figs. 3, 4, and 5).

Diagnosis

Bacillus anthracis is detectable by Gram stain of the blood, blood culture on routine media, and by ELISA, but often not until later in the course of

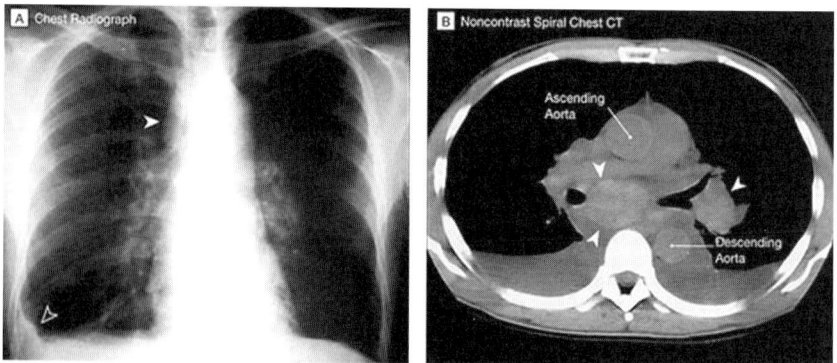

Fig. 3. Inhalational anthrax in a surviving patient. (A) Chest radiograph depicts a minimally widened mediastinum (*white arrowhead*), bilateral hilar adenopathy, moderate right pleural effusion (*black arrowhead*), and a subtle left lower lobe air-space opacity. (B) Large hyperdense lymph nodes (*arrowheads*) are depicted in the subcarinal space and left hilum on this noncontrast spiral computed tomography (CT) image. The density of the lymph nodes is equal to that of blood in the adjacent ascending and descending aorta. Bilateral pleural effusions and edema of the mediastinal fat are also presented. (*From* JAMA 2001;286:2550; Copyrighted 2001, American Medical Association.)

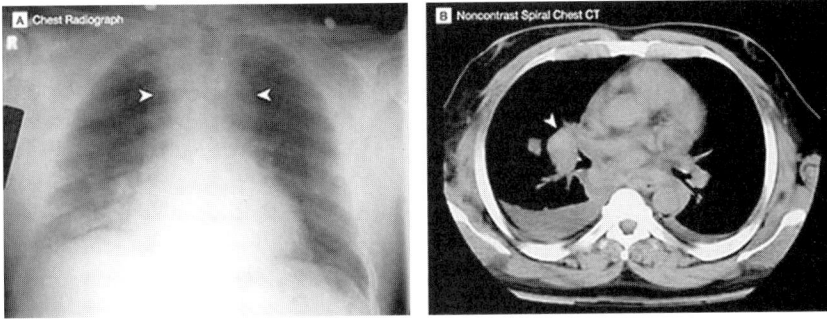

Fig. 4. Inhalational anthrax in a surviving patient. (A) Portable chest radiograph depicts a widened mediastinum (*arrowheads*), bilateral hilar fullness, a right pleural effusion, and bilateral perihilar air-space disease. (B) Noncontrast spiral computed tomography (CT) depicts an enlarged and hyperdense right hilar lymph node (*arrowhead*), bilateral pleural effusions, and edema of the mediastinal fat. (*From* JAMA 2001;286:2552; Copyrighted 2001, American Medical Association.)

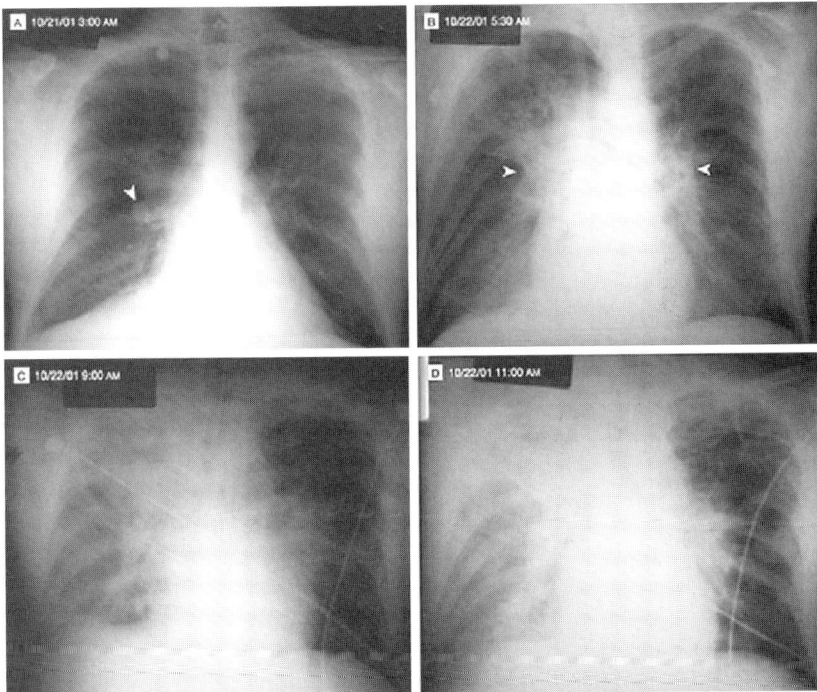

Fig. 5. Inhalational anthrax in a fatal case. Note progression of radiographic changes. (A) Initially, only subtle bilateral hilar prominence (*arrowhead*) and a right perihilar infiltrate were noted, but subsequent images (B–D) revealed a progressively widened mediastinum (B, *arrowheads*) and marked perihilar infiltrates, peribronchial cuffing, and air bronchograms. (*From* JAMA 2001;286:2555; Copyrighted 2001, American Medical Association.)

the illness. Approximately 50% of cases are accompanied by hemorrhagic meningitis, and therefore organisms may also be identified in cerebrospinal fluid (CSF) [17,28] (Fig. 6). Only vegetative encapsulated bacilli are present during infection. Spores are not found within the body unless the bacilli are exposed to ambient air. Studies of inhalational anthrax in rhesus monkeys showed that bacilli and toxin appear in the blood late on day two or early on day three post-exposure [19,33]. Toxin production parallels the appearance of bacilli in the blood, and tests are available to rapidly detect the toxin. With the appearance of symptoms, the white blood cell (WBC) count becomes elevated and remains so until death [17,27].

Infection control precautions

Standard precautions are recommended for patient care. Person-to-person spread of disease from inhalational anthrax is not known to occur. After any invasive procedure or autopsy, instruments and the local area should be disinfected with a sporicidal agent. Iodine can be used but must be of disinfectant strengths, as antiseptic-strength iodophors are not usually sporicidal. Chlorine, in the form of sodium or calcium hypochlorite, can also

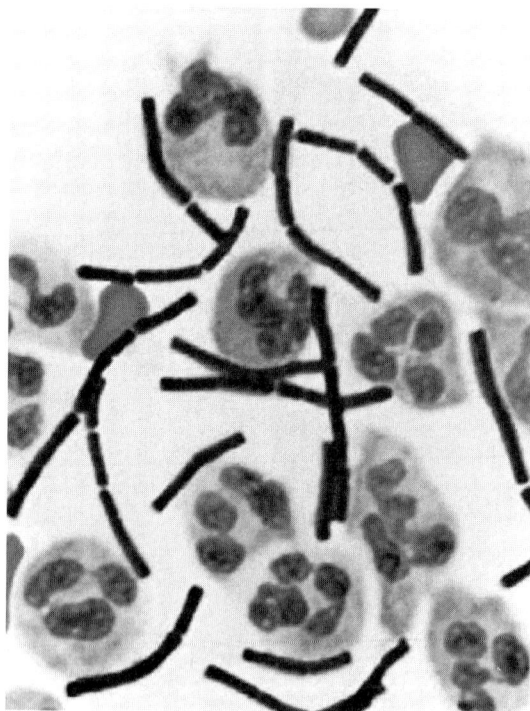

Fig. 6. Cerebrospinal fluid specimen containing many polymorphonuclear white cells and gram-positive bacilli (Gram's stain, ×1000). (*From* N Eng J Med 2001;345:1609; Copyright © 2001 Massachusetts Medical Society. All rights reserved.)

be used, but with the caution that the activity of hypochlorites is greatly reduced in the presence of organic material.

Treatment and prophylaxis

Before the events of the fall of 2001, almost all cases of inhalational anthrax in which treatment was initiated after the development of significant symptoms were fatal. Of the 11 confirmed inhalational cases resulting from bioterrorism in the fall of 2001, five were fatal (case fatality rate of 45%) [18]. This reduced mortality rate is most likely attributable to earlier and more aggressive supportive care and antibiotic therapy [18,19].

Penicillin had been regarded as the treatment of choice, with two million units given intravenously every two hours [14]. Recently, CDC advised initial therapy to begin with doxycycline or ciprofloxacin, then switch to penicillin if sensitivities allow [21]. Tetracyclines and erythromycin have been recommended in penicillin-allergic patients. Most naturally occurring anthrax strains are sensitive in vitro to penicillin. Penicillin-resistant strains do exist naturally, however, and one has been recovered from a fatal human case. Moreover, it might not be difficult for an adversary to induce resistance to penicillin, tetracyclines, erythromycin, or many other antibiotics through laboratory manipulation of organisms. All naturally occurring strains tested to date have been sensitive to erythromycin, chloramphenicol, gentamicin, and ciprofloxacin [34]. In the absence of antibiotic sensitivity data, empiric intravenous antibiotic treatment should be instituted at the earliest signs of disease. Current CDC recommendations for inhalational anthrax are noted in Table 1. In cases of cutaneous anthrax associated with bioterrorism, a full 60-day course of antibiotics is recommended instead of the usual 10–14-day course recommended in naturally occurring cutaneous anthrax [21]. Therapy may be tailored once antibiotic sensitivity is available, and in the case of inhalational anthrax it should be changed to oral therapy as the clinical condition improves. There is little clinical experience with the treatment of gastrointestinal anthrax but given the severity of the disease and often terminal course, aggressive antibiotic therapy similar to that recommended for inhalational anthrax (Table 1) is probably warranted. The primary cause of morbidity and mortality is believed to be the extreme toxin load generated by the organism. Thoracentisis with removal of infected exudate was credited with improving patient status significantly more than was predicted with increased ventilatory capacity alone.

A licensed vaccine (Anthrax Vaccine Adsorbed) is derived from sterile supernatant taken from an attenuated anthrax strain [35]. The Food and Drug Administration (FDA) licensed this vaccine in 1970 for use by workers at high risk for occupational exposure to anthrax. It was not licensed for use against inhalational exposure, although there is some limited animal data suggesting protection against doses more than 900 LD$_{50}$ [36,37]. In the 1990s the US military began a mandatory vaccination program for all active duty members in response to the threat of battlefield and rear echelon use of an anthrax biological weapon [38]. This program has come under fire by service members and Congress and there have also been production problems with the manufacturer. In February 2002 the manufacturer of anthrax vaccine was finally able to meet all FDA production and licensing requirements and has been permitted to continue full-scale vaccine production. A decision on whether to reinstitute mandatory vaccination of all active duty service members is pending.

The CDC recommends prophylaxis with ciprofloxacin (500 mg PO bid) or doxycycline (100 mg PO bid) as first-line medications for presumptive treatment of anthrax, and for prophylaxis after inhalational exposure to anthrax. More than 30,000 patients have been taking ciprofloxacin or doxycycline as postexposure prophylaxis since the bioterrorism incidents of October 2001 [39–41]. Alternatives are listed in Table 1. If confirmed that anthrax has been used as a biological weapon, antibiotics should be continued for at least 60 days in all exposed individuals, and patients should be closely followed after antibiotics are discontinued. Military doctrine also requires that service members begin active immunization with anthrax vaccine while taking postexposure antibiotics. Anthrax vaccine is not currently available for use by the general public. In response to the bioterrorism events of 2001, however, CDC offered anthrax vaccine as part of an investigational new drug (IND) protocol. This was necessary because anthrax vaccine was never licensed for use as a post-exposure treatment [37]. The CDC had no recommendation as to whether patients should or should not receive the vaccine; this led to considerable confusion and consternation among the public. Consequently, few patients chose to receive the vaccine [42,43].

On discontinuation of antibiotics, patients should be closely observed. If clinical signs of anthrax develop, empiric therapy for anthrax is indicated, pending etiologic diagnosis. Optimally, patients should have medical care available from a fixed facility with intensive care capabilities and readily available access to infectious disease consultants.

Variola major (smallpox)

History and significance

Smallpox is caused by the Variola virus, a DNA virus of the Chorodopoxviridae family of the orthopoxvirus genus. Other members of this family include vaccinia, monkeypox, cowpox, camelpox, rabbitpox, racoonpox, taterapox, and buffalopox. There are no non-human reservoirs for smallpox and no human carriers. Thus, the disease survived throughout history through continual person-to-person transmission. There are two forms of smallpox, variola major (20%–40% mortality in the unvaccinated) and variola minor (1% mortality in the unvaccinated) [44,45]. Smallpox was probably responsible for more than 100 million deaths during the twentieth century alone.

Smallpox is perhaps the most feared of potential biological warfare agents. The World Health Organization (WHO) declared the disease eradicated in 1980 and vaccination of the general population in the United States ceased shortly thereafter [46]. Vaccination in military personnel was discontinued in 1989. Researchers estimate that vaccinated individuals retain immunity for approximately 10 years, although in selected populations this may continue past 20 years [47]. Thus, most of the US population is probably susceptible to smallpox. Vaccines are in short supply; however, the Federal government has recently entered into contracts to rectify this and it is expected that 200 million doses will be produced in 2002 [48]. No proven chemotherapy exists, although several antivirals are being tested, most notably cidofovir. Finally, because few physicians are familiar with the clinical presentation of smallpox, recognizing an outbreak may be problematic.

D.A. Henderson, who led the WHO's effort to eradicate smallpox in the 1960s and 1970s has stated "...the deliberate reintroduction of smallpox as an epidemic disease would be an international crime of unprecedented proportions" [44,49]. Currently there are two WHO-approved repositories of the virus: the CDC in Atlanta and the Russian State Research Center of Virology and Biotechnology in Koltsovo, Novosibirsk Region, Russian Federation. Recent reports suggest that other countries may have clandestine stockpiles [3]. Because of the difficulty of acquiring or growing smallpox, it is unlikely that smaller terrorist groups will use this agent; however, state-sponsored terrorist organizations, or larger well-funded groups might attempt to do so [49]. According to the former deputy director of the biological weapons program in the former Soviet Union, massive amounts of smallpox have been produced since 1980, and Russia continues to attempt to genetically engineer the organism [3].

Clinical presentation

The brick-shaped smallpox virion is readily transmitted from person to person by way of respiratory particles. Virions can also remain viable on fomites for up to one week. The virus initially replicates in respiratory tract epithelial cells then migrates to regional lymph nodes. From there, a massive asymptomatic viremia ensues three to four days later and may result in focal infections involving lymphoid tissues, skin, intestines, lungs, kidneys, or brain [44]. Initial symptoms resemble an acute viral illness. Following an incubation period of approximately 12 days (range 7–17 days), a second viremia, lasting two to five days, results in high fevers, malaise, headache, backache, rigors, and vomiting. The patient may develop delirium. A rash typically develops within 48 hours, beginning in the mouth, and heralds the onset of viral shedding. The rash rapidly spreads to the hands and forearms followed by the legs and trunk (Figs. 7 and 8). Lesions are initially maculopapular, then vesicular. The rash becomes distinctive when the lesions become pustular. Around the eighth day of the rash, pustules begin to scab.

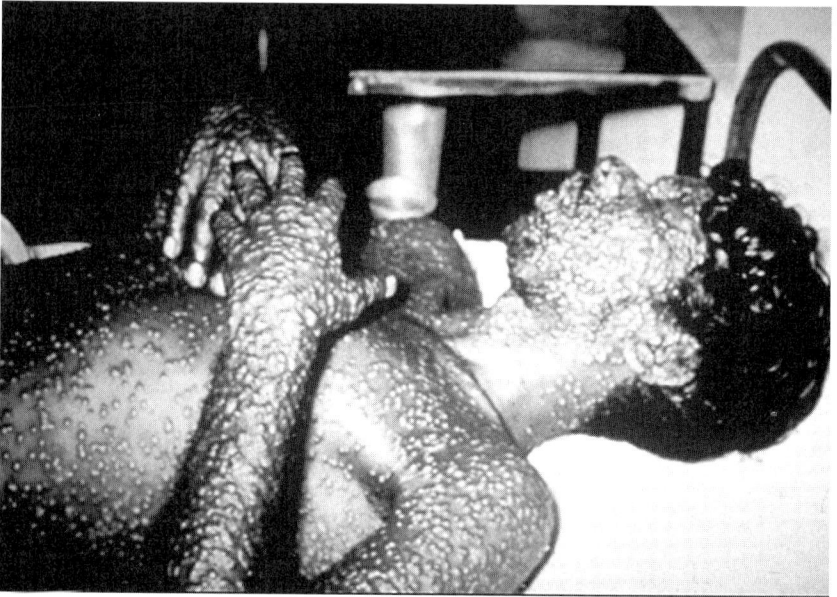

Fig. 7. Adult male with smallpox. Note density of rash and near confluence of pustules. In some patients the severity of the rash resulted in sloughing of large areas of skin. (*Courtesy of* Barbara Rice, Centers for Disease Control/NIP [public domain].)

As scabs separate and heal, deep hypopigmented scars form. Viral shedding and secondary infection cases may occur from the onset of the rash until scabs have separated [44,45]. Death usually occurs late in the first week or during the second week of the illness and is caused by the toxemia induced by the overwhelming viremia. A rare hemorrhagic form occurs with extensive bleeding into the skin and gastrointestinal tract followed almost universally by death within a few days.

During the vesicular stage, the rash may resemble chickenpox. There are two important distinctions, however. First, the rash of smallpox develops synchronously, in contrast to the asynchronous development observed with varicella. Second, the rash of smallpox is concentrated on the face and extremities, as opposed to on the trunk as occurs in chickenpox [50]. The pustules of smallpox are also notable for a characteristic central umbilication (Fig. 8).

Diagnosis

Initial diagnosis will likely be clinical, based on the characteristic rash. Diseases with similar skin manifestations must be considered in the differential diagnosis, including cutaneous lues (syphilis), meningococcemia, acute leukemia, or drug toxicity. Laboratory confirmation is extremely important, as a single case of smallpox must be treated as an international public health emergency [51]. Smallpox can be confirmed through clinical presentation and identification of the virion particles on electron microscopy of vesicular

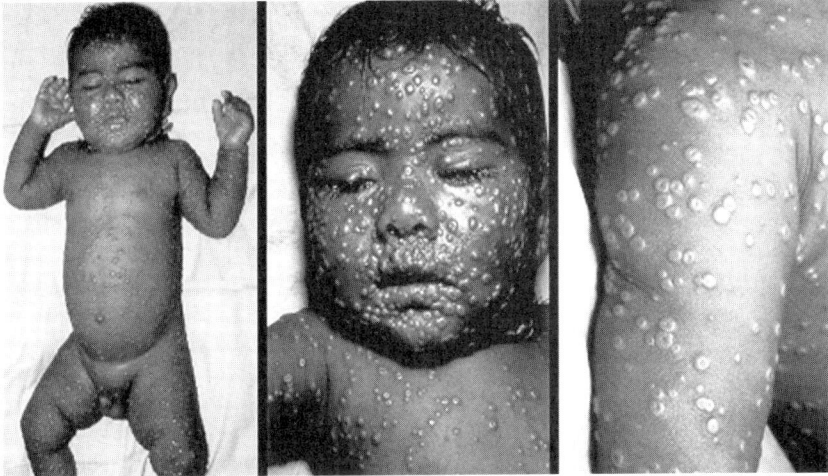

Fig. 8. Child with evolving smallpox. This series of photographs illustrates the evolution of skin lesions in an unvaccinated infant with the classic form of *Variola major*. (A) The third day of rash shows synchronous eruption of skin lesions; some are becoming vesiculated. (B) On the fifth day of rash, almost all papules are vesicular or pustular. (C) On the seventh day of rash, many lesions are umbilicated, and all lesions are in the same general stage of development. (*From* Fenner F. Henderson DA, Arita I, Jezek Z, Ladnyi ID. Smallpox and its eradication. Geneva: World Health Organization; 1988.)

fluid, although this only confirms presence of an orthopox virus. Further classification of the orthopox virus requires cell culture or growth on chorioallantoic egg membrane. Only Biosafety Level 4 containment laboratories should attempt to identify the agent [44,45].

Infection control precautions

During a small-scale attack, infected patients should be admitted to the hospital in negative-pressure isolation rooms with HEPA filtration. In larger outbreaks, home care of patients and quarantine may have to be considered [44]. The institution of a quarantine in today's society would pose numerous problems and would raise a myriad of legal issues [52]. In an attempt to address these issues, the CDC has recently published a model quarantine law that was developed after a comprehensive examination of existing state laws. The attorneys working for CDC attempted to modernize the proposed law so that it conforms to the advances in public health and medicine [53].

In addition to standard precautions (gowns, gloves, and masks), all hospital workers should use airborne and contact precautions [54]. Healthcare workers at risk should also receive immunizations (see later discussion). All contaminated material (ie, laundry and waste) should be placed in biohazard bags and should be autoclaved before incineration or washing. Standard hospital disinfecting solutions can be used to clean surfaces [44,51].

Treatment and prophylaxis

Treatment for smallpox is primarily supportive. Although no antivirals have been proven effective in humans, cidofovir has been shown to be effective in vitro [44,45]. Animal model data also demonstrate that cidofovir is active against a variety of orthopoxviruses. Data from monkeys infected with monkeypox showed that treatment after infection with clinically achievable concentrations of cidofovir was effective at reducing mortality. Human data demonstrate that achievable plasma concentrations following administration of the recommended cidofovir dose are effective against 32 human smallpox strains. Clinical disease has been reproduced in cynomolgus monkeys, but additional development and evaluation will be required before cidofovir can be directly tested in that model. An IND protocol has been submitted to the FDA for review (personal communication, John Huggins, PhD, December 2001).

Once an outbreak of smallpox is confirmed, a large-scale vaccination program will need to begin immediately. Even persons vaccinated before cessation of the program should be considered susceptible to infection [55]. Smallpox is somewhat unique in that postexposure vaccination may be effective in preventing or ameliorating disease even up to four days after infection. Anyone who has had a remote possibility of exposure should be vaccinated as soon as possible. Household members and those with face-to-face contact with the victim should be placed under surveillance and promptly isolated if they develop a fever higher than 38°C (101°F) for up to 17 days following exposure. These contacts should also be considered for postexposure immunization [44]. Because of the lack of effective treatment, the high risk for transmission by way of aerosol to hospital workers and patients, and the limited isolation capacity in hospitals, many infected victims may have to be cared for at home in the event of an attack [49]. Some patients may need to be cared for at home if the hospitals become overwhelmed with patients. This option may not be unreasonable because treatment is largely supportive and in most cases there is little that hospitalization can offer these patients. Air handling systems without HEPA filters may disseminate the infectious aerosol throughout the structure.

Vaccination is not without risk. Complications from the use of the current smallpox (vaccinia) vaccine range from the benign autoinoculation and generalized vaccinia through the more severe progressive vaccinia. The most serious complications include post-vaccinial encephalopathy and encephalitis. Before worldwide smallpox eradication, the only contraindications to vaccination were the state of pregnancy, certain immunocompromised conditions, and eczema.

Production of vaccinia vaccine was halted in the 1980s. The 15.4 million doses of vaccine available in the United States are under control of the Department of Health and Human Services (DHHS), but the diluent is outdated, requiring use of these stores under an IND protocol. Worldwide stores are estimated at approximately 50 million doses. In 2000, a study examined the "take" rate of undiluted vaccine and at a 1:10 and 1:100 dilutions. The results showed that the full-strength vaccine had maintained its potency, and that most people (70%) who received a single dose of the 10-percent vaccine developed a reaction at the scarification site and antibodies in their blood. The 1:100 dilution was not effective. Even though the 1:10 vaccine stimulated an immune response in most subjects, it will probably not protect a sufficient portion of the population to stop the spread of smallpox. A study has been designed to determine if a 1:5 (20%) vaccine combined with an alternative vaccination schedule would protect more people than did the standard dose and regimen (personal communication, John Huggins, PhD, December 2001).

The CDC has plans to increase the supply of vaccinations [23]. In late 2001, DHHS contracted with the British drug manufacturer Acambis to produce nearly 200 million doses of vaccine by the end of 2002 [48].

Yersinia pestis (plague)

History and significance

Yersinia pestis, a gram-negative bacillus, has tormented mankind throughout history. The Byzantine Empire recorded a sixth century pandemic, and the Black Death killed millions of people throughout fourteenth-century Europe. The most recent pandemic originated in China and spread worldwide at the turn of the twentieth century [56]. A new vaccine was available at that time, but was refused by the Indian populace as a British plot. As the pandemic spread across the Indian subcontinent, more than a million people died.

Plague is a zoonosis with a rodent host and a flea vector. The vector is not essential, however, and direct host-to-host transmission can occur by way of an infectious aerosol. A bite from an infected flea causes an infection in the lymphatic system leading to the bubonic form of the disease. Inhalation of aerosolized bacillus, preferred for deliberate dissemination, results in a primary pulmonary infection, known as pneumonic plague. The disease is rapidly fatal in the absence of prompt antibiotic treatment and may result in secondary contagion spread.

Y. pestis only occurs as a vegetative bacillus and is susceptible to destruction by drying, heat, and ultraviolet light. Direct weaponization is thus difficult. "Successful" attempts to use plague as a weapon in antiquity were probably related more to natural disease spread by fleas than by the practice of flinging plague-infected corpses over city walls. Modern efforts to weaponize *Y. pestis* were begun by the Japanese during World War II, but dissemination attempts met with limited success. Infected fleas were bred by the billions and then released over northern Chinese cities that had not previously recorded plague casualties. Epidemics subsequently occurred and plague has remained endemic in the region since [57]. The United States dismissed plague as a potential weapon because of its persistence in the environment and the likelihood of non-combatant and friendly casualties after an attack. The former Soviet Union's extensive biological warfare program however, reportedly included dry, antibiotic-resistant, environmentally stable forms of the plague organism that could be disseminated as an aerosol [3].

Clinical presentation

Skin penetration or direct ingestion of fewer than 10 *Y. pestis* organisms can induce an infection in humans. In research models, the minimal respiratory dose ranges from 100 to 20,000 organisms [58]. The clinical course will vary substantially with the route of exposure. If plague were used as a biological weapon, the most likely exposure route would be via inhalation.

Bubonic plague is acquired naturally through the bite of a flea after it regurgitates the contents from its *Y. pestis*-infected foregut [59]. The bacilli are phagocytized by macrophages and some of the organisms proliferate intracellularly. The organisms develop an antiphagocytic capsule, multiple new *Yersinia* outer-membrane protein (Yop) antigens, and a plasminogen activator [60]. Organisms become resistant to phagocytosis and rapidly multiply extracellularly. Spread to regional lymph nodes causes a suppurative lesion one to eight days after the initial infection, the characteristic "bubo" (Figs. 9 and 10). Without treatment, the disease most likely will progress to septicemia within days [61]. Between 5%–15% of patients will develop a secondary pneumonia and will shed infectious bacilli in droplet nuclei while coughing [62]. Because these organisms already possess an anti-phagocytic capsule in contrast to the "naked" bacilli that are delivered in the weaponized version, they are particularly virulent [63].

Toward the end of the incubation period, patients usually demonstrate malaise, headache, fever, nausea, and vomiting. Six to eight hours after the onset of symptoms, buboes become markedly enlarged and exquisitely painful. By 24 hours buboes are visible, usually in the femoral and inguinal areas from fleabites on the lower extremities. Tuberculosis, chanchroid, lymphogranuloma venereum, adenitis, and scrub typhus are included in the differential diagnosis. Plague may lead to the development of abdominal pain, confusion, oliguria, bladder distension, and obtundation. At later stages the differential diagnoses include meningitis, encephalitis, and other infectious processes. Acral necrosis of distal extremities may develop in patients with septicemic plague (Fig. 11). The massive ecchymoses and fetid odor gave the disease the name "Black Death" during the Middle Ages. Gastrointestinal plague follows a similar, rapid course. In the latter case, buboes develop in mesenteric drainage sites and early gastrointestinal symptoms predominate. Pneumonic plague presents without buboes and may progress rapidly if vegetative organisms with previously developed antiphagocytic capsules and Yop antigens have been inhaled as an aerosol [63]. Most patients develop a productive cough with blood-tinged sputum within 24 hours of the

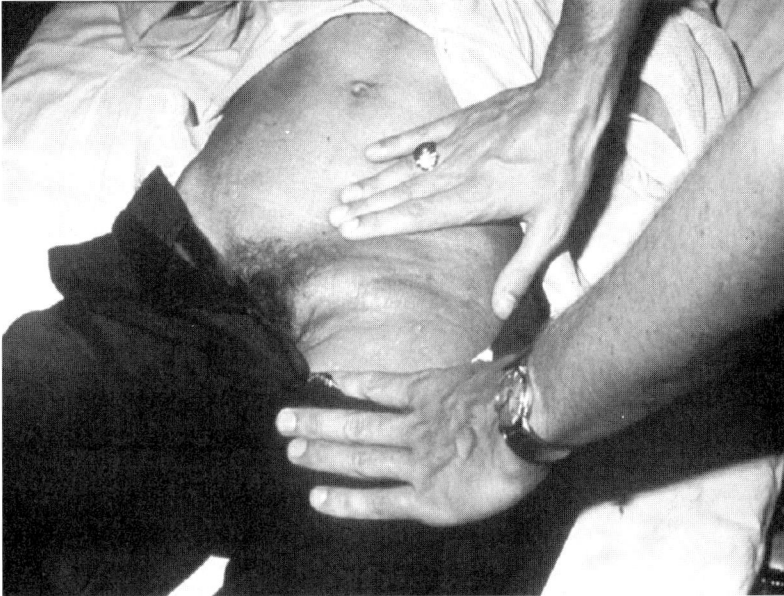

Fig. 9. Adult patient with bubonic plague. Note presence of large femoral bubo. These lesions are exquisitely tender. At this point in the disease process patients are extremely ill and may begin showing signs of sepsis. Prompt and aggressive antibiotic therapy is warranted. Incision and drainage of these lesions is not indicated. (*From* Butler T. Textbook of plague and other yersinia infections. New York: Plenum Press; 1983.)

onset of symptoms. This is an important diagnostic clue that should lead one to consider bioterrorism if many previously well patients present with this sign [59]. Chest radiographs may reveal a consolidating lobar pneumonia [64].

Diagnosis

Demonstration of the *Y. pestis* organism by way of direct fluorescent antibody staining of the capsular antigen is available [65]. Buboes may be aspirated with a small-gauge needle, but incision and drainage should not be performed because of the significant risk for aerosolization of the organism. Peripheral blood smears and sputum should be examined under Gram's, Wayson's, or Wright-Giemsa stain. The bipolar "safety pin" morphology is usually evident.

Initial hematologic studies will demonstrate a leukocytosis with a left shift. Because of hepatic involvement, bilirubin levels and serum aminotransferases are often elevated. Blood, sputum, bubo aspirate, and CSF cultures on normal blood agar media are often negative at 24 hours but positive by 48 hours [56]. The colonies of *Y. pestis* are usually one to three millimeters in diameter and have been described as having a "beaten copper" or "hammered metal" appearance.

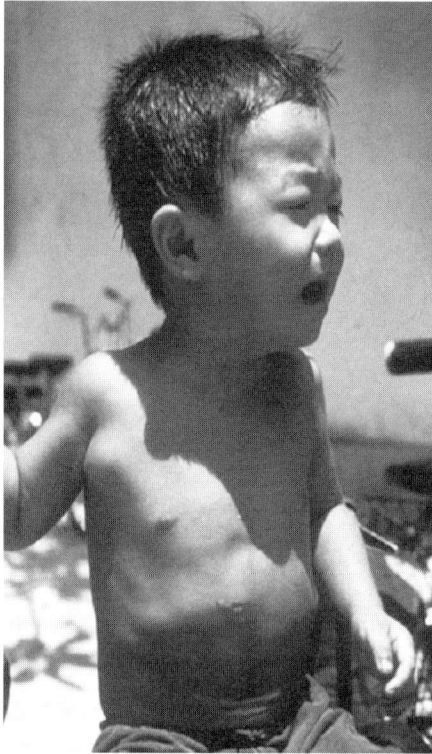

Fig. 10. Axillary bubo in a child. (*From* Butler T. Textbook of plague and other yersinia infections. New York: Plenum Press; 1983.)

Infection control precautions

Patients with bubonic plague will require body fluid precautions and segregation from other patients until completion of at least three days of appropriate antibiotics. Those patients who are suspected of having septicemia, respiratory symptoms, or pneumonic plague should be maintained under droplet precautions, including the use of eyeshields, masks, gowns, gloves, and negative-pressure isolation, until completion of four days of antibiotic therapy [56].

Treatment and prophylaxis

Historically, the antibiotic of choice for *Y. pestis* infection has been intramuscular streptomycin, 15 mg/kg bid. Buboes typically resolve after 10–14 days of therapy. Gentamicin and gentamicin-chloramphenicol combinations are acceptable alternative regimens. If meningitis is suspected, or if the patient is hemodynamically unstable, use of chloramphenicol (50–75 mg/kg/d) is mandatory. Treatment should be continued for a minimum of 10 days or for 4 days after clinical recovery. Mildly ill patients may be treated with oral tetracycline. Laboratory models demonstrate that doxycycline, ofloxacin, and ceftriaxone all have significant efficacy in the treatment of plague [56].

The primary preventive measures for bubonic plague include flea and rodent control. In epidemic or epizootic areas, intensive use of insecticides must precede any use of rodenticides. The death of many host rodents would induce infected fleas to seek alternative hosts, such as humans, and may induce or worsen an epidemic [62].

Medical personnel who practice good barrier precautions require no prophylaxis. Unprotected direct contacts should receive postexposure prophylaxis with tetracycline (15–30 mg/kg/d) or doxycycline (100mg bid) for six days. Alternatively, administration of trimethoprim/sulfamethoxazole may be used in sensitive individuals. Other persons who should be considered for prophylaxis are individuals who were known to be in the same environment as the casualties. Plague vaccine USP that was protective against bubonic plague is no longer available. Moreover, it did not protect against aerosol

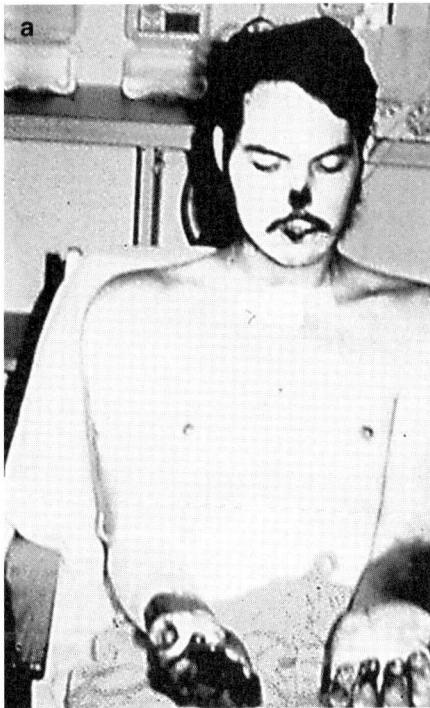

Fig. 11. This patient is recovering from bubonic plague that disseminated to the blood (septicemic form) and the lungs (pneumonic form). Note the dressing over the tracheostomy site. At one point, the patient's entire body was purpuric. Note the acral necrosis of (a) the patient's nose and fingers, and (b) the toes. (*Courtesy of* Ken Gage, PhD, Centers for Disease Control and Prevention, Fort Collins, CO [public domain].)

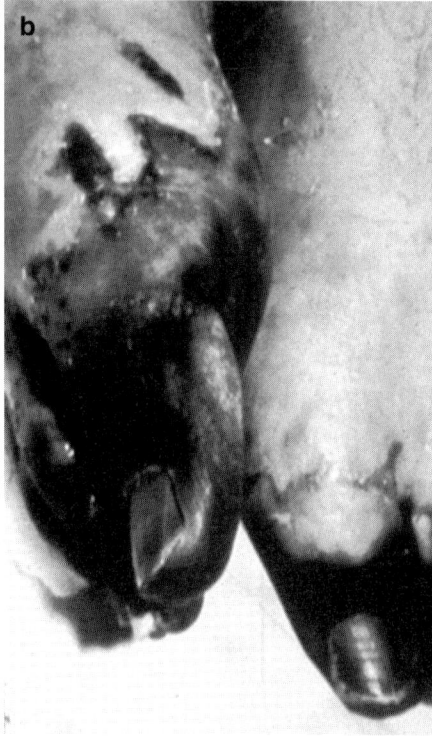

Fig. 11 (*continued*)

infection in test models [66]. A recombinant vaccine is under development and seems to protect against the pneumonic variant of plague.

Francisella tularensis (tularemia)

History and significance

Francisella tularensis, the causative agent of tularemia, is a small, aerobic, non-motile, gram-negative cocco-bacillus. Tularemia (also known as rabbit fever and deer fly fever) is a zoonotic disease that humans may acquire after skin or mucous membrane contact with tissues or body fluids of infected animals, or from bites of infected ticks, deerflies, or mosquitoes. Less commonly, inhalation of contaminated dusts or ingestion of contaminated foods or water may produce clinical disease. Respiratory exposure by aerosol would typically cause typhoidal or pneumonic tularemia. *F. tularensis* remains viable for weeks in water, soil, carcasses, hides, and for years in frozen meat. Resistant for months to temperatures of freezing and below, it is easily killed by heat and disinfectants [67].

Tularemia was recognized in Japan in the early 1800s and in Russia in 1926. In the early 1900s American workers investigating suspected plague epidemics in San Francisco isolated the organism and named it *Bacterium tularense* after Tulare County, California where the research was performed [68]. Dr. Edward Francis, USPHS, established the cause of deer fly fever as *Bacterium tularense*, and subsequently devoted his life to researching the organism and disease [69]. Hence, the organism was later renamed *Francisella tularensis*.

Francisella tularensis was weaponized by the United States in the 1950s and 1960s during the US offensive biowarfare program. Other countries are suspected to have weaponized this agent [70]. This organism could potentially be stabilized for weaponization by an adversary and produced in a wet or dried form for delivery against US forces or as a weapon of terror in a fashion similar to the other bacteria discussed in this article.

Clinical presentation

Onset of disease is usually acute and occurs after an incubation period that ranges from 1 to 21 days (average three to five days), presumably dependent on the dose of organisms received. Tularemia typically appears in one of six forms in humans, depending on the route of inoculation: typhoidal, ulceroglandular, glandular, oculoglandular, oropharyngeal, and pneumonic tularemia [71]. In humans, as few as 10 to 50 organisms may cause disease if inhaled or injected intradermally; however, approximately 10^8 organisms are required with oral challenge [72]. All ages are susceptible, and recovery is generally followed by permanent immunity.

Typhoidal tularemia (5%–15% of naturally acquired cases) occurs mainly after inhalation of infectious aerosols, but can occur after intradermal or gastrointestinal challenge. *F. tularensis* would most likely be delivered as an aerosol if used as a weapon and would primarily cause typhoidal tularemia that manifests as fever, prostration, and weight loss, but unlike most other forms of the disease, presents without lymphadenopathy. Pneumonia may be severe and fulminant and may be associated with any form of tularemia (30% of ulceroglandular cases), but it is most common in typhoidal tularemia (80% of cases) [73]. Respiratory symptoms, substernal discomfort, and a cough (productive or nonproductive) may also be present. Case fatality rates following a bioterrorist attack may be greater than the 1%–3% seen with appropriately treated natural disease. Case fatality rates are approximately 35% in untreated naturally acquired typhoidal cases

Ulceroglandular tularemia (75%–85% of cases) is most often acquired through inoculation of skin or mucous membranes by blood or fluids of infected animals and is characterized by fever, chills, headache, malaise, an ulcerated skin lesion, and painful regional lymphadenopathy. Skin lesions are usually located on the fingers or hand where contact with the agent occurs. The case fatality rate is approximately 5% without treatment [67].

Glandular tularemia (5%–10% of cases) causes fever and tender lympha-denopathy without skin ulceration.

Oculoglandular tularemia (1%–2% of cases) occurs after inoculation of the conjunctivae by contaminated hands, splattering of infected tissue fluids, or by aerosols. Patients have unilateral, painful, purulent conjunctivitis with preauricular or cervical lymphadenopathy. Chemosis, periorbital edema, and small nodular lesions or ulcerations of the palpebral conjunctiva are noted in some patients.

Oropharyngeal tularemia refers to a primarily ulceroglandular disease confined to the throat. It produces an acute exudative or membranous phar-yngotonsillitis with cervical lymphadenopathy.

Pneumonic tularemia is a severe, atypical pneumonia that may be fulmi-nant and is associated with a high case fatality rate if untreated. It occurs after inhalation of organisms (primary) or following hematogenous or sep-ticemic spread (secondary). It occurs in 30%–80% of typhoidal cases and in 10%–15% of ulceroglandular cases [67].

Diagnosis

A clue to the diagnosis of tularemia resulting from a bioterrorist attack may be a large number of temporally clustered patients presenting with sim-ilar systemic illnesses and a nonproductive cough and pneumonia. The clin-ical presentation of tularemia may be severe yet non-specific. Differential diagnoses include other typhoidal syndromes (eg, salmonella, rickettsia, malaria) or pneumonic processes (eg, plague, mycoplasma, SEB).

Radiologic evidence of pneumonia or mediastinal lymphadenopathy is most common with typhoidal disease. Approximately 50% of patients have pneumonia radiograpically, and less than 1% have hilar adenopathy without parenchymal involvement. Pleural effusions are seen in 15% of patients with pneumonia. Interstitial patterns, cavitary lesions, bronchopleural fistulae, and calcifications have also been reported [74–76].

Initial laboratory evaluations are generally nonspecific. Peripheral WBC count usually ranges from 5000 to 22,000 cells per microliter. Differential blood cell counts are normal, occasionally with a lymphocytosis late in the disease. Hematocrit, hemoglobin, and platelet levels are usually normal. Mild elevations in lactic dehydrogenase, serum transaminases, and alkaline phosphatase are common. Rhabdomyolysis may be associated with eleva-tions in serum creatine kinase and urinary myoglobin levels. Cerebrospinal fluid is usually normal, although mild abnormalities in protein, glucose, and white blood cell count have been reported [67].

Tularemia can be diagnosed by recovery of the organism in cultures of blood, ulcers, conjunctival exudates, sputum, gastric washings, and phar-yngeal exudates. Recovery may be possible even after the institution of appropriate antibiotic therapy [72]. The organism grows poorly on standard media but produces small, smooth, opaque colonies after 24–48 hours on media containing cysteine or other sulfhydryl compounds (eg, glucose cysteine blood agar, thioglycollate broth). Isolation of the organism represents a clear hazard to laboratory personnel and culture should only be attempted in a Biosafety Level 3 containment facility.

Most diagnoses of tularemia are made serologically using bacterial agglutination or enzyme-linked immunosorbent assay (ELISA) [77–79]. Antibodies to *F. tularensis* appear within the first week of infection, but levels adequate to allow confidence in the specificity of the serologic diagnosis (titer >1:160) do not appear until more than two weeks after infection [79,80]. Because cross-reactions can occur with *Brucella* species [81–83], Proteus OX19 [84], and *Yersinia* organisms, and because antibodies may persist for years after infection, the diagnosis should be made only if a fourfold or greater increase in the tularemia tube agglutination or microagglutination titer is seen during the course of the illness. Titers are usually negative during the first week of infection, become positive during the second week in 50%–70% of cases, and achieve a maximum level at four to eight weeks [85].

Infection control precautions

Neither isolation nor quarantine is required. Strict adherence to standard precautions is required, especially for draining lesions, and during disinfection of soiled clothing, bedding, and equipment [86]. Heat and disinfectants easily inactivate the organism.

Treatment and prophylaxis

Streptomycin has historically been the drug of choice for tularemia. Because it may not be readily available immediately after a large-scale bioterrorist event, however, gentamicin and other alternative drugs should be considered first [87–89]. Requests for streptomycin should be directed to the Roerig Streptomycin Program at Pfizer Pharmaceuticals in New York (800-254-4445). Another concern is that a fully virulent streptomycin-resistant strain of *F. tularensis* was developed during the 1950s and it is presumed that other countries have obtained it. This strain was sensitive to gentamicin. Gentamicin also offers the advantage of providing broader coverage for gram-negative bacteria and may be useful when the diagnosis of tularemia is considered but not confirmed.

Initial antibiotic therapy consists of either intravenous gentamicin or ciprofloxacin. Once the patient has clinically improved treatment may be changed to oral ciprofloxacin or streptomycin. Tetracycline and chloramphenicol are also effective antibiotics; however, they are associated with higher relapse rates.

An investigational live-attenuated vaccine (Live Vaccine Strain, LVS), administered by scarification, has been given to more than 5000 persons without significant adverse reactions and can prevent the typhoidal form and ameliorate the ulceroglandular form of laboratory-acquired tularemia [90]. Aerosol challenge tests in laboratory animals and human volunteers have demonstrated significant protection [91–94]. As with all vaccines, the degree of protection depends on the magnitude of the challenge dose. Vaccine-induced protection could be overwhelmed by extremely high doses of the tularemia bacteria.

Ciprofloxacin or doxycycline may confer postexposure protection against tularemia, based on in vitro susceptibilities. A two-week course is effective as postexposure prophylaxis when given within 24 hours of aerosol exposure. Chemoprophylaxis is not recommended following potential natural exposures.

Viral hemorrhagic fevers

History and significance

The viral hemorrhagic fevers are caused by a diverse group of ribonucleic acid (RNA) viruses in four separate families: Arenaviridae, Bunyaviridae, Filoviridae, and Flaviviridae. All have lipid envelopes, limited geographic ranges, are highly infectious by way of the aerosol route (except Dengue), and are believed to have animal reservoirs with arthropod vectors. Terrorist groups have attempted to weaponize agents from this class [95]. Each disease is characterized by its own unique characteristics, but all have a final common pathway of diffuse hemorrhage and bleeding diathesis.

Yellow fever and dengue (Flaviviridae) are probably the archetypical diseases of this group, but are not considered significant biological warfare threat agents. Hantavirus (Bunyaviridae) is enzootic in rodents. West Africa's Lassa fever, and Argentine, Bolivian, Brazilian, and Venezuelan hemorrhagic fevers (Arenaviridae) are also enzootic in rodents within their respective areas. The most publicized viral hemorrhagic fevers are the Ebola and Marburg (Filoviridae) viruses. These viruses produce grotesquely lethal diseases making them favorites with the popular media (Fig. 12). The reservoir and natural transmission of Ebola and Marburg are unknown but they are readily transmittable by infected blood and tissue. Aerosols may be formed naturally when infectious body fluids are expelled or in the case of hantavirus when rodent feces and urine are resuspended by movement in the area. Laboratory cultures can yield sufficient concentrations of organisms to provide a credible terrorist weapon if disseminated as an aerosol.

Clinical presentation

The presentation of each type of hemorrhagic fever can vary significantly. Some of the factors that influence presentation include the route of infection, the virulence of the virus, the specific viral strain, the health of the individual patient, vaccination status, and quantity of the inoculum. The main

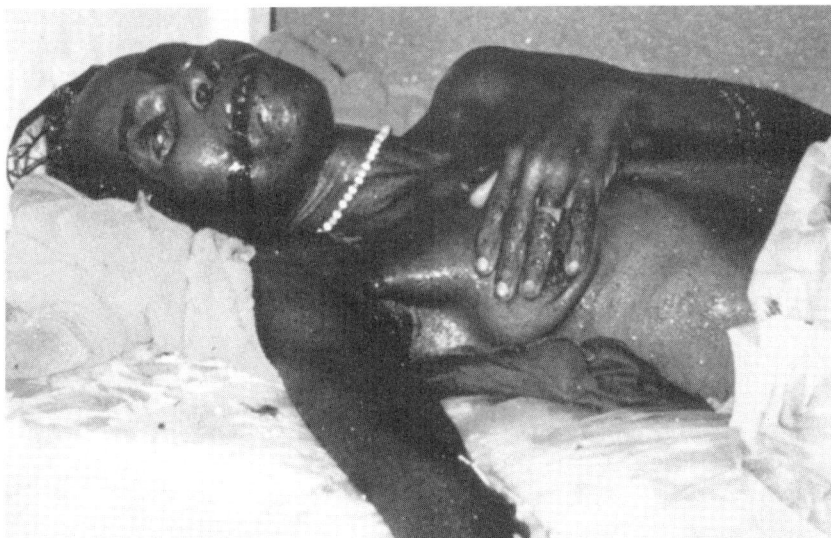

Fig. 12. Gravely ill African female with Ebola virus infection. Note extensive hemorrhage from mouth. This photo was taken during the Zaire outbreak of 1995. (*Courtesy of* Ken Gage, PhD, Centers for Disease Control and Prevention, Fort Collins, CO [public domain].)

differences among the diseases are their primary organ targets, but the end result is a bleeding diathesis. A viral hemorrhagic fever should be suspected in any patient presenting with a severe febrile illness and evidence of vascular involvement [96].

Lassa fever presents as a mild or subclinical disease in up to 90% of cases. Most patients present with cough, chest pain, pharyngitis, proteinuria, abdominal pain, and vomiting. Less than 20% develop mucosal hemorrhages. In endemic areas, the combination of proteinuria, retrosternal pain, fever, and pharyngitis is considered 70% specific for diagnosis [96]. Children seem to be more susceptible to development of severe morbidity and mortality. Patients developing hypotension, peripheral vasoconstriction, oliguria, and facial or pulmonary edema often develop mucosal hemorrhages. Survivors often develop eighth nerve deafness.

The immunologically distinct Argentine (Junin), Bolivian (Machupo), and other South American hemorrhagic fevers have similar clinical presentations, with mortality between 15%–30% [96]. Myalgia, low back pain, fever, and malaise herald the onset of illness. Subsequently, photophobia, conjunctival injection flushing, and orthostatic hypotension may develop. The petechial exanthem, retro-orbital pain, and lymphadenopathy yield to encephalopathy and vascular disease with marked microvascular damage and increased capillary permeability. Mucous membranes become hemorrhagic and shock ensues. The development of seizures and cerebellar dysfunction herald a fatal outcome.

The Marburg and Ebola viruses (Filoviridae) are most commonly transmitted by contaminated needles in medical facilities or by the preparation of bodies for burial. Body fluids may contain high concentrations of virus and are extremely hazardous. Skin tissues are heavily laden with virus during the active disease phase. The incubation period is usually 5 to 10 days with the onset of disease marked by fever, myalgia, and headache. Symptoms progress to include chest pain, abdominal pain, nausea, vomiting, diarrhea, cough, and pharyngitis. Photophobia, conjunctival injection, and pancreatitis may develop. Later stages include hemorrhages, petechiae, and extensive areas of ecchymosis (Fig. 13). By day five most patients develop a maculopapular rash. During the second week, defervescence occurs and the patient either deteriorates into shock with multi-system organ failure and disseminated intravascular coagulopathy or begins to recover. The filoviruses have been detected in all body fluids including semen of survivors [96]. Consequently negative viral cultures should be obtained before release of the patient.

Diagnosis

In a bioterrorism scenario, aerosol dissemination would result in many patients who shared a common location approximately three to eight days before presentation. Specific disease identification requires ELISA detection of antiviral IgM antibodies or direct culture of the viral agent from blood or tissue samples. If the agent remains unknown, it may be visualized by electron microscopy followed by immunohistochemical techniques [97]. During the clinical course of each of the diseases, hepatocellular enzymes are often elevated. Appropriate precautions should be observed in collection, handling, and processing of diagnostic samples, which should be sent to a Level D laboratory that currently exist only at the CDC or USAMRIID.

Infection control precautions

Because all of the viral hemorrhagic fever viruses (except the dengue fever virus) may be transmitted by way of an infectious aerosol, aerosol precautions should be strictly maintained. All body fluids should be considered contagious. Under ideal conditions, each patient should be cared for in a private room. The room should be entered through an adjoining anteroom that is used for decontamination and handwashing. Staff should be provided a changing area and suitable protective equipment. The room should be maintained under negative air pressure and the air should be filtered and vented, not recirculated. Even in the absence of signs during the pre-clinical phase, a negative airflow room is recommended to avoid having to transfer the patient later. Normal barrier protective garments should be adequate protection for staff, but HEPA-filtered positive pressure masks combined with impermeable Level A protective suits would provide an added level of protection [96].

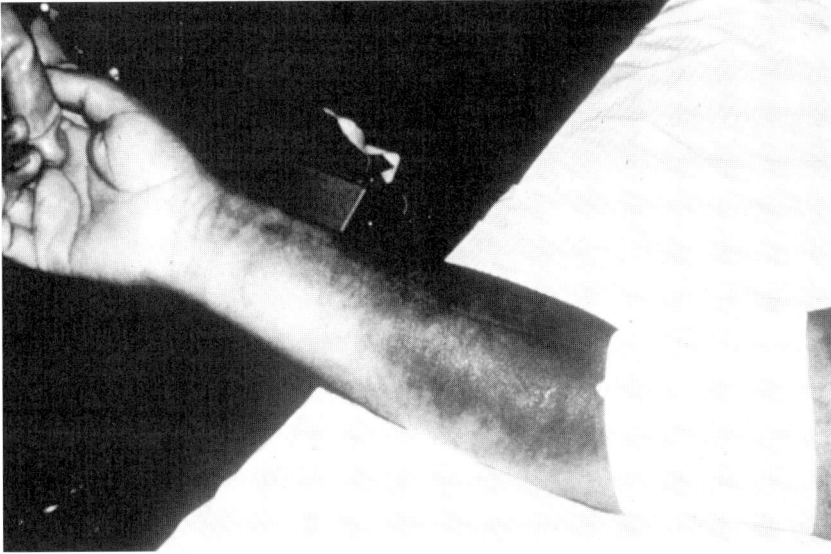

Fig. 13. Massive cutaneous ecchymosis associated with late-stage Crimean-Congo hemorrhagic fever virus infection, 7 to 10 days after clinical onset. Ecchymosis indicates multiple abnormalities in the coagulation system, coupled with loss of vascular integrity. Epistaxis and profuse bleeding from puncture sites, hematemesis, melena, and ecchymoses may occur anywhere on the body as a result of needlesticks or other minor trauma. The sharply demarcated proximal border of this patient's lesion is not explained. (*Courtesy of* Pierre Rollin, Centers for Disease Control and Prevention, Special Pathogens Section, Atlanta, GA [public domain].)

Treatment and prophylaxis

All therapy is supportive. No specific treatment has been demonstrated as safe and effective for any of the hemorrhagic fevers. The goal of therapy is to maintain function and allow recovery in casualties where possible. Ribaviran is under human investigational trials and shows promise in the treatment of Congo-Crimean hemorrhagic fever, hantavirus, and Lassa fever infections [98]. Close personal contacts of patients or medical personnel exposed to blood or secretions from a patient with a viral hemorrhagic fever should be monitored for signs and symptoms during the incubation period. Oral ribaviran may be effective in the prophylaxis of high-risk contacts [96].

Clostridium botulinum toxin (botulism)

History and significance

Clostridium botulinum is a gram-positive, spore-forming, anaerobic bacillus found in soil around the world. Botulism is the syndrome caused by botulinum toxin produced by this bacterium, or in rare cases, *Clostridium butyricum* and *Clostridium baratii*. Cases have historically been categorized according to transmission as foodborne illness (from ingestion of the toxin in home-canned goods, poorly heated vegetables, or meats), wound botulism (secondary to soil-contaminated wounds, drug abuse, and C-section deliveries), and infantile illness (from ingestion of spores) [99]. A fourth form, adult intestinal colonization botulism, has recently been described [100]. It occurs in the presence of colitis, after bowel surgery, or in association with local or widespread disruption in the normal intestinal flora [100]. In 1999, there were 154 cases of botulism reported to the CDC, with the infantile form predominating (92 cases) [101].

Botulinum toxin is one of the most toxic substances known, with an LD_{50} of 0.001 μg/kg [102,104], making it 100,000 times more toxic per microgram than the nerve agent sarin [99]. Seven distinct types of toxin exist, identified by antigenicity and referred to as types A–G. Types A, B, and E are most often responsible for human disease, whereas types C and D cause disease only in other animals. Spores can survive several hours at 100°C, but toxins are heat labile, and become inactivated after one minute at 85°C. Theoretically there is enough toxin present in a single gram of crystallized Botulinum toxin to kill more than one million people [99]. Botulinum toxin could be used to sabotage food supplies, although a more likely scenario would involve dissemination as an aerosol [104]. During the Gulf War, Iraq produced 20,000 L of botulinum toxin, 12,000 liters of which were used in field-testing and to fill warheads [4]. Scientists in the former Soviet Union and the Aum Shinrikyo cult in Japan also experimented with botulinum toxin [3,12]. Despite these efforts to produce an effective botulinum toxin weapon, most authorities agree that it is unlikely this toxin could ever be effectively deployed as a weapon of mass destruction. Aerosol delivery over a battlefield or a defined geographic region populated by civilians would require a precisely orchestrated effort. Large quantities of toxin would have to be delivered to the area at the optimal time because botulinum toxin quickly degrades in the environment and is therefore rendered non-lethal to the intended target minutes after release. Even municipal water reservoirs are most likely safe from contamination by terrorist actions because literally ton quantities of toxin would be necessary because of the effects of dilution. In addition, botulinum toxin is not stable for extended periods in water and chlorination provides an effective means of destruction.

Clinical presentation

All seven neurotoxins act through the same mechanism. Botulinum toxin binds to receptors on presynaptic terminals of cholinergic synapses where it is internalized into vesicles and released into the cytosol. It then acts to prevent exocytosis and to permanently impair acetylcholine release. Recovery occurs when the axon sprouts a new terminal to replace the toxin-damaged one. Chemical effects are seen at the neuromuscular junction and cholinergic sites resulting in cranial nerve deficits and descending skeletal muscle weakness that are the clinical hallmarks of all forms of botulism [99,104].

The classic presentation for botulism occurs 12–72 hours following exposure. The patient complains first of visual changes and bulbar symptoms including (eg, mydriasis and diplopia, photophobia, dysarthria, dysphagia, and dysphonia). Physical examination demonstrates an awake, afebrile patient with a normal mental status who may complain of a dry mouth or sore throat. The pupils may be dilated and possibly fixed. The gag reflex is diminished or absent. Extraocular muscle palsies or ptosis may be evident (Fig. 14). The patient exhibits varying degrees of symmetric descending muscle weakness or paralysis without a sensory deficit. Respiratory depression or failure may ensue, leading to mental status changes from retention of carbon dioxide. Should the disease progress to this point, death will occur secondary to respiratory failure if ventilatory support is not provided [99,104].

The differential diagnosis includes neuromuscular disorders such as myasthenia gravis, Guillain-Barré (ascending paralysis), poliomyelitis, or tick paralysis (ascending paralysis). An edrophonium test, used to detect myasthenia, may be falsely positive, but electromyography differentiates between the two [99].

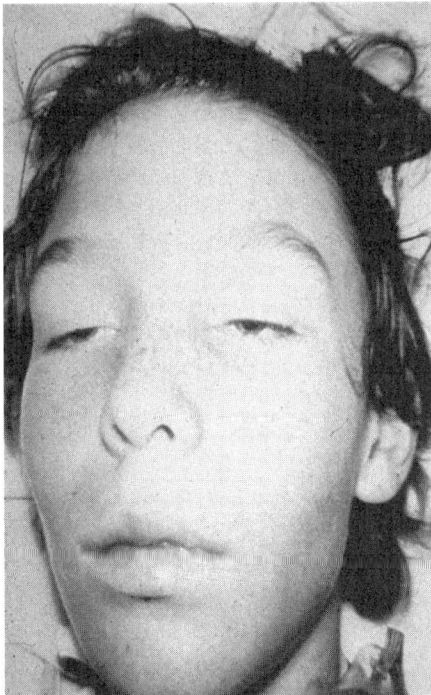

Fig. 14. Adolescent female with wound botulism. Note marked ptosis and absence of facial expression. (*Courtesy of* Robert Swanepoel, PhD, DTVM, MRCVS, National Institute of Virology, Sandringham, South Africa.)

Diagnosis

In the emergency setting the diagnosis of botulism intoxication will be clinical. An influx of patients with descending muscle paralysis and bulbar findings may herald a bioterrorist event or a natural outbreak of foodborne botulism. No routine laboratory tests will aid in the diagnosis. Specialized tests (ie, mouse bioassay) often require days to complete. The toxin may be detected by assays of serum or gastric contents. Specimens should be examined by appropriately designated laboratories [99,104].

Infection control precautions

Botulism is not transmitted from person to person. Healthcare workers should be instructed to use standard precautions. Isolation is unnecessary. Decontamination with soap and water should be performed after an acute exposure to aerosolized toxin [99,104]. Clothes should be removed, bagged, and preserved as potential criminal evidence [103].

Treatment and prophylaxis

Treatment of the patient with botulinum toxin poisoning relies on ventilatory support because respiratory failure secondary to muscle paralysis is the most serious complication. Intubation and mechanical ventilation are usually necessary. The patient may require weeks to months of intensive care and it may take up to one year for patients to fully recover [99].

Three different antitoxin preparations are available in the United States. A trivalent equine botulinum antitoxin, containing antibodies to Types A, B, and E, is available through the CDC and some state health departments [105]. A monovalent human antiserum (type A) is available from the California Department of Health Services for infant botulism, and a despeciated equine heptavalent antitoxin against all seven serotypes is available from the US Army Medical Research Institute of Infectious Diseases (USAMRIID) (www.uamriid.army.mil). This latter product is available only under IND protocol.

Antitoxin may prevent progression or shorten the course of the illness. It acts by neutralizing toxin not yet bound to nerve terminals and has a circulating half-life of five to eight days. Untreated patients show free toxin in serum for up to 28 days. It should therefore be given as soon as possible after the clinical diagnosis. There is no indication at present for use of botulinum antitoxin as a prophylactic modality. Skin testing for sensitivity to horse serum must be performed before administration of the antitoxin [99,104].

A pentavalent toxoid of *Clostridium botulinum* toxin types A, B, C, D, and E is available as an IND product for pre-exposure prophylaxis. The currently recommended primary series of 0, 2, and 12 weeks, followed by a 1-year booster, induces protective immunity in greater than 90% of vaccinees after one year.

Physicians are encouraged to call their state epidemiologists as soon as a case of botulism is suspected, to facilitate expedient investigation. Epidemiologists can work in concert with the CDC to coordinate acquisition of the antitoxin and offer recommendations for laboratory testing and patient management [105].

Summary

Although once considered unlikely, bioterrorism is now a reality in the United States since the anthrax cases began appearing in the fall of 2001. Intelligence sources indicate there are many countries and terrorist organizations that either possess biological weapons or are attempting to procure them. In the future it is likely that we will experience additional acts of bioterrorism. The CDC category A agents represent our greatest challenge because they have the potential to cause grave harm to the medical and public health systems of a given population. Thus, it is imperative that plans be developed now to deal with the consequences of an intentional release of any one or more of these pathogens.

References

[1] Okumura T, Takas N, Ishimatsu S, et al. Report on 640 victims of the Tokyo subway sarin attack. Ann Emerg Med 1996;28(2):129–35.

[2] Suzuki J, Kohno T, Tsukagosi M, et al. Eighteen cases exposed to sarin in Matsumoto. Japan Int Med 1997;36(7):466–70.

[3] Alibek K. Biohazard. New York: Random House; 1999.

[4] Zilinskas RA. Iraq's biological weapons, the past as future? JAMA 1997;278(5):418–24.

[5] Centers for Disease Control and Prevention. Biological and chemical terrorism: strategic plan for preparedness and response. Recommendations of the CDC Strategic Planning Workgroup. Morb Mortal Wkly Rep 2000;49(RR-4):1–4.

[6] Simon JD. Biological terrorism, preparing to meet the threat. JAMA 1997;278(5):428–30.

[7] Eitzen EM. Education is the key to defense against bioterrorism. Ann Emerg Med 1999; 34(2):221–3.

[8] Look for syndromes in absence of cultures. Hosp Inf Control 2000;27(3):36.

[9] Carter A, Deutsch J, Zelicow P. Catastrophic terrorism. Foreign Aff 1998;77:80–95.

[10] Brown D. Canadian study shows anthrax's easy spread: one letter could cause many deaths. Washington Post, December 12, 2001. p. A27.

[11] Pile JC, Malone JD, Eitzen EM, et al. Anthrax as a potential biological warfare agent. Arch Intern Med 1998;158:429–34.

[12] Christopher GW, Cieslak TJ, Pavlin JA, et al. Biological warfare, a historical perspective. JAMA 1997;278(5):412–7.

[13] Cole LA. The specter of biological weapons. Sci Am 1996;December:60–5.

[14] Barnes JM. Penicillin and B anthracis. J Pathol Bacteriol 1947;194:113–25.

[15] Meselson M, Guillemin J, Hugh-Jones M, et al. The Sverdlovsk anthrax outbreak of 1979. Science 1994;266:1202–8.

[16] WuDunn S, Miller J, Broad W. How Japan germ terror alerted world. New York Times, May 26, 1998. p. 1–6.

[17] Bush L, Abrams B, Beall A, Johnson C. Index case of fatal inhalational anthrax due to bioterrorism in the United States. N Engl J Med 2001;345:1607–10.

[18] Jernigan J, Stephens D, Ashford D, et al. Bioterrorism-related inhalational anthrax: the first 10 cases reported in the United States. Emerg Infect Dis 2001;7:933–44.

[19] Borio L, Frank D, Mani V, et al. Death due to bioterrorism-related inhalational anthrax: report of 2 patients. JAMA 2001;286:2554–9.

[20] Centers for Disease Control and Prevention. Investigation of bioterrorism-related anthrax, 2001. Morb Mortal Wkly Rep 2001;50:1008–10.

[21] Centers for Disease Control and Prevention. Update: investigation of bioterrorism-related anthrax and interim guidelines for exposure management and antimicrobial therapy, October 2001. Morb Mortal Wkly Rep 2001;50(42):909–19.

[22] Centers for Disease Control and Prevention. Update: investigation of bioterrorism-related anthrax – Connecticut, 2001. Morb Mortal Wkly Rep 2001;50:1077–9.

[23] Centers for Disease Control and Prevention gearing up rapid vaccine response plans for smallpox bioterror. Hosp Inf Control 2000;27(3):29–35.

[24] Centers for Disease Control and Prevention. Update: investigation of bioterrorism-related inhalational anthrax – Connecticut, 2001. Morb Mortal Wkly Rep 2001;50(47):1049–51.

[25] Mayer T, Bersoff-Matcha S, Murphy C, et al. Clinical presentation of inhalational anthrax following bioterrorism exposure: report of 2 surviving patients. JAMA 2001;286: 2549–53.

[26] Cieslak TJ, Eitzen EM. Clinical and epidemiologic principles of anthrax. Emerg Infect Dis 1999;5:1–5.

[27] Swartz M. Recognition and management of anthrax – an update. N Engl J Med 2001; 345:1621–6.

[28] Friedlander A. Anthrax. In: Sidell FR, Takafuji ET, Franz DR, editors. Textbook of military medicine: medical aspects of chemical and biological warfare. Washington, DC: TMM Publications; 1997. p. 467–78.

[29] Glassman HN. Industrial inhalation anthrax. Bacteriol Rev 1958;30:657–9.

[30] Centers for Disease Control and Prevention. Considerations for distinguishing influenza-like illness from inhalational anthrax. Morb Mortal Wkly Rep 2001;50:984–6.

[31] Abramova FA, Grinberg LM, Yampolskaya OV, et al. Pathology of inhalational anthrax in 42 cases from the Sverdlovsk outbreak of 1979. Proc Natl Acad Sci 1993;90:2291–4.

[32] Vessal K, Yeganehdoust J, Dutz W, et al. Radiologic changes in inhalation anthrax. Clin Radiol 1975;26:471–4.

[33] Henderson DW, Peacock S, Belton FC. Observations on the prophylaxis of experimental pulmonary anthrax in the monkey. J Hyg 1956;54:28–36.

[34] Lightfoot NF, Scott RJ, Turnbull PC. Antimicrobial susceptibility of *Bacillus anthracis:* proceedings of the international workshop on anthrax. Salisbury Med Bull 1990;68:95–8.

[35] Turnbull PC. Anthrax vaccines: past, present and future. Vaccine 1991;9:533–9.

[36] Ivins BE, Fellows P, Pitt ML, et al. Efficacy of standard human anthrax vaccine against *Bacillus anthracis* aerosol spore challenge in rhesus monkeys. Salisbury Med Bull 1996;87: 125–6.

[37] Michigan Department of Public Health. Anthrax vaccine adsorbed. Lansing, Michigan: Department of Public Health; 1978.

[38] US Department of Defense. Anthrax vaccine, military use in Persian Gulf region [press release]. Washington, DC; September 8, 1998.

[39] Centers for Disease Control and Prevention. Evaluation of *Bacillus anthracis* contamination inside the Brentwood Mail Processing and Distribution Center – District of Columbia, October 2001. Morb Mortal Wkly Rep 2001;50:1129–33.

[40] Centers for Disease Control and Prevention. Investigation of bioterrorism-related anthrax and adverse events from antimicrobial prophylaxix. Morb Mortal Wkly Rep 2001;50:973–6.

[41] Centers for Disease Control and Prevention. Update: adverse events associated with anthrax prophylaxis among postal employees – New Jersey, New York City, and the District of Columbia Metropolitan Area, 2001. Morb Mortal Wkly Rep 2001;50(47): 1051–4.

[42] Altman L, Kolata G. Anthrax missteps offer guide to fight next bioterror battle. New York Times January 6, 2002.

[43] Weiss R. Perpetrator; motive remain elusive in anthrax case. Washington Post, December 23, 2001. p. A20.

[44] Henderson DA, Inglesby TV, Bartlett JG, et al. Smallpox as a biological weapon: medical and public health management. JAMA 1999;281(22):2127–37.

[45] McClain DJ. Smallpox. In: Sidell FR, Takafuji ET, Franz DR, editors. Medical management of biological casualties. 3rd edition. Washington, DC: TMM Publications; 1998. p. 58–64.

[46] World Health Organization. The global eradication of smallpox: final report of the Global Commission for the Certification of Smallpox Eradication. Geneva: WHO; 1980.

[47] Henderson DA, Moss B. Smallpox and vaccinia. In: Plotkin SA, Orenstein WA, editors. Vaccines. Philadelphia, PA: WB Saunders; 1999 [chapter 6].

[48] Beck E. Acambis, Baxter win smallpox vaccine deal (UPI) at MedLine Plus information, National Library of Medicine. http://www.medserv.dk/print.php?sid-1293. Accessed 21 May 2002.

[49] Henderson DA. Risk of a deliberate release of smallpox virus: its impact on virus destruction. Presented World Health Organization ad hoc Committee on Orthopoxvirus Infections. Geneva, Switzerland. January 14 and 15, 1999.

[50] Henderson DA. Smallpox: clinical and epidemiologic features. Emerg Inf Dis 1999;5(4): 537–9.

[51] Smallpox. A single case is a medical emergency. Hosp Inf Control 2000;27(3):33.

[52] Barbera J, MacIntyre A, et al. Large-scale quarantine following biological terrorism in the United States: scientific examination, logistic and legal limits, and possible consequences. JAMA 2001;286(21):2711–7.

[53] Gostin LO, Terret, SP, Burris S, Vernick JS. Model state emergency health powers act. Center for Law and the Public's Health, Johns Hopkins and George Washington Universities. December 21, 2001. Available at: http://www.publichealthlaw.net.

[54] Many hospitals unprepared for a bioterrorism event. Hosp Inf Control 2000;27(3):35–9.

[55] Downie AW, McCarthy K. The antibody response in man following infection with viruses of the pox group, 111: antibody response in smallpox. J Hyg 1958;56:479–87.

[56] McGovern TW, Friedlander AM. Plague. In: Sidell FR, Takafuji ET, Franz DR, editors. Medical aspects of chemical and biological warfare. Washington, DC: TMM Publications; 1989. p. 479–502.

[57] Williams P, Wallace D. Unit 731: Japan's secret biological warfare in World War II. New York: The Free Press; 1989.

[58] Speck RS, Wolochow H. Studies on the experimental epidemiology of respiratory infections, VIII: experimental pneumonic plague in Macacus rhesus. J Infect Dis 1955;96:138–44.

[59] Cavanaugh DC, Cadigan FC, Williams JE, et al. Plague. In: Ognibene AJ, Barrett O'n, editors. General medicine and infectious diseases. Vol 2. Washington, DC: Office of the Surgeon General and Center of Military History; 1982.

[60] Brubaker RR. Factors promoting acute and chronic diseases caused by Yersiniae. Clin Microbiol Rev 1991;4(3):309–24.

[61] Conrad FG, LeCocq FR, Krain R. A recent epidemic of plague in Vietnam. Arch Intern Med 1968;122(3):193 0.

[62] Poland JD. Plague. In: Hoeprich PD, editor. Infectious diseases: a guide to the understanding and management of infectious processes. New York: Harper and Row; 1972.

[63] Poland JD. Plague. In: Hoeprich PD, Jordan MC, editors. Infectious diseases: a modern treatise of infectious processes. Philadelphia: JB Lippincott; 1989.

[64] Alsoform DJ, Mettler FA Jr, Mann JM. Radiographic manifestations of plague in New Mexico, 1975–1980: a review of 42 proved cases. Radiology 1981;139:561–5.

[65] Tikomirov EV, Gratz NA, editors. World Health Organization plague manual. 3rd edition. Fort Collins, CO: Centers for Disease Control and Prevention; 1996.

[66] Ehrenkranz NF, Meyer KF. Studies on immunization against plague, VIII: study of three immunizing preparations in protecting primates against pneumonic plague. J Infect Dis 1955;96:138–44.

[67] Evans ME, Friedlander AM. Tularemia. In: Sidell FR, Takafuji ET, Franz DR, editors. Medical aspects of chemical and biological warfare. Washington, DC: TMM Publications; 1997. p. 503–12.

[68] McCoy GW. Plague-like disease in rodents. Public Health Bull 1911;43:53–71.

[69] Francis E. Tularemia (Francis 1921), I: the occurrence of tularemia in nature as a disease of man. Pub Health Rep 1921;36:1731–51.

[70] Defense Intelligence Agency. Soviet biological warfare threat, publication DST-161OF-057–86. Washington, DC: US Department of Defense; 1986.

[71] Pullen RL, Stuart BM: Tularemia: analysis of 225 cases. JAMA 1945;129:495–500.

[72] McCrumb FR Jr, Snyder MJ, Woodward TE. Studies on human infection with Pasteurella tularensis: comparison of streptomycin and chloramphenicol in the prophylaxis of clinical disease. Trans Assoc Am Physicians 1957;70:74–80.

[73] Franz DR, Jahrling PB, Friedlander A, et al. Clinical recognition and management of patients exposed to biological warfare agents. JAMA 1997;278:399–411.

[74] Archer VW, Blackford SD, Wissler JE. Pleuropulmonary manifestations in tularemia: a roentgenographic study based on thirty-four unselected cases. JAMA 1935;104:897–8.

[75] Dennis JM, Bourdreau RP. Pleuropulmonary tularemia: its roentgen manifestations. Radiology 1957;68:25–30.

[76] Rubin SA. Radiographic spectrum of pleuropulmonary tularemia. Am J Roentgenol 1978;131:277–81.

[77] Grunow R, Splettstoesser W, McDonald S, et al. Detection of Francisella tularensis in biological specimens using a capture enzyme-linked immunosorbent assay, an immunochromatographic handheld assay, and a PCR. Clin Diagn Lab Immunol 2000;7:86–90.

[78] Guarner J, Greer PW, Bartlett J, et al. Immunohistochemical detection of Francisella tularensis in formalin-fixed paraffin embedded tissue. Appl Immunohistochem Mol Morphol 1999;7:122–6.

[79] Syrja la H, Koskela P, Ripatti T, et al. Agglutination and ELISA methods in the diagnosis of tularemia in different clinical forms and severities of the disease. J Infect Dis 1986; 153:142–5.

[80] Sato T, Fujita H, Ohara Y, et al. Microagglutination test for early and specific serodiagnosis of tularemia. J Clin Microbiol 1990;28:2372–4.

[81] Francis E, Evans AC. Agglutination, cross-agglutination reaction in tularemia. J Infect Dis 1941;69:193–205.

[82] Ransmeier JC, Ewing CL. The agglutination reaction in tularemia. J Infect Dis 1941;69: 193–205.

[83] Saslaw S, Carlisle HN. Studies with tularemia vaccines in volunteers challenged with Pasteurella tularensis. Am J Med Sci 1961;242:166–72.

[84] Warring WB, Ruffin JS. A tick-borne epidemic of tularemia. N Engl J Med 1946;234: 137–40.

[85] Bevanger L, Macland JA, Naess AI. Agglutinins and antibodies to Francisella tularensis outer membrane antigens in the early diagnosis of disease during an outbreak of tularemia. J Clin Microbiol 1988;26:433–7.

[86] Garner JS. Hospital Infection Control Practices Advisory Committee. Guidelines for isolation precautions in hospitals. Epidemiology 1996;17:53–80, and Am J Infect Control 1996;24:24–52.

[87] Russell P, Eley SM, Fulop MJ, et al. The efficacy of ciprofloxacin and doxycycline against tularemia. J Antimicrob Chemother 1998;41:461–5.

[88] Sawyer WD, Dangerfield HG, Hogge AL, et al. Antibiotic prophylaxis and therapy of airborne tularemia. Bacteriol Rev 1966;30:542–8.

[89] Syrja la H, Schildt R, Ra isa inen S. In vitro susceptibility of *Francisella tularensis* to fluoroquinolones and treatment of tularemia with norfloxacin and ciprofloxacin. Eur J Clin Microbiol Infect Dis 1991;10:68–70.

[90] Saslaw S, Eigelsbach HT, Wilson HE, et al. Tularemia vaccine study, I: intracutaneous challenge. Arch Intern Med 1961;107:121–33.

[91] Hornick RB, Eigelsbach HT. Aerogenic immunization of man with live tularemia vaccine. Bacteriol Rev 1966;30:532–8.

[92] McCrumb FR Jr. Commission on epidemiological survey review of tularemia: studies on tularemia vaccine 1960–62. In: Annual Report. Washington, DC: Armed Forces Epidemiological Board; 1962. p. 81–6.

[93] McCrumb FR Jr. Aerosol infection in man with *Pasteurella tularensis*. Bacteriol Rev 1961;25:262–7.

[94] Saslaw S, Eigelsbach HT, Prior JA, et al. Tularemia vaccine study, II: respiratory challenge. Arch Intern Med 1961;107:134–46.

[95] Carus WS. The illicit use of biological agents since 1900 [working paper]. In: Bioterrorism and biocrimes. Washington DC: National Defense University; February 2001.

[96] Jarhling PB. Viral hemorrhagic fevers. In: Sidell FR, Takafuji ET, Franz DR, editors. Medical aspects of chemical and biological warfare. Washington, DC: TMM Publications; 1997. p. 591–602.

[97] Jarhling PB, Geisbert TW, Dalgard DW, et al. Preliminary report: isolation of Ebola virus from monkeys imported to the USA. Lancet 1990;335:502–5.

[98] Centers for Disease Control and Prevention: Management of patients with suspected viral hemorrhagic fever. Morb Mortal Wkly Rep 1988;37(Suppl 3):1–16.

[99] Arnon SS, Schechter R, Inglesby TV, et al. Botulinum toxin as a biological weapon: medical and public health management. JAMA 2001;285(8):1059–70.

[100] McCroskey LM, Hatheway CL. Laboratory findings in four cases of adult botulism suggest colonization of the intestinal tract. J Clin Microbiol 1988;26(5):1052–4.

[101] Centers for Disease Control and Prevention. Summary of notifiable diseases, United States, 1999. Morb Mortal Wkly Rep 2001;48(53):1–104.

[102] Török TJ, Tauxe RV, Wise RP, et al. A large community outbreak of salmonellosis caused by intentional contamination of restaurant salad bars. JAMA 1997;278(5):389–95.

[103] Moran GJ. Biological terrorism part 1: are we prepared? Emerg Med 2000;32:14–38.

[104] Middlebrook JL, Franz DR. Botulism. In: Sidell FR, Takafuji ET, Franz DR, editors. Medical management of biological casualties. 3rd edition. Washington, DC: TMM Publications; 1998. p. 86–94.

[105] Shapiro RL, Hatheway C, Becher J, et al. Botulism surveillance and emergency response. JAMA 1997;278(5):433–5.

EMERGENCY
MEDICINE
CLINICS OF
NORTH AMERICA

Emerg Med Clin N Am
20 (2002) 311–330

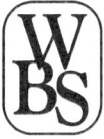

Threats in bioterrorism II:
CDC category B and C agents

Gregory J. Moran, MD, FACEP

*University of California Los Angeles, School of Medicine,
Department of Emergency Medicine and Division of Infectious Diseases,
North Annex, Olive View–UCLA Medical Center,
14445 Olive View Drive, Sylmar, CA 91342, USA*

A wide range of microorganisms could be used as weapons of mass destruction. The ideal agent for biological terrorism (BT) would be capable of producing illness in a large percentage of those exposed, would be disseminated easily to expose many people (eg, by way of aerosol), would remain stable and infectious despite environmental exposure, and would be available to terrorists for production in adequate amounts. Fortunately, few agents have these characteristics.

As part of their preparations for a possible BT event, the Centers for Disease Control and Prevention (CDC) identified several organisms believed to have the greatest potential for creating such events [1]. Those deemed top priority because of their potential for weaponization and lethality are discussed in the chapter in this issue on category A agents.

Several other organisms are assigned lower priority for specific preparations, but they are recognized as having potential for use as BT agents. These category B agents (Table 1) would be moderately easy to disseminate, would cause moderate morbidity and low mortality, and would require specific enhancements of the CDC's diagnostic capacity and disease surveillance capabilities.

The agents classified as category C by the CDC (Table 2) are emerging pathogens that could be engineered for mass exposure in the future because of availability, ease of production and dissemination, and potential for high morbidity and mortality. Preparedness for category C agents requires ongoing research to improve disease detection, diagnosis, treatment, and prevention. It is not possible to know in advance which newly emergent pathogens terrorists might use. For detection and response to these agents,

---

E-mail address: gmoran@ucla.edu (G.J. Moran).

Table 1
Category B agents: moderately easy to disseminate; cause moderate morbidity and low mortality; and require specific enhancements of CDC's diagnostic capacity and enhanced disease surveillance

Coxiella burnetti (Q fever)
Brucella species (brucellosis)
Burkholderia mallei (glanders)
Alphaviruses:
  Venezuelan encephalomyelitis
  Eastern and western equine encephalomyelitis
Ricin toxin from *Ricinus communis* (castor beans)
Epsilon toxin of *Clostridium perfringens*
Staphylococcus enterotoxin B
Food-borne or waterborne agents:
  Salmonella species
  Shigella dysenteriae
  Escherichia coli O157:H7
  Vibrio cholerae
  Cryptosporidium parvum

a strong public health infrastructure is essential. It is also important that physicians notify the local health department if unusual patterns of illness are observed.

The potential for these agents to be turned into weapons varies considerably. Some of them are highly lethal but are designated lower priority agents because they are unstable in the environment or would be difficult to disseminate effectively. Many of these agents cause non-lethal illness. Although highly lethal infections would create the most terror in the population, agents causing non-lethal illness could certainly provide significant social disruption that would suit the aims of terrorists.

This article discusses some of the agents in categories B and C, including the characteristics of these organisms and toxins and their potential for use as BT agents. It also describes their clinical features and management, and diagnostic testing and infection control.

Table 2
Category C agents: emerging pathogens that could be engineered for mass dissemination in the future because of availability; ease of production and dissemination; and potential for high morbidity and mortality and major health impact

Nipah virus
Hantaviruses
Tickborne hemorrhagic fever viruses
Tickborne encephalitis viruses
Yellow fever
Multidrug-resistant tuberculosis

Coxiella burnetii (Q fever)

Q fever is an acute or chronic zoonotic illness caused by the rickettsial organism *Coxiella burnetii*. The illness was described during a 1935 outbreak in Queensland, Australia, and was called Q (query) fever because the etiology was not identified at that time.

Q fever occurs worldwide and usually results from exposure to infected livestock such as sheep, cattle, or goats. Infected animals are usually asymptomatic; parturient animals may have large numbers of organisms present in the placenta, resulting in environmental contamination. Humans typically become infected by inhalation of aerosols containing *C. burnetii*. The organism proliferates in the lung and then spreads by way of the bloodstream.

C. burnetii has a spore-like form that can survive for weeks or months in the environment. The organism can survive heat and drying and can be disseminated by airborne spread. *C. burnetii* is highly infectious to humans— a single viable organism is adequate to cause infection. Because of these characteristics, it is considered suitable for use as a bioweapon.

Clinical presentation

The presenting symptoms of Q fever are nonspecific. In fact, it seems that many infections are asymptomatic. In those individuals who become ill, the most common findings are fever, chills, and headache. Onset may be sudden or gradual, and the incubation period can vary considerably from approximately 10 days up to several weeks. Most patients have a self-limited febrile illness that resolves within one or two weeks. Overall mortality is low—2.4% in one large series of hospitalized patients [2]. Many patients report malaise and fatigue that persist for months, however.

Q fever may manifest as pneumonia. Many Q fever patients have radiographic evidence of pneumonia but no cough. If cough is present, it is usually nonproductive. Severe headache is frequently associated with Q fever pneumonia. Hepatic transaminase levels are frequently elevated, but the peripheral white blood cell count is usually normal. Some patients have a rapidly progressing pneumonia syndrome similar to Legionnaire's disease. Although Q fever pneumonia may have a variety of radiographic appearances, multiple rounded opacities (often pleural-based) are a suggestive pattern. Pleural effusion (usually small) is found in approximately one third of cases [3].

Q fever also can have a variety of chronic manifestations, including endocarditis, intravascular infection, hepatitis, and osteomyelitis. Endocarditis typically involves abnormal or prosthetic valves but can sometimes develop in normal valves. *C. burnetii* will not grow in routine blood cultures, so culture-negative endocarditis is a typical clinical picture. Liver involvement may manifest as acute hepatitis or as a fever of unknown origin, with granulomas found on liver biopsy.

Diagnostic testing

Most laboratories do not have the facilities to isolate *C. burnetii*. Serologic testing by complement fixation, indirect fluorescent antibody (IFA), or enzyme-linked immunosorbent assay (ELISA) is the mainstay of diagnosis for Q fever. Titers may not be elevated until two to three weeks into the illness, however. Convalescent titers characteristically show a four-fold increase two or three months after onset of illness.

Infection control precautions

Human-to-human spread of Q fever does not appear to occur, so isolation is not required. Tissues from patients with Q fever may pose a threat to laboratory workers, however, and should be processed under biosafety level 3 conditions.

Treatment and prophylaxis

Several antibiotics have activity against *C. burnetii* and seem to shorten the duration of illness. Antibiotics also seem to prevent illness when given during the incubation period [4]. Tetracyclines are most commonly used for treatment. Other drugs that have been used include macrolides, quinolones, chloramphenicol, rifampin, and trimethoprim-sulfamethoxazole. The optimal duration of therapy is unclear. Treatment for uncomplicated infections or prophylaxis is generally given for five to seven days. Prolonged combination treatment (eg, doxycycline plus a quinolone or rifampin) is usually given for chronic infection such as endocarditis. A vaccine against Q fever is in use in Australia but is not licensed in the United States [5].

Brucella species (brucellosis)

Brucellosis is a zoonotic infection that can have a variety of manifestations in humans. *Brucella* species are small, aerobic, slow-growing gram-negative coccobacilli. The genus *Brucella* is divided into several species by preferred animal hosts and other features. The main manifestations in animals are abortion and sterility. Humans can become infected by direct contact with animal secretions through breaks in the skin, through infected aerosols, or by ingestion of unpasteurized dairy products. Brucellae are facultative intracellular pathogens, and replication and spread seem to occur by way of lymphatics and hematogenous dissemination. *Brucella* species can survive for many weeks in soil or water. *B. suis* was weaponized by the United States in the 1940s and 1950s; other countries are also suspected to have weaponized brucellae. The organism could be spread as a slurry in bomblets or as a dry aerosol [5].

Clinical presentation

Clinical symptoms of brucellosis are varied and nonspecific. Symptoms generally begin two to four weeks after exposure, but the incubation period can be eight weeks or more. The infection tends to localize in tissues with large numbers of macrophages, such as lung, spleen, liver, central nervous system (CNS), bone marrow, and synovium. Symptoms vary because of the widespread nature of infection. Symptoms often persist for weeks or months but the infection is rarely fatal. Fever, chills, sweats, anorexia, headache, and malaise are common manifestations. Although patients may complain of many symptoms, physical findings are often lacking.

Liver involvement is common, although transaminase levels are usually only mildly elevated. Hepatic granulomas are characteristic of some species (eg, *B. abortus*). Several skeletal complications are also found, including arthritis, osteomyelitis, and tenosynovitis. Large, weight-bearing joints (sacroiliac, hips, knees, ankles) are most commonly involved. Hematologic findings include anemia, leukopenia, and thrombocytopenia. The rare, serious complications of brucellosis include endocarditis and CNS infection. Although depression and difficulty concentrating are common complaints in patients with brucellosis, direct invasion of the CNS (meningitis, encephalitis) occurs in less than 5% of infected individuals [6]. Endocarditis occurs in less than 2% of cases but is responsible for most deaths.

Diagnostic testing

Brucellosis can be diagnosed by isolation of the organism in cultures or by serology. Because brucellae are slow growing, the laboratory should be alerted to hold culture specimens for at least four weeks if brucellosis is suspected. Cultures of bone marrow have a higher yield than blood. Rapid bacterial identification systems used by many laboratories may reduce the time to isolation, but misidentification of brucellae with these systems has been reported [7]. A presumptive diagnosis can be made by high or rising antibody titers. Most patients with infection have titers higher than 1:160. "Febrile agglutinin" tests are not adequately sensitive. Polymerase chain reaction (PCR) techniques may soon yield a rapid method of diagnosing brucellosis.

Infection control precautions

Human-to-human transmission seems to be rare, so isolation is not necessary; however, the organisms are highly infectious by aerosol, and culture specimens may pose a threat to laboratory workers. The laboratory should be notified if brucellosis is suspected; laboratory biosafety level 2 or 3 precautions are recommended. Contact isolation should be used for patients with open, draining lesions.

Treatment and prophylaxis

Although most patients recover without treatment, antibiotics reduce the severity and duration of illness. Many antibiotics have in vitro activity, but those with good intracellular penetration are most effective clinically. Combination treatment is most effective. Doxycycline plus rifampin for six weeks is the most commonly used regimen. Gentamicin or streptomycin is sometimes included in the regimen for more severe infections such as endocarditis. There is no effective human vaccine for brucellosis.

It is likely that antibiotics would prevent disease if given before the onset of symptoms, although the optimal regimen is unknown. Because of the long incubation period, the opportunity for prophylaxis is greater with brucellosis than for some other agents with shorter incubation periods such as anthrax or tularemia. An economic model estimated that the economic impact of a bioterrorist attack with brucellosis on a population of 100,000 people would be approximately$478 million. Timely intervention with antibiotic prophylaxis could reduce the economic impact by preventing illness [8].

Burkholderia mallei (glanders)

Glanders is a disease of horses, mules, and donkeys caused by the bacterium *Burkholderia mallei* (previously known as *Pseudomonas mallei*). The infection also can occur in humans and other animals. Human infection is rare but can be severe. *B. mallei* is a nonmotile, gram-negative bacillus. The route of naturally occurring infection is unclear, but it is believed that infection can occur through broken skin or nasal mucosa contaminated with infected material. It seems that infection can also occur by way of an aerosol route, as demonstrated by infections in laboratory workers from routine handling of cultures [9,10]. The potential for causing serious illness and the ability to infect by way of aerosol indicate potential use of *B. mallei* in biological terrorism. In fact, this organism has been used as a bioweapon—animals were deliberately infected with glanders during World War I [11].

Melioidosis is a human illness caused by *Burkholderia pseudomallei* that is clinically similar to glanders but does not seem to be particularly infectious by way of aerosol.

Clinical presentation

Infection by way of inoculation through a break in the skin typically results in a tender nodule with local lymphangitis. Inoculation of the eyes, nose, and mouth can result in mucopurulent discharge with ulcerating granulomas. With systemic invasion, a generalized papular or pustular eruption is frequent. This septicemic form is often fatal within 7 to 10 days. The incubation period after infection by way of inhalation (most likely in a BT event) is approximately 10 to 14 days. The most common manifestations include fever, myalgias, headache, and pleuritic chest pain. Lymphadenopathy or splenomegaly may be present. The disease often manifests as pneumonia [9].

Diagnostic testing

The organism can be difficult to identify. Blood cultures are usually negative, except in the terminal stages of septicemia. Automated bacterial identification systems used in many laboratories may not correctly identify *B. mallei*. Serologic tests will usually show an increase in titers by the second week, but agglutination titers are not specific. Complement fixation titers are more specific but less sensitive. Serologic tests are not standardized or widely available. *B. mallei* and *B. pseudomallei* cannot be distinguished morphologically, but a PCR procedure that can distinguish the two has been developed [12].

Infection control precautions

Because person-to-person transmission can occur, isolation is indicated. Culture specimens pose a threat to laboratory personnel, so the laboratory should be notified if *B. mallei* is suspected. Biosafety level 3 precautions are indicated.

Treatment and prophylaxis

The paucity of human cases has prevented any systematic study of treatment. Sulfadiazine has been effective in experimental animal infections and in humans. Agents known to be effective for human melioidosis include tetracyclines, trimethoprim sulfamethoxazole, amoxicillin clavulanate, and chloramphenicol. In vitro, *B. mallei* is susceptible to aminoglycosides, macrolides, quinolones, doxycycline, piperacillin, ceftazidime, and imipenem [13]. No vaccine is available.

Alphaviruses: Venezuelan encephalomyelitis and eastern and western equine encephalomyelitis

Venezuelan equine encephalomyelitis and eastern and western equine encephalomyelitis (VEE, EEE, and WEE) are mosquito-borne viral infections found in North and South America. EEE occurs primarily along the eastern and gulf coasts of the United States. Although human illness is rare, the case-fatality rate can be as high as 50%–70%. WEE viruses are found primarily west of the Mississippi. During an epidemic, WEE infection rates are much higher than for EEE, but the case-fatality rate is much lower (approximately 3%–4%). Outbreaks occur primarily in the summertime, and equine cases greatly outnumber human cases. VEE occurs in many areas of South and Central America, and outbreaks have occurred in North America.

These alphaviruses are limited in their geographic distribution by the mosquito vector, so finding these viruses outside the endemic areas should arouse suspicion of an intentional release. All of these viruses are highly infectious by aerosol. Because they are stable during storage and can be produced in large amounts with unsophisticated equipment, they are regarded as having potential for weaponization [5].

Clinical presentation

Most infections with these viruses result in nonspecific symptoms of fever, headache, and myalgia. Only a fraction of those individuals infected will progress to frank encephalitis. Viral encephalitides should be included in the differential of nonspecific viral syndromes following a possible BT event. Reports of ill horses in the vicinity would obviously suggest an equine encephalitis virus. It is not known whether aerosol exposure as in a BT event would lead to a different pattern of symptoms than the mosquito-borne illness.

EEE is the most severe of these infections, with high mortality rates and high rates of neurologic sequelae [14]. WEE and VEE have lower rates of progression to neurologic symptoms. Infants and the elderly are more prone to developing encephalitis. In people in whom encephalitis develops, the initial viral prodrome is followed by confusion and somnolence that may progress to coma. Peripheral blood counts often reveal a leukopenia in the early stages of illness that can progress to leukocytosis. Cerebrospinal fluid (CSF) protein is elevated, and a lymphocytic pleocytosis is usually present.

Diagnostic testing

Virus can sometimes be isolated from blood during the early stages of illness, but viremia has usually resolved by the time symptoms of encephalitis develop. Virus can sometimes be isolated from CSF, or it can be isolated from post-mortem brain tissue. The specific viral pathogen is generally identified by serologic testing of the CSF or serum (or both), but these results will not be available until later. Virus-specific IgM antibodies can be detected by ELISA [15]. Subsequent testing of convalescent serum may confirm the diagnosis but will not be helpful in initial management. Physicians should attempt to obtain enough CSF for specialized testing if encephalitis is a diagnostic possibility. Experimental PCR assays have been developed for several viral pathogens and will likely become more standardized and readily available in the future.

Infection control precautions

Person-to-person transmission does not occur, so isolation is not necessary.

Treatment and prophylaxis

There is no specific treatment for these viral encephalitides. Treatment is supportive. Inactivated vaccines are available for EEE, WEE, and VEE. None is in widespread use because of problems with poor immunogenicity and need for multiple doses. A live attenuated vaccine is available for VEE but has a high incidence of side effects such as fever, headache, and malaise. Newer vaccines using recombinant technology are in development.

Ricin toxin from *Ricinus communis* (castor beans)

Ricin is a protein toxin derived from the castor bean plant. Castor beans are easily obtained worldwide and it is easy to extract the toxin. One million tons of castor beans are processed annually in the production of castor oil worldwide; the waste mash from this process is approximately 5% ricin by weight. Ricin was used in the assassination of Bulgarian exile Georgi Markov in London in 1978. Markov was attacked with a specially engineered weapon disguised as an umbrella that implanted a ricin-containing pellet into his leg [16].

Ricin toxin is somewhat less toxic by weight compared with botulinum toxin or staphylococcal enterotoxin B, but it can be produced in large quantities easily. Ricin toxin is stable and can be disseminated as an aerosol. It is toxic by several routes of exposure, including respiratory and gastrointestinal.

Clinical presentation

Ricin toxin acts by inhibiting protein synthesis. When inhaled as an aerosol, the toxin can produce symptoms within four to eight hours. Typical symptoms include fever, chest tightness, cough, dyspnea, nausea, arthralgias, and profuse sweating. With a sub-lethal dose of toxin, the symptoms should improve within several hours. In animal studies, lethal doses produced necrosis of the respiratory tract and alveolar filling in 36–72 hours after exposure.

When ingested, ricin causes severe gastrointestinal symptoms such as nausea, vomiting, and diarrhea. With large toxin exposures this may be associated with gastrointestinal hemorrhage and hepatic, splenic, and renal necrosis. Death can occur from hypovolemic shock [17]. Ricin toxin may also cause disseminated intravascular coagulation, microcirculatory failure, and multiple organ failure if given intravenously in laboratory animals.

Diagnostic testing

Diagnosis of ricin poisoning would be primarily clinical and epidemiologic. ELISA testing can be done on serum, but this would not be widely available in most laboratories [18]. Acute and convalescent sera could be obtained from survivors for measurement of antibody response to confirm the diagnosis.

Infection control precautions

There is no potential for person-to-person spread of this toxin-mediated syndrome. Patients who are grossly contaminated may require a change of clothes and washing with soap and water.

Treatment and prophylaxis

Treatment of ricin poisoning is supportive. Respiratory support may be needed for pulmonary edema. Gastric decontamination with charcoal may have some benefit for ingestions. Fluids may be required to replace gastrointestinal losses. Vaccines against ricin toxin are currently under development [19].

Epsilon toxin of *Clostridium perfringens*

Clostridium perfringens is an anaerobic, gram-positive, spore-forming bacillus. This ubiquitous organism is present in soil throughout the world and has been found in the stool of virtually every vertebrate organism ever tested [20]. *Clostridium* species can produce a variety of toxins and these are responsible for illness. Enterotoxin-producing strains of *C. perfringens* type A cause a mild form of food poisoning that is common worldwide. It would be possible to produce large amounts of this toxin for use in intentional exposure.

Clinical presentation

Within hours of exposure, gastrointestinal symptoms such as watery diarrhea, nausea, and abdominal cramps will develop. Fever is rare. Spontaneous resolution typically occurs within a day and fatalities are rare. The *C. perfringens* enterotoxin can act as a superantigen and is a potent stimulator of human lymphocytes. It is possible that gross exposure by way of aerosol or ingestion could lead to more severe systemic symptoms.

Diagnostic testing

Enterotoxin can be detected in stool by latex agglutination or ELISA, but these tests are not widely available. Cultures are not of value because *C. perfringens* is normally found in stool.

Infection control precautions

Because this is a toxin-mediated syndrome, there is no potential for person-to-person spread.

Treatment and prophylaxis

Treatment is supportive.

Staphylococcus **Enterotoxin B**

Staphylococcal enterotoxin B (SEB) is a common cause of food poisoning caused by a heat-stable toxin produced by the ubiquitous organism *Staphylococcus aureus*. The toxin is stable in aerosols (more stable than botulinum toxin); even low doses can cause symptoms when inhaled. Although rarely fatal, it could render a high percentage of exposed individuals seriously ill within a few hours. It could also be used to contaminate food or water supplies.

Clinical presentation

SEB is a potent activator of T cells and most of the clinical manifestations are mediated by the patient's own immune system. Symptoms begin 3 to 12 hours after exposure. Typical symptoms are high fever, headache, myalgia, prostration, and dry cough. Vomiting and diarrhea may result from swallowed toxin. Patients may be incapacitated for up to two weeks. In severe cases, pulmonary edema or adult respiratory distress syndrome may develop. In rare cases, death occurs from dehydration.

Diagnostic testing

The diagnosis of SEB intoxication is primarily clinical and epidemiologic. Practically speaking, a specific diagnosis of SEB would be difficult. The symptoms are nonspecific and overlap with many other clinical syndromes, including those of other BT agents. Because of the short incubation period, this agent is more likely to lead to a sudden cluster of cases in a localized area compared with many other BT agents. The toxin may be identified by ELISA of nasal swabs after aerosol exposure, or the antigen can be detected in urine [5]. Neither of these tests is readily available.

Infection control precautions

Because this is a toxin-mediated syndrome, there is no potential for person-to-person spread. If patients are grossly contaminated after a recent exposure, however, healthcare workers could be exposed to the toxin on skin or clothing. A simple change of clothes and shower with soap and water would provide adequate decontamination.

Treatment and prophylaxis

Treatment is supportive. Some patients may require rehydration for fluid losses, though care must be taken to avoid pulmonary edema in more severe intoxications. Ventilatory support may be required in severe cases. Vaccines are under development.

Food-borne and waterborne pathogens

Although most agents considered likely to be used for BT would be disseminated by way of aerosol, it would also be possible to use food-borne or waterborne agents. In fact, *Shigella* and *Salmonella* have already been used in intentional exposures in the United States. *Shigella* was used to contaminate donuts given to fellow workers by a disgruntled employee and caused 12 cases of diarrhea [21]. *Salmonella* was used by a religious commune in Oregon to contaminate local salad bars, leading to more than 750 cases of gastroenteritis [22].

The use of food-borne and waterborne agents would be less likely than airborne agents in a large-scale attack, because it is difficult to expose many people. Standard treatment of municipal water supplies would preclude survival of most biological agents. Food-borne outbreaks are generally limited to small groups of people. More centralized processing of foods for mass marketing may however increase the potential for widespread food-borne outbreaks, as has been shown by multistate outbreaks of *Listeria* and *Salmonella* resulting from contamination in food-processing facilities [23,24].

Salmonella species, *Shigella dysenteriae*, *Escherichia coli* O157:H7, and *Vibrio cholerae* are all bacterial causes of food-borne gastroenteritis. *Salmonella*, *Shigella*, and *E. coli* all cause illness sporadically in the United States [25]. Cholera is a cause of severe gastroenteritis in developing countries but is only occasionally imported into the United States.

Cryptosporidium parvum is a protozoal organism that is also associated with diarrhea. *C. parvum* can be spread by contamination of food or water and has been involved in outbreaks related to swimming pools. Because it is resistant to chlorine, *C. parvum* can survive in swimming pools and municipal water supplies. *C. parvum* was associated with a massive outbreak caused by contamination of the municipal water supply in Milwaukee, Wisconsin in 1993 [26]. More than 400,000 people became ill, resulting in more than 40,000 healthcare visits and 4000 hospitalizations.

Clinical presentation

These infections generally present as diarrhea, sometimes associated with nausea, vomiting, fever, and abdominal cramps. The incubation period is approximately one to three days. Gastroenteritis caused by *Shigella* is often associated with blood or mucus in the stool. *Salmonella typhi* and *S. paratyphi* can produce a typhoidal syndrome with gradual onset of fever, headache, malaise, myalgias, and constipation. Diarrhea is uncommon. Cholera is associated with severe watery diarrhea that can cause death from dehydration within hours.

E. coli O157:H7 is notable for being associated with bloody diarrhea, but *Salmonella* or *Shigella* can also be associated with this condition. *E. coli* O157:H7 produces a shiga toxin associated with development of hemolytic uremic syndrome (HUS) [27]. HUS is characterized by hemolytic anemia, thrombocytopenia, and renal insufficiency. Approximately 6% of people with bloody diarrhea caused by *E. coli* O157:H7 develop HUS, but the rate is higher (approximately 10%) in children younger than 10 years of age. The mortality associated with HUS is 3%–5%.

C. parvum typically causes watery diarrhea associated with crampy abdominal pain. The incubation period is usually approximately a week but can sometimes extend to several weeks. Illness can sometimes last for many weeks.

Diagnostic testing

Routine stool cultures for enteropathogens will identify agents such as *Salmonella* and *Shigella*. Many laboratories do not routinely test for *E. coli* O157:H7, so the laboratory should be notified if this agent is suspected (eg, if the patient has bloody diarrhea). *E. coli* O157:H7 appears as a colorless colony on sorbitol MacConkey agar. These colonies can be tested for O157 antigen using a commercial kit. It is also possible to test stool cultures directly for shiga toxin using a commercial kit. *V. cholerae* requires special media to grow, so the laboratory should be notified if cholera is suspected. *C. parvum* can be identified with a modified acid-fast stain of stool.

Infection control precautions

Standard body fluid precautions should prevent spread of these organisms. Patients should be instructed to be extra vigilant about handwashing after using the bathroom.

Treatment and prophylaxis

Treatment of these infections is generally supportive. Most infections with *Salmonella* and *Shigella* are self-limited and will resolve without specific treatment within a few days. If patients have severe or persistent symptoms, antimicrobial treatment may reduce the duration and severity of symptoms. *Salmonella* is susceptible to quinolones, azithromycin, and third-generation cephalosporins. Resistance to Trimethoprim-sulfamethoxazole (TMP/SMX) seems to be increasing, and it seems likely that antimicrobial-resistant organisms would be used in a BT event. *Shigella* is susceptible to quinolones, TMP/SMX, and azithromycin. *E. coli* O157:H7 infection should not be treated with antimicrobials or antimotility agents, because treatment may increase toxin production and thereby increase the risk for HUS. Treatment of cholera typically requires large amounts of intravenous fluids and replacement of electrolytes. Oral administration of ciprofloxacin or doxycycline is effective for cholera. No antimicrobial agent has proven efficacy for *C. parvum* infection, although paromomycin and azithromycin have been used in AIDS patients with chronic diarrhea caused by this organism.

Nipah virus

In April 1999, an outbreak of 257 cases of encephalitis (100 fatal) was reported in Malaysia [28]. A previously unrecognized paramyxovirus called Nipah was identified as the cause. It appeared that pigs were the primary source of human infection in this outbreak.

Clinical presentation

Patients in the reported outbreak presented with fever, headache, and myalgias, and eventually developed signs of meningitis or encephalitis. A few patients had respiratory symptoms.

Diagnostic testing

Identification of Nipah virus requires specialized testing in a reference laboratory such as the CDC or the US Army Medical Research Institute of Infectious Diseases (USAMRIID). IgM antibodies can be detected in blood and CSF. Better diagnostic tests for this recently discovered agent are under development [29].

Infection control precautions

Person-to-person spread of Nipah virus has not been identified. Virus has been isolated from respiratory secretions and urine of patients with Nipah virus infection [30]. Pending further study of the potential for person-to-person spread, it would be prudent to use strict isolation for patients with suspected infection with this virus.

Treatment and prophylaxis

Treatment is primarily supportive. A small, open-label trial conducted during the outbreak in Malaysia demonstrated a 36% reduction of mortality among patients with acute Nipah virus encephalitis with ribavirin [31].

Hantaviruses

Hantaviruses are in the family Bunyaviridae that also contains California encephalitis virus and several hemorrhagic fever viruses. Hantaviruses are found in many rodent species worldwide. Hantavirus and several related viruses cause a syndrome of fever, thrombocytopenia, and renal insufficiency; the disease occurs primarily in Eastern Asia. Sin nombre virus (SNV), a similar virus, was identified as the cause of several cases of severe pulmonary edema and shock (Hantavirus pulmonary syndrome) in the southwestern United States in 1993 [32]. Aerosols of virus-contaminated rodent urine or feces appeared to be the mechanism of transmission in these cases. Because aerosol transmission is possible, the virus is believed to have potential for weaponization.

Clinical presentation

Hantavirus pulmonary syndrome (HPS) begins with a viral prodrome of fever and myalgias. Respiratory symptoms, including cough and dyspnea, begin after several days. Laboratory investigations may reveal an elevated hematocrit, leukocytosis, mild thrombocytopenia, and elevated liver transaminases. In severe cases the illness progresses to pulmonary edema with respiratory failure and shock [33].

Diagnostic testing

Hantaviruses are difficult to isolate in viral culture. In the acute phase of the disease, the clinical diagnosis may be confirmed by serology or by PCR. ELISA and IFA are available to identify antibody to hantaviruses [34]. An immunoblot assay is also available.

Infection control precautions

Person-to-person transmission of naturally occurring SNV in the United States has not been identified. It has been identified in Argentina, including a fatal infection in a physician who also transmitted the virus to his family [35,36]. Because of the potential for person-to-person spread of a virus used in an intentional attack, it would be prudent to use respiratory isolation for persons with suspected HPS related to a BT event.

Treatment and prophylaxis

Treatment of HPS is primarily supportive. Extracorporeal membrane oxygenation has been used in severe cases [37]. An open-label trial of ribavirin for HPS failed to show any benefit. Controlled trials of ribavirin are ongoing. Vaccines are under development.

Other agents

Several arthropod-borne viruses might have potential for use as bioweapons. These include the flaviviruses that cause yellow fever and tick-borne encephalitis. Person-to-person transmission of flaviviruses does not seem to occur except by way of the arthropod vectors.

Yellow fever is a mosquito-borne virus of historical interest because of large outbreaks that played a role in development of the Americas. The dis-

Table 3
Category B and C agent characteristics

Disease	Clinical presentation	Transmit man to man	Isolation precautions	Incubation period	Duration of illness	Lethality (approximate case fatality rates)	Persistence of organism	Diagnostic testing	Treatment	Prophylaxis	Vaccine
Q Fever	Fever, chills, headache, pneumonia	Rare	Standard	10–40 days	2–14 days	Very low	For months on wood and sand	Serology	Tetracycline or doxycycline	Tetracycline or doxycycline × 5d	Single dose inactivated whole cell, not licensed in US
Brucellosis	Fever, chills, anorexia, malaise	No	Standard	5–60 days (usually 1–2 months)	Weeks to months	<5% untreated	Very stable	Blood culture or serology	[Doxycycline or quinolone] plus rifampin × 6 wks	[Doxycycline or quinolone] plus rifampin	No vaccine
Glanders	Tender skin nodules, septicemia, pneumonia	Low	Standard	10–14 days via aerosol	Death in 7–10 days in septicemic form	>50%	Very stable	Blood culture or serology	Doxycycline, TMP/SMX, chloramphenicol	Doxycycline, TMP/SMX, macrolides	No vaccine
Venezuelan equine encephalitis	Fever, headache, myalgia, rare encephalitis	Low	Standard	2–6 days	Days to weeks	Low	Relatively unstable	Serology	Supportive	None	Live vaccine, high incidence of side effects
Ricin	Fever, dyspnea, vomiting, diarrhea, shock	No	Standard	4–24 hours	Days. Death within 10–12 days for ingestion	High	Stable	Serology (not widely available)	Supportive	None	No vaccine
C. perfringens toxin	Diarrhea, nausea, cramps	No	Standard	Hours	1 day	Very low	Stable	ELISA or latex agglutination test of stool	Supportive	None	No vaccine
Staph enterotoxin B	Fever, headache, myalgias, vomiting, diarrhea, dry cough	No	Standard	3–12 hours after inhalation or ingestion	Hours	<1%	Resistant to freezing	Urine antigen, ELISA of nasal swab (not widely available)	Supportive	None	No vaccine
Salmonella	Fever, nausea, ±diarrhea	Yes	Standard	1–3 days	1–3 days	Very low	Relatively stable in food or water	Stool culture	Usually supportive, quinolones, azithromycin	Quinolones, azithromycin	Vaccine for S typhi: inactivated parenteral, and live attenuated oral

Disease	Clinical features	Person-to-person	Isolation	Incubation	Duration	Mortality	Environmental stability	Diagnosis	Treatment	Prophylaxis	Vaccine
Shigella	Fever, nausea, cramps, diarrhea ± blood	Yes	Standard	1–3 days	1–3 weeks	Very low	Relatively stable in food or water	Stool culture	Usually supportive, quinolones, TMP/SMX, azithromycin	Quinolones, TMP/SMX, azithromycin	Experimental live, attenuated vaccines
E coli O157:H7	Bloody diarrhea, fever, HUS in about 6%	Yes	Standard	1–3 days	1–3 days	Low	Relatively stable in food or water	Stool culture on sorbitol MacConkey agar	Supportive, avoid antibiotics or anti-motility agents, watch for HUS	Quinolones may be effective	No vaccine
Cholera	Severe watery diarrhea	Rare	Standard	4 hours–5 days (usually 2–3 days)	≥1 week	Low with treatment, high without	Unstable in aerosols and fresh water; stable in salt water	Stool culture with special media	Fluids, ciprofloxacin, doxycycline	Ciprofloxacin, doxycycline	2-dose vaccine, not highly effective
Cryptosporidium	Diarrhea, cramps	Yes	Standard	1–3 weeks	1–3 weeks	Very low	Stable, resists chlorination	Acid fast stain of stool	Supportive; azithromycin or paromomycin may be effective	Azithromycin or paromomycin may be effective	No vaccine
Nipah virus	Encephalitis	Very low	Respiratory/contact	1–2 weeks	2–4 weeks	Moderate	Unstable	Blood, CSF serology in specialized labs	Supportive; ribavirin possibly effective	None	No vaccine
Hantavirus	Fever, myalgias, dyspnea	Very low	Standard	Few days	Days to weeks	High	Unstable	Serology, PCR	Supportive	None	No vaccine
Tickborne encephalitis	Fever, headache, rare encephalitis	No	Standard	1–4 weeks	Weeks	Very low, 20% with encecephalitis	Unstable	Serology	Supportive	None	Inactivated vaccines licensed in Europe
Yellow fever	Fever, headache, myalgias, hepatitis	No	Standard	3–6 days	Weeks	Moderate	Unstable	Serology; virus occasionally isolated from blood	Supportive	None	Attenuated vaccine 95% effective
MDR-TB	Cough, fever	Yes	Respiratory	Weeks to years	Weeks to years	Moderate, even with treatment	Relatively stable in aerosol, but killed by UV light	Sputum acid fast stain and culture	Combination therapy with 2nd-line TB agents	Combination therapy with 2nd-line TB agents	BCG vaccine not highly effective

ease has been greatly diminished by mosquito control and vaccination, though sporadic outbreaks still occur. The severity of illness can range from a mild self-limited viral syndrome to a fatal hemorrhagic fever [38]. After an incubation period of several days, symptoms begin as fever, headache, and myalgias. Conjunctivitis, relative bradycardia, and leukopenia may be present. Jaundice occurs secondary to hepatitis, and gastrointestinal bleeding may also occur. Death can occur 7 to 10 days after onset. Treatment of yellow fever is supportive. The illness is preventable with the attenuated 17D vaccine that produces immunity in approximately 95% of those vaccinated.

Tick-borne encephalitis occurs in many areas of Europe and Asia. Infection can also occur from consumption of unpasteurized milk products. Most infections are asymptomatic or only mildly symptomatic, but a small fraction of infected individuals can develop encephalitis. Approximately 1% of encephalitis cases are fatal, mostly in the elderly [39]. There is no specific therapy for flavivirus encephalitis.

Multidrug-resistant tuberculosis has become a significant problem in many areas of the world over the past several decades. Although the illness tends to progress slowly and person-to-person transmission occurs slowly, the ability to disseminate by aerosol and the difficulty in treating multi-drug-resistant strains could make the organism attractive as a bioweapon. Treatment options for highly resistant strains are severely limited [40].

Summary

A variety of agents have potential for use as weapons of biological terrorism. Knowledge of the likely organisms may be useful in preparations to mitigate the effects of a BT event. Recognition of the clinical presentation of these organisms could help physicians identify them quickly, allowing more appropriate management and possible prophylaxis of others who may have been exposed. Although many of these agents do not have specific treatments, it is important to recognize those that do. It is also important to know which infections require isolation because of potential for person-to-person spread. Table 3 summarizes important features of the CDC category B and C agents.

The list of agents discussed in this article is by no means exhaustive. It is always possible that some "mad scientist" could modify an existing organism or engineer some new agent for use in biological terrorism. The possibilities are limited only by the ingenuity and depravity of those individuals who would take part in such an attack.

References

[1] Centers for Disease Control and Prevention. Biological and chemical terrorism: strategic plan for preparedness and response. Morb Mortal Wkly Rep 2000;49(RR04):1–14.

[2] Dupont HT, Raoult D, Brouqui P, et al. Epidemiologic features and clinical presentation of acute Q fever in hospitalized patients: 323 French cases. Am J Med 1992;93:427–34.

[3] Millar JK. The chest film findings in Q fever—a series of 35 cases. Clin Radiol 1978;329: 371–5.

[4] Raoult D. Treatment of Q fever. Antimicrob Agents Chemother 1993;37:1733–6.

[5] Franz DR, Jahrling PB, Friedlander AM, et al. Clinical recognition and management of patients exposed to biological warfare agents. JAMA 1997;278(5):399–411.

[6] Young EJ. Overview of brucellosis. Clin Infect Dis 1995;21:283–9.

[7] Barham WB, Church P, Brown JE, et al. Misidentification of Brucella species with use of rapid bacterial identification systems. Clin Infect Dis 1993;17:1068–9.

[8] Kaufmann AF, Meltzer MI, Schmid GP. The economic impact of a bioterrorist attack: are prevention and postattack intervention programs justifiable? Emerg Infect Dis 1997;3: 83–94.

[9] Centers for Disease Control and Prevention. Laboratory-acquired human glanders—Maryland, May 2000. Morb Mortal Wkly Rep 2000;49:532–5.

[10] Srinivasan A, Kraus CN, DeShazer D, Becker PM, Dick JD, Spacek L, Bartlett JG, Byrne WR, Thomas DL. Glanders in a military research microbiologist. N Engl J Med 2001;345: 256–8.

[11] Mobley JA. Biological warfare in the twentieth century: lessons from the past, challenges for the future. Mil Med 1995;160(11):547–53.

[12] Bauernfeind A, Roller C, Meyer D, Jungwirth R, Schneider I. Molecular procedure for rapid detection of Burkholderia mallei and Burkholderia pseudomallei. J Clin Microbiol 1998;36:2737–41.

[13] Heine HS, England MJ, Waag DM, Byrne WR. In vitro antibiotic susceptibilities of Burkholderia mallei (causative agent of glanders) determined by broth microdilution and E-test. Antimicrob Agents Chemother 2001;45:2119–21.

[14] Deresiewicz RL, Thaler SJ, Hsu L, Zamani AA. Clinical and neurologic manifestations of eastern equine encephalitis. N Engl J Med 1997;336:1867–74.

[15] Calisher CH, El-Kafrawi AO, Al-Deen Mahmud MI, et al. Complex-specific immunoglobulin M antibody patterns in humans infected with alphaviruses. J Clin Microbiol 1986;23: 155–9.

[16] U.S. Army Medical Research Institute of Infectious Diseases. Ricin. In: Medical management of biological casualties. 4th edition. February 2001.

[17] Challoner KR, McCarron MM. Castor bean intoxication. Ann Emerg Med 1990;19:1177–83.

[18] Leith AG, Griffiths GD, Green MA. Quantification of ricin toxin using a highly sensitive avidin/biotin enzyme-linked immunosorbent assay. J Forensic Sci Soc 1988;28:227–36.

[19] Yan C, Rill WL, Malli R, et al. Intranasal stimulation of long-lasting immunity against aerosol ricin challenge with ricin toxoid vaccine encapsulated in polymeric microspheres. Vaccine 1996;14:1031–8.

[20] Lorber B. Gas gangrene and other clostridium-associated diseases. In: Mandell GL, Bennett JE, Dolin R, editors. Principles and practice of infectious diseases. 5th edition. Philadelphia: Churchill Livingstone; 2000. p. 2549–61.

[21] Kolavic SA, Kimura A, Simons SL, et al. An outbreak of Shigella dysenteriae type 2 among laboratory workers due to intentional food contamination. JAMA 1997;278:396–8.

[22] Torok TJ, Tauxe RV, Wise RP, et al. A large community outbreak of salmonellosis caused by intentional contamination of restaurant salad bars. JAMA 1997;278:389–95.

[23] Centers for Disease Control and Prevention. Emerging infectious diseases: outbreak of Salmonella enteritidis associated with nationally distributed ice cream products–Minnesota, South Dakota, and Wisconsin, 1994. Morb Mortal Wkly Rep 1994;43:740–1.

[24] Centers for Disease Control and Prevention. Multistate outbreak of listeriosis–United States, 2000. Morb Mortal Wkly Rep 2000;49:1129–30.

[25] Centers for Disease Control and Prevention. Diagnosis and management of foodborne illnesses: a primer for physicians. Morb Mortal Wkly Rep 2001;50(RR02):1–69.

[26] Mac Kenzie WR, Hoxie NJ, Proctor ME, et al. A massive outbreak in Milwaukee of Cryptosporidium infection transmitted through the public water supply. N Engl J Med 1994;331:161–7.

[27] Mead PS, Griffin PM. Escherichia coli O157:H7. Lancet 1998;352:1207–12.

[28] Centers for Disease Control and Prevention. Update: outbreak of Nipah virus, Malaysia and Singapore, 1999. Morb Mortal Wkly Rep 1999;48:335–7.

[29] Daniels P, Ksiazek T, Eaton BT. Laboratory diagnosis of Nipah and Hendra virus infections. Microbes Infect 2001;3(4):289–95.

[30] Chua KB, Lam SK, Goh KJ, et al. The presence of Nipah virus in respiratory secretions and urine of patients during an outbreak of Nipah virus encephalitis in Malaysia. J Infect 2001;42(1):40–3.

[31] Chong HT, Kamarulzaman A, Tan CT, et al. Treatment of acute Nipah encephalitis with ribavirin. Ann Neurol 2001;49(6):810–3.

[32] Nichol ST, Spiropoulou CF, Morzunov S, et al. Genetic identification of a hantavirus associated with an outbreak of acute respiratory illness. Science 1993;262:914–7.

[33] Duchin JS, Koster F, Peters CJ, et al. Hantavirus pulmonary syndrome: clinical description of disease caused by a newly recognized hemorrhagic fever virus in the southwestern United States. N Engl J Med 1994;330:949–55.

[34] Koraka P, Avsic-Zupanc T, Osterhaus AD, Groen J. Evaluation of two commercially available immunoassays for the detection of hantavirus antibodies in serum samples. J Clin Virol 2000;17:189–96.

[35] Padula PJ, Edelstein A, Miguel SD, et al. Hantavirus pulmonary syndrome outbreak in Argentina: molecular evidence for person-to-person transmission of Andes virus. Virology 1998;241:323–30.

[36] Wells RM, Sosa Estani S, Yadon ZE, et al. An unusual hantavirus outbreak in southern Argentina: person-to-person transmission? Emerg Infect Dis 1997;3:171–4.

[37] Fabbri M, Maslow MJ. Hantavirus pulmonary syndrome in the United States. Curr Infect Dis Rep 2001;3:258–65.

[38] Monath TP. Yellow fever: a medically neglected disease. Rev Infect Dis 1987;9:165–75.

[39] Tsai TF. Flaviviruses. In: Mandell GL, Bennett JE, Dolin R, editors. Principles and practice of infectious diseases. 5th edition. Philadelphia: Churchill Livingstone; 2000. p. 1714–36.

[40] Small PM, Fujiwara PI. Management of tuberculosis in the United States. N Engl J Med 2001;345:189–210.

EMERGENCY
MEDICINE
CLINICS OF
NORTH AMERICA

Emerg Med Clin N Am
20 (2002) 331–350

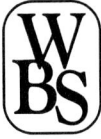

Diagnostic analyses of biological agent-caused syndromes: laboratory and technical assistance

Julie A. Pavlin, MD, MPH[a],*, Mary J.R. Gilchrist, PhD[b],
Gary D. Osweiler, DVM, PhD, MS[c],
Neal E. Woollen, DVM, PhD[d]

[a]*Walter Reed Army Institute of Research, 503 Robert Grant Avenue,
Silver Spring, MD 20910, USA*
[b]*University Hygienic Laboratory, University of Iowa, 102 Oakdale Campus,
Iowa City, IA 52242, USA*
[c]*Veterinary Diagnostic Laboratory, Iowa State University, 1600 South 16th Street,
Ames, IA 50011, USA*
[d]*Diagnostic Systems Division, US Army Medical Research Institute of Infectious Diseases,
1425 Porter Street, Fort Detrick, MD 21702, USA*

Early diagnosis and treatment are central to saving victims of a bioterrorism incident. Without quick and accurate diagnoses, most of the initial victims of such an attack will go unrecognized until after many more patients present with similar symptoms, or until their illness proves fatal. Accurate biologic agent identification will also prevent unnecessary or inappropriate treatment. Between April 1997 and June 1999 approximately 200 mailed or telephoned hoaxes, usually claiming that anthrax had been released, resulted in more than 13,000 potential victims being inappropriately treated by emergency responders [1]. To diagnose and manage victims most effectively, the emergency physician must have access to a clinical laboratory that is knowledgeable regarding biologic agent diagnostic techniques, and competent to test for these infections or refer them to a laboratory with appropriate capabilities.

Bioterrorism, the re-emergence of infectious diseases, and changes in healthcare market forces have produced new challenges for clinical laboratories. In light of the changing balance between the clinical laboratory and clinicians, it is of utmost importance that clinicians, and particularly

---

* Corresponding author.
E-mail address: julie.pavlin@amedd.army.mil (J.A. Pavlin).

0733-8627/02/$ - see front matter © 2002, Elsevier Science (USA). All rights reserved.
PII: S 0 7 3 3 - 8 6 2 7 (0 1) 0 0 0 0 4 - 9

emergency physicians, make the extra effort to communicate with the laboratory and know the structure and hierarchy under which the laboratory operates. First line physicians should cultivate a close working relationship with their hospital laboratory to obtain appropriate specimens and to understand the needs and limitations of the laboratory. Laboratory personnel must in turn appreciate the demanding environment and special needs of emergency physicians and their patients. The clinical laboratory will play a vital role in supporting the health care provider, especially in cases of suspected bioterrorism.

Current challenges to clinical laboratories

The recent incidents involving anthrax terrorism has dramatically emphasized our reliance on sophisticated laboratory support to provide efficient and effective care for our patients. However, this reliance is not limited to bioterrorism. From 1980 to 1992, infectious diseases increased 58% as a leading cause of death in the United States, to rank third, up from fifth at the beginning of this period [2]. In addition, antimicrobial resistance patterns are rapidly changing, and physicians and other health care providers need to be aware of these changes.

Challenges in communication between health care providers, laboratorians, and public health practitioners have been highlighted by recent outbreaks. For example, the West Nile virus encephalitis outbreak in New York City demonstrated the need for close communication between hospital, public health, and veterinary laboratories and the human and animal health care providers that use them [3].

Laboratory capacity is another challenge. The shift from fee-for-service to managed care has created a general restructuring of hospital-based laboratories, with many laboratories consolidated and centralized in an attempt to cut costs, with the attendant overall reduction in community laboratory capacity [4]. Participants in the West Nile outbreak response effort stressed the need for increased numbers of Biosafety Level 2 (BL2) laboratory facilities and the ability to quickly access these laboratories by the health care community [3]. The recent anthrax incidents also reinforced the need for critical laboratory capacity locally and nationally.

Another essential component of a comprehensive biodefense strategy is laboratory capability. Microorganisms and toxins associated with bioterrorism are rarely encountered and may require sophisticated laboratory capabilities in testing and containment. These capabilities are often beyond those of existing local laboratories.

Concerns regarding these challenges prompted the Infectious Disease Society of America (IDSA) to develop policy statements and an action plan on the use of the clinical microbiology laboratory in the United States [5]. A survey performed during the IDSA review listed poor communication between physicians and laboratory personnel as the most significant detrimental effect of the consolidation of laboratories [5]. In addition, recent statements from the Mayo Clinic in Rochester, Minnesota note that improving identification and control of antibiotic-resistant strains of bacteria depends on a well-staffed and equipped microbiology laboratory that maintains close contact with clinicians [6].

Laboratory component in bioterrorism agent identification

The role of the clinical laboratory in bioterrorism is no different than with any other patient scenario—to detect, recover, characterize, and identify any infectious agent and to determine sensitivity to antimicrobial agents [7]. However, laboratory workers may be unfamiliar with many bioterrorism agents, some of which may pose a greater health hazard to laboratory staff.

A recent blind survey of laboratories in New Mexico revealed that the private laboratory community does not routinely recognize and report the anthrax bacillus [8]. Among the genus *Bacillus* are a variety of common contaminants, and thus from a historical perspective, the laboratory community has become accustomed to not identifying or reporting their presence, especially because human illness caused by *Bacillus anthracis* has been so rare in the United States. With the recent advent of bioterrorism, laboratory strategies must change. Collaboration between the front line physician and the laboratory staff will serve health care providers and the system well by more quickly alerting all to the possibility of a bioterrorist agent.

Because bioterrorism exposures may occur in relative isolation or in airports, subways, and public gatherings, from which exposed individuals may widely disperse during the incubation period, a cluster of sick people appearing at emergency departments may not signal an unusual event. More likely, initial symptomatic individuals will seek healthcare from a variety of settings, such as emergency departments, urgent care centers, or private physicians' offices. If initial clinical symptoms resemble a flu-like syndrome or other usually benign condition, laboratories may not receive orders to test for unusual pathogens, much less a bioterrorism agent. Thus, the laboratorian must be able to recognize key microorganisms without prior prompting from physicians. As the medical community prepares for acts of bioterrorism, improvement in supporting clinical laboratory capability is essential [9].

The Laboratory Response Network

To assist laboratories in bioterrorism detection, the Association of Public Health Laboratories and the Centers for Disease Control and Prevention (CDC) have created a multilevel Laboratory Response Network (LRN) [10,11].

The LRN is a pyramidal structure in which the lowest (Level A) of four levels of laboratories provides initial sample referrals to increasingly more sophisticated laboratories [7,12]. Each level has different responsibilities in the detection, confirmation, and typing of specimens, and different requirements to save suspected or known bioterrorism agent isolates. Capabilities of each level are found in Table 1. The network is evolving rapidly as the plans and procedures are developed and distributed. An understanding of

Table 1
Functions and biosafety levels of LRN laboratories

Laboratory level	Functions of bioterrorism laboratories in the Laboratory Response Network (LRN)	Biosafety level (practices/ facility)
A Front line (hospital, clinic)	Evaluate specimens from patients not suspected of bioterrorism Rule out bioterrorism agents or refer to B, C labs Refer specimens from patients suspected of bioterrorism and provide patient information	2/2
B Referral (public health)	Confirmation of identification of A lab referrals Routine isolation and identification of agents Training and education of A labs Susceptibility testing of isolates	3/2
C Advanced capacity (public health)	Evaluate molecular tests for application in other labs Molecular typing of isolates Toxigenicity testing Routine isolation and identification of agents Training and education of A labs	3/3 (3 + for VEE)
D CDC, DOE, USAMRIID	Develop new molecular tests for all agents Provide molecular characterization of isolates Archive isolates for later comparison and typing Develop educational materials, lab protocols	4/4

Abbreviations: CDC, Centers for Disease Control and Prevention; DOE, Department of Energy; USAMRIID, US Army Medical Research Institute of Infectious Diseases.
Adapted from Gilchrist MJR: A national laboratory network for bioterrorism: evolution from a prototype network of laboratories performing routine surveillance. Military Medicine; International Journal of AMSUS 2000;165(Suppl 2):28–31.

the LRN and collaboration with clinical laboratories to quickly mobilize available resources will greatly increase the ability to recognize a bioterrorism attack and implement appropriate curative and post-exposure disease prevention measures. Additional information about the LRN, including laboratory protocols, is available through the CDC web site, found at http://www.bt.cdc.gov.

Level A laboratories

The LRN architecture relies on the hospital microbiology laboratory, designated Level A, as the key filter for the detection of agents in covert bioterrorism events. Level A laboratories are expected to routinely screen cultures for the presence of bioterrorism agents by simple methods, employing an algorithmic logic. (Examples of clinical Level A laboratory protocols can be found on the CDC website at http://www.bt.cdc.gov/Agent/Agentlist.asp.) Screening should be done routinely (ie, without prompting from the physician) although an alert from the ordering clinician would enhance sensitivity. The local laboratory should forward unidentifiable microorganisms to Level B or Level C laboratories—state public health laboratories that are equipped for rapid, specific identification.

Level A laboratory staff members must also report this information to the clinician, who is then expected to revisit the patient's clinical picture and monitor or provide prophylaxis, pending identification of the agent. Until there is specific identification reported by the Level B or Level C laboratory, or until there are clusters of patients with consistent symptoms, notification to local authorities is not required. The initial laboratory report is meant to alert but not alarm.

Level B and C laboratories

When bioterrorism is strongly suspected or is known to have occurred, suspect samples should be sent directly to a Level B or Level C laboratory, for at least two reasons. First, methods available at Level B or C laboratories are more rapid and reliable. Second, although Level A laboratories are able to safely handle some bioterrorism agents, many isolates pose a significant risk to laboratory workers and should be deferred to laboratories with higher biosafety containment capability. Orders for cultures from patients believed to be part of a bioterrorism cluster can be sent to the hospital laboratory with instructions that the specimens be delivered immediately to a Level B or C laboratory.

During a large outbreak caused by bioterrorism, Level B and C laboratories throughout the nation may be called on to supply surge capacity to the affected state public health laboratory [11]. This capability exists in many but not all state laboratories. The greatest problem may occur in addressing the concerns of people close to the suspected exposure event who may believe that they are ill or who worry that they will become ill [11]. Laboratory capacity may become overwhelmed by the ill alone, much less these concerned but unaffected individuals.

Level D laboratories

In addition to identification, these higher-level laboratories will be able to test for toxins and type the isolates for comparison studies that may aid in linking seemingly separate outbreaks. Laboratory and clinical characteristics and methodologies of identification of potential bioterrorism agents are found in Table 2. Developing new assays, evaluating available assays, and typing and archiving isolates are also the purview of the Level D laboratories [12]. An additional function is the characterization of isolates using molecular techniques. The federal laboratories at CDC, the US Army Medical Research Institute of Infectious Diseases (USAMRIID), and the Department of Energy (DOE) are functioning at this level in the LRN.

Diagnosis of illnesses caused by toxins

Several toxins may be used by bioterrorists, including botulinum toxin, ricin, and staphylococcal enterotoxin B (SEB). Local hospital laboratories do not generally have capabilities to detect or confirm the presence of such toxins. The physician must therefore request that confirmation be supplied directly from a Level C or D laboratory. Toxins usually have shorter incubation periods than those of infective microorganisms, and clinical effects are fairly characteristic. Thus, clusters of similarly affected individuals will likely appear, rapidly raising the suspicion of an abnormal event. Under these circumstances, the local laboratory is less critical.

Collection of the proper sample for submission to a Level C or D laboratory is important. Urine samples can be diagnostic for patients suffering from the effects of exposure to SEB, and face or nasal swabs may be of value when considering exposure to ricin, SEB, or botulinum toxin, although the clinical sensitivity of this approach has not been established [13]. Antibody assays are available for testing acute and convalescent sera as a means of confirming the clinical diagnosis but will not assist the clinician in selecting appropriate treatment strategies. Proteolytic degradation of toxins can be rapid. It is important to refrigerate or freeze samples immediately after collection and transport them to the laboratory quickly, with maintenance of the cold-chain. Table 3 provides recommendations on sample collection for biologic threat agents.

When to notify the laboratory of suspicion of bioterrorism

Knowledge of basic epidemiologic principles is the key to help decide whether an acutely ill patient could be the victim of a biologic attack. This

Table 2
Clinical and laboratory characteristics of potential bioterrorism agents

Biological agent	Biosafety level[a]	Incubation period/duration of illness	Initial clinical symptoms after aerosol exposure	Clinical hallmarks	Important agent identity markers	Clinical specimens	Diagnostic assays
Bacillus anthracis	2	1–6 days Duration: 3–5 days	Fever, cough, malaise, headache	Mediastinitis Fatal untreated	Gram-positive rods Spore-former Non-hemolytic Gammaphage sensitive Capsule	Nasal swab Feces Lesion Exudate Acute and convalescent sera	Non-hemolytic on 5% sheep blood agar, 35°C (18–24 h). Gammaphage FA PCR Capsule demonstration
Yersinia pestis	2	2–3 days Duration: 1–6 days	Fever, cough, malaise, headache, bloody sputum	Pneumonia Fatal untreated	Gram-negative coccobacilli Bipolar staining Non-lactose fermenter	Nasal swab Sputum Bubo aspirate Acute and convalescent sera	5% sheep blood agar, chocolate agar, Casman blood agar, cystine heart blood agar, or MacConkey agar, 35°C (24–48 h) FA PCR

(continued on next page)

Table 2 (*continued*)

Biological agent	Biosafety level[a]	Incubation period/duration of illness	Initial clinical symptoms after aerosol exposure	Clinical hallmarks	Important agent identity markers	Clinical specimens	Diagnostic assays
Brucella sp.	2	5–60 days Duration: weeks to months	Fever, cough, malaise, headache	Sepsis, abscess Low mortality	Gram-negative coccobacilli Aerobic Non-motile Non-fermenter	Whole blood Bone marrow Acute and convalescent sera	Blood culture Tryptose agar with 5% bovine sera, Thayer-Martin, chocolate agar with VCNT, 35°C, 5–10% CO_2 (10 days) FA PCR
Burkholderia sp.	2	10–14 days Duration: weeks to months	Fever, cough, malaise, headache	Pneumonia, sepsis, abscess High mortality with fulminant sepsis	Gram-negative rods Motile (except *B. mallei*)	Whole blood Acute and convalescent sera Lesion exudate	5% sheep blood agar, MacConkey agar. 35°C (24–48 h) PCR
Francisella tularensis	2	1–21 days Duration: 2–4 weeks	Fever, cough, malaise, headache	Pneumonia Moderate lethality	Gram-negative Obligate aerobe	Nasal swab Acute and convalescent sera	Glucose cystine heart blood agar, thioglycolate, 35°C (48–72 h) FA PCR
Botulinum toxin	2	1–5 days Duration: death in 24–72 h, lasts months if not lethal	Blurred vision Generalized weakness	Flaccid paralysis Fatal untreated	150 kDal protein neurotoxin	Nasal swab Acute and convalescent sera	Immunoassay Mouse neutralization

Agent	BSL	Incubation/Duration	Symptoms	Clinical features	Agent	Specimen	Diagnostic tests
Ricin	2	18–24 hours Duration: 10–12 days	Cough, flu-like illness	Airway necrosis Moderate lethality	66 kDal protein toxin	Nasal swab Acute and convalescent sera	Immunoassays for antigen Serology
Staphylococcal enterotoxin B	2	3–12 hours Duration: hours to days, cough for weeks	Cough, flu-like illness	Febrile respiratory syndrome Low lethality	23–29 kDal protein superantigens	Nasal swab Urine Acute and convalescent sera	Immunoassays for antigen Serology
Variola virus	4	7–17 days Duration: 4 weeks	Fever, cough, malaise, headache	Pustules High lethality	Brick morphology	Nasal swab Throat swab Lesion exudate Acute and convalescent sera	Viral culture[b] Electron microscopy PCR
Venezuelan equine encephalitis virus	2	1–5 days Duration: days to weeks	Fever, cough, malaise, headache	Encephalitis Low lethality	Enveloped RNA virus	Nasal swab Throat swab Acute and convalescent sera	Viral culture Virus neutralization RT-PCR
Viral hemorrhagic fever viruses	4	4–21 days Duration: 7–16 days	Fever, cough, malaise, headache	Endothelial damage Hemorrhage Fatal	Enveloped RNA viruses	Nasal swab Acute and convalescent sera	Viral culture[b] RT-PCR

[a] Biosafety level descriptions are contained in *Biosafety in Microbiological and Biomedical Laboratories*.

[b] Not recommended except by qualified laboratory with appropriate biosafety equipment.

From Henchal EA, Teska JD, Ludwig GV. Current laboratory methods for biological threat agent identification. Laboratory aspects of biological warfare in clinics in laboratory medicine 2001;21(3):661–78.

Table 3
Medical sample collection for biological threat agents

Early post-exposure	Bacteria and rickettsia	
	Clinical	Convalescent/terminal/postmortem
Anthrax		
Bacillus anthracis		
0–24 h	24–72 h	3–10 d
Nasal and throat swabs, induced respiratory secretions for culture, FA, and PCR	Serum (TT, RT) for toxin assays	Serum (TT, RT) for toxin assays
	Blood (E, C, H) for PCR	Blood (BC, C) for culture
	Blood (BC, C) for culture	Pathology samples
Plague		
Yersinia pestis		
0–24 h	24–72 h	>6 d
Nasal swabs, sputum, induced respiratory secretions for culture, FA, and PCR	Blood (BC, C) and bloody sputum for culture and FA (C), F-1 Antigen assays (TT, RT), PCR (E, C, H)	Serum (TT, RT) for IgM and later for IgG
		Pathology samples
Tularemia		
Francisella tularensis		
0–24 h	24–72 h	>6 d
Nasal swabs, sputum, induced respiratory secretions for culture, FA and PCR	Blood (BC, C) for culture	Serum (TT, RT) for IgM and later for IgG, agglutination titers
	Blood (E, C, H) for PCR	Pathology samples
	Sputum for FA and PCR	
Glanders		
Burkholderia mallei		
0–24 h	24–72 h	>6 d
Nasal swabs, sputum, induced respiratory secretions for culture and PCR	Blood (BC, C) for culture	Blood (BC, C) and tissues for culture
	Blood (E, C, H) for PCR	Serum (TT, RT) for immunoassays
	Sputum and drainage from skin lesions for PCR and culture	Pathology samples
Brucellosis		
Brucella abortus, suis, and *melitensis*		
0–24 h	24–72 h	>6 d
Nasal swabs, sputum, induced respiratory secretions for culture and PCR	Blood (BC, C) for culture	Blood (BC, C) and tissues for culture
	Blood (E, C, H) for PCR	Serum (TT, RT) for immunoassays
		Pathology samples

Q-fever
Coxiella burnetii

Early post-exposure	Clinical	Convalescent/terminal/postmortem
0–24 h	2–5 d	>6 d
Nasal swabs, sputum, induced respiratory secretions for culture and PCR	Blood (BC, C) for culture in eggs or mouse inoculation Blood (E, C, H) for PCR	Blood (BC, C) for culture in eggs or mouse inoculation Pathology samples

	Toxins	
Early post-exposure	Clinical	Convalescent/terminal/postmortem
Botulism Botulinum toxin from *Clostridium botulinum*		
0–24 h	24–72 h	>6 d
Nasal swabs, induced respiratory secretions for PCR (contaminating bacterial DNA) and toxin assays	Nasal swabs, respiratory secretions for PCR (contaminating bacterial DNA) and toxin assays	Usually no IgM or IgG Pathology samples (liver and spleen for toxin detection)
Serum (TT, RT) for toxin assays	Serum (TT, RT) for toxin assay	
Ricin intoxication Ricin toxin from Castor beans		
0–24 h	36–48 h	>6 d
Nasal swabs, induced respiratory secretions for PCR (contaminating castor bean DNA) and toxin assays	Serum (TT, RT) for toxin assay	Serum (TT, RT) for IgM and IgG in survivors
Serum (TT) for toxin assays	Tissues for immunohistological stain in pathology samples	
Staph enterotoxicosis *Staphylococcus* enterotoxin B		
0–3 h	2–6 h	>6 d
	Urine for immunoassays	Serum for IgM and IgG

(*continued on next page*)

Table 3 (*continued*)

Toxins

Early post-exposure	Clinical	Convalescent/terminal/postmortem
Nasal swabs, induced respiratory secretions for PCR (contaminating bacterial DNA) and toxin assays Serum (TT, RT) for toxin assays	Nasal swabs, induced respiratory secretions for PCR (contaminating bacterial DNA) and toxin assays Serum (TT, RT) for toxin assays	
T-2 toxicosis 0–24 h postexposure Nasal and throat swabs, induced respiratory secretions for immunoassays, HPLC/mass spectrometry (HPLC/MS)	1–5 d Serum (TT, RT), tissue for toxin detection	>6 d postexposure Urine for detection of toxin metabolites

Viruses

Early post-exposure	Clinical	Convalescent/terminal/postmortem
Equine encephalomyelitis VEE, EEE and WEE viruses 0–24 h Nasal swabs and induced respiratory secretions for RT-PCR and viral culture	24–72 h Serum and throat swabs for culture (TT, RT), RT-PCR (E, C, H, TT, RT) and antigen ELISA (TT, RT), CSF, throat swabs up to 5 d	>6 d Serum (TT, RT) for IgM Pathology samples plus brain
Ebola 0–24 h Nasal swabs and induced respiratory secretions for RT-PCR and viral culture	2–5 d Serum (TT, RT) for viral culture	>6 d Serum (TT, RT) for viral culture Pathology samples plus adrenal gland
Pox (smallpox, monkey pox) *Orthopoxvirus* 0–24 h	2–5 d	>6 d

Nasal swabs and induced respiratory secretions for PCR and viral culture	Serum (TT, RT) for viral culture	Serum (TT, RT) for viral culture Drainage from skin lesions/scrapings for microscopy. EM, viral culture, PCR Pathology samples.

Abbreviations: BC, Blood culture bottle; C, Citrated blood (3-ml); E, EDTA (3 ml); H, Heparin (3-ml); TT, Tiger-top (5–10 ml); RT, Red top if no TT. Proper collection of specimens is dependent on the time-frame following exposure. Sample collection time is described for "Early post-exposure," "Clinical," and "Convalescent/Terminal/Postmortem" but is not rigid and will vary according to the concentration of agent, agent strain, and predisposing health factors of the patient.

Early post-exposure: when it is known that an individual has been exposed to a bioagent aerosol; aggressively attempt to obtain samples as indicated

Clinical: samples from those individuals presenting with clinical symptoms

Convalescent/Terminal/Postmortem: samples taken during convalescence, the terminal stages of infection or toxicosis, or postmortem during autopsy

Shipping samples: Most specimens sent rapidly (less than 24 h) to analytical labs require only blue or wet ice or refrigeration at 2–8°C. If the time span increases beyond 24 h, however, contact the receiving laboratory for specific shipping instructions.

Blood samples: Several choices are offered—only one sample is required. Centrifuged tiger-top tubes are preferred over red-top clot tubes with serum removed from the clot. Blood culture bottles are also preferred over citrated blood for bacterial cultures.

Pathology samples: Routinely include liver, lung, spleen, and regional or mesenteric lymph nodes. Possible additional samples include brain tissue for encephalomyelitis cases and the adrenal gland for Ebola.

awareness should prompt the notification of the clinical laboratory of this possibility. The clinician should also alert the laboratory if a sample requires special attention. The possibility of biologic terrorism, or any infection requiring immediate individual and public health action, should always be contemplated when seeing a patient with a presentation compatible with an acute infectious disease. By remembering some simple axioms for the behavior of biologic terrorism agents, the health care provider can maintain an index of suspicion and properly alert the laboratory to any irregularities.

Any suspected disease that is unusual for a given geographic area or transmission season, or that is normally transmitted by a vector that is not present in that area, should be investigated and the laboratory alerted. This especially includes any potential disease process caused by an uncommon agent such as a hemorrhagic fever virus or *Variola major* (smallpox virus). The laboratory can also assist with detecting unusual strains or variants of organisms or antimicrobial resistance patterns different from those currently circulating in the area. Level D laboratories may be able to determine similar genetic types isolated from distinct sources at different times or locations, thus alerting authorities to the possibility of a bioterrorism incident.

Any time there is an unusual presentation of a disease (eg, abnormal demographics, a sudden severe illness in a previously healthy patient, or a cluster of patients with similar signs and symptoms in a short period of time), the health care provider should consider contacting the local health department to determine if similar cases have presented elsewhere. The laboratory should also be notified of a potential outbreak of disease. Multiple ill patients with similar exposures but no direct contact with other patients is especially worrisome. There may also be evidence of a similar illness occurring in non-contiguous areas or in animals. Close contact with the local public health department and a continual information flow between the clinician and the laboratory will assist in identifying clues of a bioterrorism event.

Need for close contact with the laboratory regarding patient status

Smallpox and hemorrhagic fever viruses are two significant bioterrorism candidates. Smallpox may initially present in an atypical or milder fashion in previously vaccinated individuals and may be confused with disease caused by one of the herpes viruses. Manipulation of these viruses is dangerous and will put the laboratorian at increased risk if they are not aware of the need for increased safety standards. Handling of culture-amplified viruses that may be present in much greater numbers than usually dispersed by a patient is also dangerous without adequate precautions. When there is an unknown virus whose characteristics do not conform to those of a conventional virus, the laboratory should ascertain the patient's clinical condition. With some viruses such as smallpox, a rapid confirmation will allow vaccination of laboratory workers. The physician should thus also notify laboratory staff regarding any change in patient status.

Environmental sampling

In the event of a known or suspected bioterrorism incident, environmental samples will be under the supervision of the Federal Bureau of Investigation (FBI). A chain of custody must be maintained so that results may be used as evidence in subsequent legal proceedings. Sampling for these purposes is a law enforcement, not a medical, issue. No Level A laboratory or individual physician should be expected to culture or collect environmental samples. Requests for such sampling should be referred to the Incident Command Center.

Veterinary diagnostic laboratory support for animal-related bioterrorism

Animal diseases may be transmitted to humans and have been investigated for use as biologic warfare agents. There is currently an effort to improve networking and interactions among federal and state veterinary laboratories to improve response to potentially large or explosive disease outbreaks or bioterrorism attacks involving animals as victims or as sentinels for human outbreaks [14].

Veterinary laboratories already recognize the need to ensure a complete range of testing for diagnosis of potential animal bioterrorism attacks or widespread outbreaks of foreign animal disease. A search engine and database are being developed to provide rapid and secure access to updated and reliable information about veterinary testing laboratories and procedures in North America, and to provide a roster of available experts for diseases of particular concern [14].

A centralized federal laboratory system within the US Department of Agriculture, Animal and Plant Health Inspection Services (APHIS), aids in detection of foreign animal diseases and diseases targeted for eradication in the United States [15]. Veterinary medical first responders including local veterinary practices, public health departments, veterinary colleges, and veterinary diagnostic laboratories which, if well prepared and actively networking, could help in effectively responding to large scale accidental or intentional epizootics.

The Ames Laboratory, Department of Energy, and the Federal Bureau of Investigation collaboratively support a veterinary laboratory response capability that can detect and assist in responding to a potential bioterrorism attack. Iowa State University is developing a coordinated database and search engine to document veterinary laboratory capabilities and to identify experienced laboratory personnel as an aid to rapid field response [16]. This database could be used to assist medical and public health communities in their response to acts of domestic bioterrorism involving people. The stated goal is to create a secure communication system among appropriate agencies and laboratories, followed by collection of as much information as possible on the type of testing available, specific methodologies, and documentation of quality control, precision, sensitivity, and specificity. The database will be key in better organizing local resources against animal-related bioterrorism.

Technical components of agent identification

Following Operation Desert Storm, Department of Defense efforts to develop more robust detection and diagnostic capabilities for biologic warfare agents escalated. Advances in technology have provided several new tools for defense against these agents. Such technologies include high volume air-samplers capable of concentrating airborne particulate material and performing presumptive identification of specific agents, easy-to-use rapid hand-held immunoassays for presumptive identification, and immunoassays and gene amplification assays for laboratory identification and confirmation [17,18]. Still, a great deal of research and improvements are needed in this crucial area. More information about Department of Defense biologic agent defense systems is available at the Joint Program Office for Biological Defense website, found at http://www.jpobd.net.

Successful diagnosis of clinically ill patients and a risk assessment of potentially exposed individuals can be influenced by type of sample collected, mode of collection, and subsequent sample management. Immediate post-exposure risk may be determined by analyzing swabs collected from the face or nares of potentially exposed individuals [13,19]. Collection to support clinical diagnosis will vary, depending on the suspected agent. Sampling of blood, sputum, stool, urine, vesicular fluids, scabs, bronchial washings, lymph node aspirates, biopsies, swabs from wounds, and vomitus or gastric contents have all been described to aid in diagnostics [7,20]. Table 3 provides a guide to sample collection in the event of a suspected bioterrorism attack.

There are important principles to remember when sampling. Synthetic swabs are recommended over cotton swabs because of a greater recovery rate of the biologic agent during laboratory extraction procedures (personal communication, Dr. Fred Knauert, Fort Detrick, Maryland, March 1999). Facial and nasal swabs are only recommended for 18–24 hours post-exposure [21]. Anthrax spores may be recoverable from feces for as long as 48 hours post-exposure [13]. For all samples, it is important to expeditiously cool and maintain refrigeration throughout transport. A sample from an individual's face, nares, or blood may also contain enzymes capable of degrading the targeted antigens and nucleic acid sequences, compromising subsequent identification. Refrigerating or freezing the samples will slow this process, resulting in a higher quality sample. Freezing is not routinely recommended unless delivery will be significantly delayed (personal communication, Dr. John Ezzell, Fort Detrick, Maryland, March 1999), and efforts should always be taken to minimize the time between sample collection and analysis. These issues may all be factors in data review for preventive medicine and treatment decision-making.

Microbiology laboratories may use one or more of three principle diagnostic systems: culture, immunodiagnostic assays, and gene amplification assays. All have distinct advantages and disadvantages.

Culture is the most readily available technology and is available throughout the nation's public health laboratory system. It requires the presence of viable microorganisms in the sample and maintenance of their viability throughout sample transportation. Laboratory personnel may require additional training to recognize uncommon agents, and some agents may require selective media. Culture also requires considerable time to produce a final result [13]. Virus culture may only be available in specialized laboratories.

Immunoassays target agent-specific antigens and antibodies [13], and generally are not dependent on agent viability. The technology is diverse and antigen-detection antibodies can be produced to detect structural components and metabolic by-products associated with the microorganism. They are well suited for demonstrating the presence of a toxin [13,22]. Antibody detection can be an important adjunct to confirming patient diagnoses. Many infections caused by biologic threat agents, however, may cause death before measurable antibody production [13].

Gene amplification assays target microbial or plant (ricin) DNA or RNA, do not require the presence of viable microorganisms, and are rapid and sensitive. If used for identifying a toxin, one must consider that the DNA is a contaminant from the microorganism or plant that produced the toxin and may not be present in the sample. Gene amplification assays work best with purified nucleic acids that may require 2–6 hours of sample preparation time before the reaction.

In general, immunoassays are less sensitive than gene amplification assays (ie, PCR), and gene amplification assays will be slightly less sensitive than culture techniques [13]. There are, however, several factors that may alter those generalizations. Confidence in results is partially dependent on the sensitivity and specificity of the analysis system. Limit of detection is a product of sample quality, sample processing, and the sensitivity of the assay being used. An integrated use of the various technologies described will produce the highest level of confidence.

New technologies for rapid detection of biologic threat agents are under development. Until they have been approved for clinical diagnostic use, most clinical laboratory analyses will be conducted using standard approved microbiologic techniques. The more advanced technologies will initially be available only in reference laboratories. New PCR technology development is producing some alternatives that may be available soon in a hospital laboratory. These include the smaller bench-top and field deployable systems such as the Ruggedized Advanced Pathogen Identification System (RAPID™) (Idaho Technologies, Salt Lake City, Utah), Smart Cycler™ (Cepheid, Sunnyvale, California), and Light Cycler™ (Roche Biomedical, Indianapolis, Indiana). These technologies enhance sensitivity by amplifying targeted nucleic acid sequences and may also enhance specificity by using an agent-specific probe that targets a unique nucleic acid sequence [13,23]. Electrochemiluminesence (ECL) assays are also under development and will enhance the sensitivity, specificity, and speed of immunodiagnostics. These assays have demonstrated 100- to 1000-times greater sensitivity when compared with comparable enzyme-linked immunosorbent assays (ELISA) [13,22].

Hand-held lateral flow immunoassays have been developed for environmental detection of biologic threat agents, but none are approved for medical use [13]. It is important to understand their limits of detection and specificity when considering results as part of the patient history from a suspect exposure. They may lack the sensitivity and specificity required to accurately estimate a patient's risk for exposure [13].

Importance of rapid identification of a bioterrorist agent

Clinicians and other health professionals may be faced with a flood of information surrounding suspect bioterrorist incidents. They do not need to become experts on the various technologies used to identify the various agents. They should, however, have a working knowledge of sampling methods, diagnostic capabilities and limitations, and interpretation of results so that an appropriate level of confidence can be applied in making decisions for patient evaluation and treatment, including preventive medicine risk assessments. In doing so, they can more effectively use all possible laboratory options to diagnose the potential bioterrorist victim as rapidly as possible. Many of the agents that could be used in a biologic attack are not commonly seen, and their treatments may be different than those most health care providers commonly use. Early diagnosis of these diseases will allow rapid, correct treatment of the patient. In addition, many potential bioterrorist agents have preventive measures that can be instituted immediately, such as anthrax and smallpox vaccination, to prevent those exposed from developing disease. For potentially contagious diseases, appropriate quarantine can also be instituted.

During a major bioterrorism event, it is hoped that Incident Command Centers will provide guidance to physicians serving in the epicenters of the outbreaks. Pending such guidance, physicians may consider sending cultures from those patients deemed unlikely to have been exposed to a bioterrorist agent to their local diagnostic laboratories, because they are less likely to need rapid results and the specimens are unlikely to present a hazard to the laboratory staff. Some agents may have prolonged incubation periods, however, during which an infected patient would be asymptomatic. Extended prophylaxis of exposed individuals therefore may still be required. At this time, initial cultures are unlikely to successfully guide prophylaxis. The local public health director, in concert with experts in bioterrorism, should provide guidance on prophylaxis based on exposure history and availability of prophylactic antibiotics.

Education in all aspects of bioterrorism diagnosis and treatment is crucial in combating resultant epidemics. The Working Group for Civilian Biodefense is attempting to increase awareness among the medical and public health communities. Reports from this group consistently stress early recognition and prophylaxis when available [24–28]. As health professionals use information in their decision-making process, they must also understand the confidence level that should be applied to information at each level of the integrated system.

Summary

The impact of a bioterrorism attack can be greatly reduced by collaboration among primary healthcare providers, laboratories, the veterinary community, public health officials, and emergency response personnel. Improved communication and coordination are essential to make this happen. As a first-line provider, the emergency physician must keep in mind the possibility of bioterrorism and alert the laboratory so that samples can be processed in the correct fashion. New and exciting developments in laboratory organization, communication, and diagnostic capabilities will ensure that all patients receive the best possible care.

References

[1] Cole LA. Bioterrorism threats: learning from inappropriate responses. J Public Health Manag Pract 2000;6(4):8–18.

[2] Pinner RW, Teutsch SM, Simonsen L, et al. Trends in infectious diseases mortality in the United States. JAMA 1996;275:189–93.

[3] Fine A, Layton M. Lessons for the West Nile viral encephalitis outbreak in New York City, 1999: implications for bioterrorism preparedness. Clin Infect Dis 2001;32:277–82.

[4] Skeels M: Laboratories and disease surveillance. Mil Med 2000;165(Suppl 2):16–9.

[5] Peterson LR, Hamilton JD, Baron EJ, et al. Role of the clinical microbiology laboratories in the management and control of infectious diseases and the delivery of health care. Clin Infect Dis 2001;32:605–11.

[6] Virk A, Steckelberg JM. Clinical aspects of antimicrobial resistance. Mayo Clin Proc 2000;75:200 14.

[7] Klietmann WF, Ruoff KL. Bioterrorism: implications for the clinical microbiologist. Clin Microbiol Rev 2001;14(2):364–81.

[8] Horensky D. Blind submissions of the avirulent Sterne strain of *Bacillus anthracis* to New Mexico clinical laboratories [paper Y-5]. In: Abstracts of the 101st General Meeting of the American Society for Microbiology, Orlando, Florida, 2001. Available at: http://www.asmusa.org/pcsrc/gm2001/34250.htm. Accessed 15 Aug 2001.

[9] Jortani SA, Snyder JW, Valdes Jr. R. The role of the clinical laboratory in managing chemical or biological terrorism. Clin Chem 2000;46(12):1883–93.

350   J.A. Pavlin et al / Emerg Med Clin N Am 20 (2002) 331–350

[10] Khan AS, Levitt AM, Sage MJ. Biological and chemical terrorism: strategic plan for preparedness and response. Morb Mortal Wkly Rpt 2000;49(RR-4):1–14.
[11] Snyder JW, Check W. Bioterrorism threats to our future: the role of the clinical microbiology laboratory in detection, identification, and confirmation of biological agents. American Academy of Microbiology, Washington, DC, 2000. Available at: http://www.asmusa.org. Accessed 15 Aug 2001.
[12] Gilchrist MJR. A national laboratory network for bioterrorism: evolution from a prototype network of laboratories performing routine surveillance. Mil Med 2000;165(Suppl 2): S28–31.
[13] Henchal EA, Teska JD, Ludwig GV, et al. Current laboratory methods for biological threat agent identification. Clin Lab Med 2001;21(3):661–78.
[14] US Department of Agriculture. Available at: http://www.aphis.usda.gov/vs/safeguard.htm. Accessed September 30, 2001.
[15] US Department of Agriculture. Available at: http://www.aphis.usda.gov. Accessed September 30, 2001.
[16] Iowa State University. College of Veterinary Medicine, Veterinary Diagnostic Laboratory. Available at: http://www.vdpam.iastate.edu/VDL/default.htm. Accessed September 30, 2001.
[17] Kortepeter MG, Cieslak TJ, Eitzen EM. Bioterrorism. J Environ Health 2001;63(6):21–4.
[18] O'Brien T, Johnson LH III, Aldrich JL, et al. The development of immunoassays to four biological threat agents in a bidiffractive grating biosensor. Biosens Bioelectron 2000; 14(10–11):815–28.
[19] Hail AS, Rossi CA, Ludwig GV, et al. Comparison of noninvasive sampling sites for early detection of Bacillus anthracis spores from rhesus monkeys after aerosol exposure. Mil Med 1999;164(12):833–7.
[20] Franz DR, Jahrling PB, Friedlander AM, et al. Clinical recognition and management of patients exposed to biological warfare agents. JAMA 1997;278(5):399–411.
[21] Eitzen E, Pavlin J, Cieslak T, et al, editors. Medical management of biological casualties handbook. 3rd edition. Fort Detrick, Maryland: US Army Medical Research Institute of Infectious Diseases; 1998.
[22] Kijek TM, Rossi CA, Moss D, et al. Rapid and sensitive immunomagnetic-electrochemiluminescent detection of staphylococcal enterotoxin B. J Immunol Methods 2000;236(1–2): 9–17.
[23] Higgins JA, Ezzell J, Hinnebusch BJ, et al. 5' nuclease PCR assay to detect Yersinia pestis. J Clin Microbiol 1998;36(8):2284–8.
[24] Arnon SS, Schechter R, Inglesby TV, et al. Botulinum toxin as a biological weapon: medical and public health management. JAMA 2001;285(8):1059–70.
[25] Dennis DT, Inglesby TV, Henderson DA, et al. Tularemia as a biological weapon: medical and public health management. JAMA 2001;285(21):2763–73.
[26] Henderson DA, Inglesby TV, Bartlett JG, et al. Smallpox as a biological weapon: medical and public health management. JAMA 1999;281(22):2127–37.
[27] Inglesby TV, Dennis DT, Henderson DA, et al. Plague as a biological weapon: medical and public health management. JAMA 2000;283(17):2281–90.
[28] Inglesby TV, Henderson DA, Bartlett JG, et al. Anthrax as a biological weapon: medical and public health management [published erratum appears in JAMA, 283(15):1963, 2000]. JAMA 1999;281(18):1735–45.

EMERGENCY
MEDICINE
CLINICS OF
NORTH AMERICA

Emerg Med Clin N Am
20 (2002) 351–364

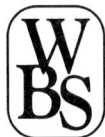

Medical management of the suspected victim of bioterrorism: an algorithmic approach to the undifferentiated patient

Fred M. Henretig, MD, FACEP[a],*,
Theodore J. Cieslak, MD, FAAP[b],
Mark G. Kortepeter, MD, MPH, FACP[c],
Gary R. Fleisher, MD[d]

[a]Division of Emergency Medicine, Children's Hospital of Philadelphia,
34th Street and Civic Center Boulevard, Philadelphia, PA 19104, USA
[b]Department of Pediatrics, Ft. Sam Houston, TX 78234, USA
[c]US Army Medical Research Institute of Infectious Diseases, Fort Detrick, MD 21702, USA
[d]Division of Emergency Medicine, Children's Hospital, 300 Longwood Ave.,
Boston, MA 02115, USA

The increasing threat of biological and chemical terrorism has gained considerable attention of late, and appropriately so given the recent cluster of anthrax incidents associated with contaminated mail that America has experienced. Accompanying this threat is an obvious significant preparedness and defense requirement. A comprehensive strategy for preparation and response against an attack using bioweapons will provide America with an ability to deter or mitigate any incident. Central to any response plan is early detection. Early detection will initiate a quicker guided response. A faster response will result in more lives saved, less damage to our critical infrastructure, and maintenance of society's well-being. In this article, we focus on the initial emergency department (ED) evaluation and management of patients who are suspected victims of bioterrorism.

Various working groups have determined which agents have the potential to cause mass casualties in the absence of appropriate preparedness [1–3].

* Corresponding author.
E-mail address: henretig@email.chop.edu (F.M. Henretig).

The opinions and assertions contained herein are the private views of the authors and are not to be construed as official or as necessarily reflecting the views of the Department of Defense, the US Army, the US Army Medical Research Institute of Infectious Diseases, or Brooke Army Medical Center.

Table 1
Primary survey: one (or first) patient

Mnemonic	Interpretation/assessment and action[a]
A	Airway with cervical spine precautions Assess for air movement, stridor, etc. Effect positioning, suction, OP/NP airway, ETT, crichothyrotomy, etc.
B	Breathing Assess color, respiratory rate, pulse oximetry, etc. Effect ventilation support prn: mouth-mouth, bag-valve mask, bag-ETT, etc.
C	Circulation Assess cardiac activity, skin perfusion, capillary refill, pulses, blood pressure, cardiac monitor Effect chest compressions prn, IV access, fluids, ACLS meds prn
D	Disability Assess responsiveness to stimulation, pupil size, reaction Consider ETT, hyperventilation, etc., for severe compromise
E	Expose the patient/environmental assessment for hypo- or hyperthermia Undress, log-roll, assess temperature Rapid cooling or warming prn *Epidemiology* *"Exposure" history—visible cloud, delivery device, explosion, known* *threat, etc.?* *"Epidemic" numbers of patients with acute onset, or tight cluster?* *"Exotic" diseases, clinical syndromes?* *If positive, consider biologic terrorism attack—go to Biological Attack Secondary Survey 2 (Table 2)*

[a] Italics indicate addition to conventional paradigm.

Abbreviations: OP/NP, oropharyngeal/nasopharyngeal; ETT, endotracheal tube; IV, intravenous; ACLS, advanced cardiac life support.

According to the recommendations of a strategic planning workgroup organized by the Centers for Disease Control and Prevention (CDC) [1], a comprehensive public health response to a biological attack with such agents should involve epidemiologic investigation, medical treatment and prophylaxis, and the initiation of disease prevention measures. Providing prompt and effective medical treatment and prophylaxis to victims of an attack with biological agents would likely be problematic, however. Many factors account for this: (1) several of the agents considered as high threats (and their diagnostic modalities) are unfamiliar to most emergency health care providers (EHCPs), (2) many EHCPs have not yet received adequate training in biological defense to recognize or even suspect a biological event, (3) unlike conventional weapons, explosives, and chemical agents, biological agents have incubation periods that will cause victims to present for care far-removed in time and space from the time an agent was released, (4) early signs and symptoms are likely to be non-specific in initial presentation, and (5) stockpiles of many therapeutic drugs are not yet readily available. Moreover, when EHCPs receive training, it is often agent-specific, pre-supposing a definitive diagnosis has already been made. We propose an algorithmic approach (Tables 1 and 2; Fig. 1) to guide EHCPs in the early recognition and initial management of a potential attack with an unknown biological agent.

A conceptual model: Advanced Trauma Life Support

For individual EHCPs, the first challenge of preparedness is knowing when to suspect a bioterrorist event. EHCPs continually evaluate and treat febrile patients manifesting vague systemic complaints and signs. Even the most well-trained and vigilant clinician is unlikely to correctly diagnose the initial patients of a bioterrorist attack who present with non-specific febrile syndromes. To enable early recognition, an educational plan must link the heightened awareness level of physicians who have received biological defense training to appropriate epidemiologic clues. This plan is best carried out in a context that is familiar to health care professionals, one that parallels more common clinical paradigms.

Table 2
Biological attack secondary survey (for suspected biological weapon incidents, subsequent patients, mass casualties)

Step	Mnemonic	Interpretation/assessment and action
1	A	*A*nticipate biological weapons incident (pattern recognition, multiple casualties, etc.)
2	B	*B*e careful (personal protection issues)
		–Standard precautions for most scenarios
		–When in doubt, use a mask and protect mucus membranes. If known plague, VHF, or smallpox, see specific measures below (E_1) and in text
3	C	*C*ontinue life support prn
4	D	*D*econtaminate, isolate patient as warranted
5	D_2	*D*iagnosis
		–*Succinct history*: acuity of onset, exposure history, multiple patients, febrile prodrome, respiratory, neurologic, or dermatologic symptoms?
		–*Focused physical examination*: vital signs; cardiorespiratory, neurologic, and dermatologic findings?
		–*Laboratory testing*: chest radiograph; CBC, coagulation studies
		–Diagnostic impressions (Table 4, Fig. 1)
6	D_3	(*D*rugs) treatment (Fig. 1)
7	E_1	*E*pidemic infection control
		Plague: droplet precautions
		VHFs: contact droplet (consider airborne) precautions
		Smallpox: airborne contact precautions
		All others: standard precautions
8	E_2	*E*pidemic reporting to law enforcement, public health
9	E_3	*E*pidemiologic investigation
10	E_4	*E*ducate others

Abbreviations: CBC, complete blood count; VHFs, viral hemorrhagic fevers.

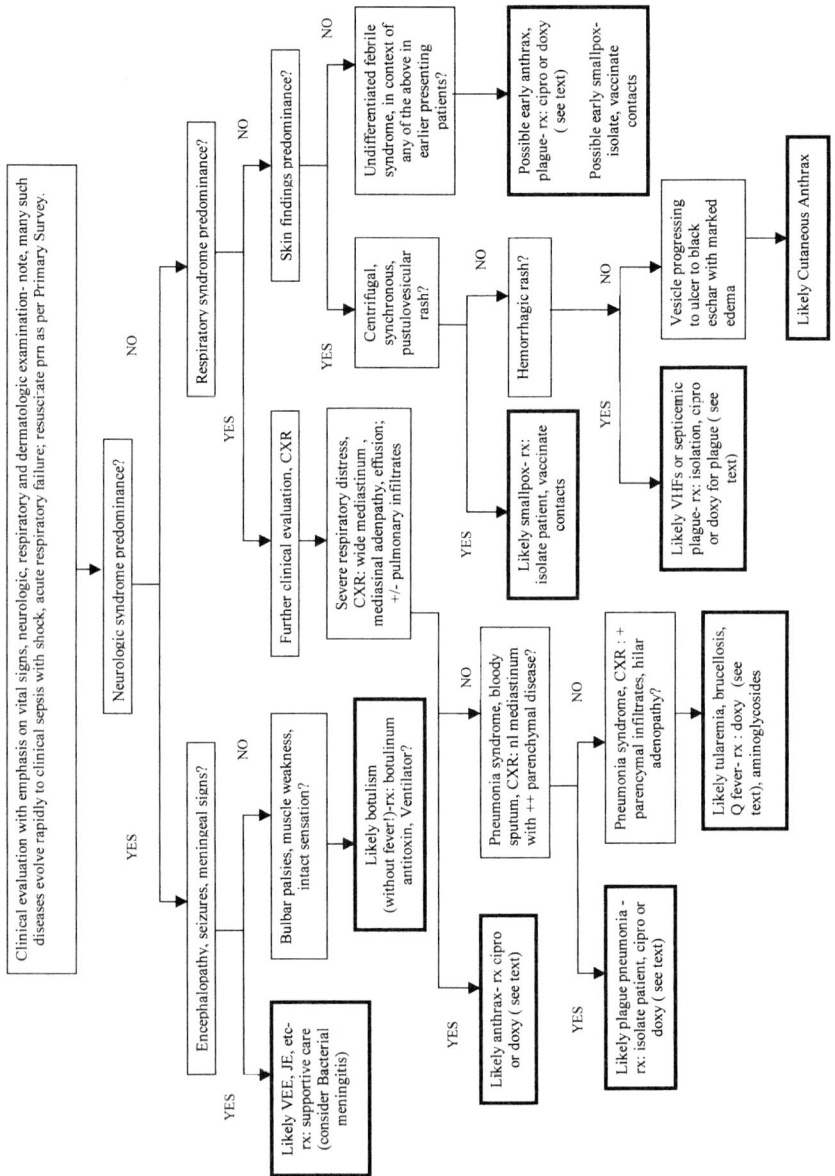

Clinical evaluation with emphasis on vital signs, neurologic, respiratory and dermatologic examination- note, many such diseases evolve rapidly to clinical sepsis with shock, acute respiratory failure; resuscitate prn as per Primary Survey.

Neurologic syndrome predominance?

YES — NO

Encephalopathy, seizures, meningeal signs?

YES — Likely VEE, JE, etc- rx: supportive care (consider Bacterial meningitis)

NO — Bulbar palsies, muscle weakness, intact sensation?

Likely botulism (without fever?)-rx: botulinum antitoxin, Ventilator?

YES — Likely anthrax- rx cipro or doxy (see text)

NO — Pneumonia syndrome, bloody sputum, CXR: nl mediastinum with ++ parenchymal disease?

YES — Likely plague pneumonia - rx: isolate patient, cipro or doxy (see text)

NO — Pneumonia syndrome, CXR : + parenchymal infiltrates, hilar adenopathy?

Likely tularemia, brucellosis, Q fever- rx : doxy (see text), aminoglycosides

Respiratory syndrome predominance?

YES — Further clinical evaluation, CXR

Severe respiratory distress, CXR: wide mediastinum, mediasinal adenpathy, effusion; +/- pulmonary infiltrates

NO — Skin findings predominance?

Centrifugal, synchronous, pustulovesicular rash?

YES — Likely smallpox- rx: isolate patient, vaccinate contacts

NO — Hemorrhagic rash?

YES — Likely VHFs or septicemic plague- rx: isolation, cipro or doxy for plague (see text)

NO — Vesicle progressing to ulcer to black eschar with marked edema — Likely Cutaneous Anthrax

NO — Undifferentiated febrile syndrome, in context of any of the above in earlier presenting patients?

Possible early anthrax, plague- rx: cipro or doxy (see text)
Possible early smallpox- isolate, vaccinate contacts

One model that is well known to EHCPs and that applies to a major class of critically ill patients is Advanced Trauma Life Support (ATLS) [4]. ATLS offers a 2-stage process of early diagnosis and treatment for multiple trauma victims that builds on the traditional ABCs of cardiopulmonary resuscitation. The ATLS model conceptualizes trauma as a "disease," potentially involving multiple organ systems in which critical interventions made within a short period of time post-incident (the "golden hour") will have a major impact in reducing mortality. Simultaneous recognition and correction of the most immediately life-threatening injuries are emphasized first, followed by a more comprehensive evaluation to detect important causes of delayed morbidity—the "Primary Survey/Secondary Survey" concept.

Victims of a biological agent attack might be similarly thought of as critically injured, or at least at risk for injury. The potential agents of biological terrorism typically cause life-threatening manifestations, including multi-organ system dysfunction. Delay in recognition of traumatic injury increases mortality. By analogy, delay in recognition of biological agent infection can have dire consequences, because several specific measures exist, which, if instituted early could substantially reduce mortality. Such interventions include empiric, and sometimes unconventional, antibiotic therapy for large numbers of undifferentiated febrile patients, used early and before the evolution of characteristic clinical syndromes or the receipt of confirmatory laboratory results. Furthermore, institution of isolation and personal protection measures on a hospital- or community-wide basis might be required in certain cases. Notification of public health authorities and the subsequent initiation of large-scale immunization procedures might likewise be warranted.

It is imperative that the ECHP, especially in the setting of a mass-casualty event, has a method to integrate his or her thinking about potential bioterrorism victims into a familiar approach employed in the management of other, more conventional, patients. As noted earlier, the earliest presenting patients in a bioterrorist incident would likely be difficult to recognize, because many of the most likely agents present with an undifferentiated febrile illness. Even with advanced disease, other more common diagnoses would likely be considered. By linking the epidemiologic clues of a biological attack to the usual mnemonic for trauma patients, individual emergency physicians, nurses, and emergency medical services (EMS) personnel may be able to recognize and manage the first wave of victims earlier. Further, with just slight modifications to this well-practiced paradigm, EHCPs may be able to rapidly adjust their clinical practice into a mass casualty mode, with earlier hospital and community disaster protocol initiation. Most authorities in this field believe that in the context of a significant bioterrorism incident, even

Fig. 1. Algorithm for initial approach to victims of biologic attack (steps 5–7 of Biological Weapon Secondary Survey). *Abbreviations*: VEE, Venezuelan equine encephalitis; JE, Japanese encephalitis; CXR, chest radiograph; cipro, ciprofloxacin; doxy, doxycycline; nl, normal; rx, treatment; VHFs, viral hemorrhagic fevers.

several hours to a day of earlier recognition, notification, treatment, and prophylaxis might have an enormous impact on limiting epidemic spread and overall mortality [5].

From the perspective of the individual ECHP, any epidemic will begin with the first patient seeking care at the ED. Critically ill patients may be approached using the traditional ABCs, and many physicians already use and teach a modified ATLS model for additional categories of critical medical conditions, especially those with acute onset and multi-organ system involvement, such as acute intoxications [6]. We propose an expanded "Primary Survey" that will trigger early anticipation and recognition of a biological mass casualty incident, without hampering the appropriate assessment and treatment of more conventional critical illness or injury. If such an incident is suspected, an expanded "Secondary Survey" guides early diagnosis, empiric treatment, and the institution of epidemic control measures.

Expanding the traditional Primary Survey

Most EHCPs are familiar with the traditional ATLS Primary Survey paradigm (Table 1). The fifth step in this paradigm, "E," refers to *Exposure* of the patient's body surface to search for occult injuries and to assess and mitigate any *Environmental* insult (eg, hypo- or hyperthermia). Our model proposes this simple adjunct: a third "E" for *Epidemiology*. This is further delineated using subcategories represented by three small "*e*"s: *exposure* history, an *epidemic* of patients, and *exotic* disease presentations. A careful exposure history might elicit the observation of a visible cloud at a mass gathering, the discovery of a delivery device, reports of an explosion, or other unusual occurrences. A thorough exposure history might also include information from law enforcement or intelligence agencies.

The EP might recognize an epidemic number of patients presenting with similar clinical syndromes. When evaluating a situation for the possibility of an as yet unrecognized epidemic, the threshold might vary with routine patient volume fluctuations for time of year and by type of clinical syndrome. With this in mind, certain characteristics of the larger than usual influx of patients might raise suspicions that a sinister or intentional event might have occurred. These might include a tight clustering of severely ill patients seeking care, especially if their illness was of acute onset, or a recognizable geographic commonality among the victims [7].

Exotic diseases might be suggested by any unusual clinical syndromes, particularly if fulminant disease progression occurred in otherwise healthy persons. Moreover, a preponderance of respiratory disease or a finding of diseases unusual for a given geographic region might provoke consideration of an intentional outbreak. The ECHP who keeps this third "E" in mind during routine, daily care of critical patients will be ready to anticipate the occurrence of a biological attack and can proceed to the more detailed Secondary Survey.

The expanded Secondary Survey

This represents an expansion of the traditional Secondary Survey, admittedly contrived to fit into a 10-step mnemonic (Table 2). We begin with a repetition of the A-B-C-D paradigm designed to reinforce the three basic principles (three "p"s) of prompt recognition, personal protection, and patient life support (Table 2, Steps 1–4), and then proceed to more specific diagnosis and early treatment. Although there are some redundancies with the Primary Survey, we believe this is acceptable considering the anticipated rarity of an EHCP facing an actual bioterrorist incident, and the need to keep the practitioner focused on optimal care of each patient.

Steps 1–4: prompt recognition, EHCP protection, and patient life support

The first step is *"A"—Anticipation.* The EHCP will already have some degree of suspicion regarding the possibility of a biological attack if he or she has headed down this pathway. Consideration of pertinent epidemiologic features [7], however, might help to convince EHCPs that the threat is real (even if not yet confirmed) and thus allow them to cross the psychologic threshold beyond routine practice mode and to "sound the alarm." An extraordinary number or acuity of patients might be the first clue. The epidemic might be further characterized by noting timing, place, and routes of exposure, and the particular clinical findings of the ill patients. The disease pattern typically observed after a natural infectious disease outbreak is that of a gradual increase in disease incidence. In contrast, victims of a biological attack would likely be exposed at the same time, and thus become ill and present in a compressed time frame. Diseases that are rare or not endemic to the given region would also obviously be suspect. A few additional clues to a bioterrorist incident would include an especially high infection rate among exposed persons, a higher incidence of respiratory forms of disease than usual, especially severe morbidity, several simultaneous epidemics, infected and dying animals, and of course the discovery of suspicious actions or delivery systems (eg, strangely-lettered envelopes contaminated with anthrax spores!).

Additional clues may be afforded by recognizing the characteristic features of advanced disease caused by the most feared biological agents. Several of these are sufficiently exotic and distinct as to have a limited differential diagnosis. Inhalational anthrax victims may develop fever, toxicity, severe respiratory distress, and a widened mediastinum on chest radiograph. Cutaneous anthrax begins as a papular lesion that progresses to vesicle then ulcer, and finally becomes a depressed black eschar with marked surrounding edema and limited tenderness. Botulism victims develop a characteristic descending, symmetric, flaccid paralysis, with intact sensation and mental status. Plague victims may exhibit fulminant pneumonia with hemoptysis, an uncommon finding in previously healthy young people. Smallpox presents initially with high fever, prostration, and a few days later with a unique exanthem. Unfortunately, by the time these hallmark findings develop, treatment is likely to be ineffective; therefore, it is desirable to make a diagnosis during the prodromal stage of illness, when signs and symptoms are much less specific in nature for many of the biological agent-induced diseases. This will prove difficult if not impossible for the index patient, but it is hoped that early recognition may benefit subsequent victims after just one or two such patients have declared themselves (Table 3). Moreover, many potential biological-agent diseases such as tularemia, brucellosis, Q-fever, and Venezuelan equine encephalitis (VEE) are likely to present simply as undifferentiated febrile illnesses, and may never progress further. Prompt diagnosis is possible only when EHCPs maintain a high index of suspicion based on the epidemiologic features of the outbreak as outlined in the discussion earlier.

The second step, *"B,"—Be Careful*—reminds EHCPs that they must protect themselves. Although full personal protective ensembles (Level C or greater) may be necessary when approaching certain chemical-agent victims, it should be kept in mind that most potential agents of bioterrorism are not contagious. Standard (formerly known as universal) precautions suffice for personal protection against most biological-agent diseases. Exceptions include smallpox, pneumonic plague, and, to a lesser degree, certain viral hemorrhagic fevers that require additional precautions detailed in the section on infection control. Prophylactic antibiotics are recommended for health care providers after close contact with pneumonic plague patients [8], and immediate vaccination would be indicated for smallpox exposure [9].

With self-protection accomplished, EHCPs should apply the third step: *C—"Continue the Primary Survey."* This requires continual reassessment

Table 3
Critical triggering events

Number[a]	Events or syndromes	Diseases
1	Critically ill patient with characteristic pustulovesicular rash	Smallpox
2–3	Weakness, bulbar palsy	Botulism
	Pneumonia, hemoptysis, rapid progression to death	Plague
	Respiratory symptoms (fever, severe dyspnea), pleural effusion, wide mediastinum	Anthrax
	Septic shock, fever, and purpuric rash	Plague, VHFs
	Encephalitis syndrome	VEE, JE, other (eg, WNV)
>3	Severe or bloody diarrhea	*C. perfringens*, Staphylococcal enterotoxin, *Salmonella*, *Shigella*

[a] Number of cases within a limited timeframe, such as 4–24 hours, or confirmed diagnoses of a specific disease that should trigger sufficient suspicion of a bioterrorist incident (or emerging infectious disease outbreak) to prompt notification of appropriate authorities and institution of protective measures. Epidemiologic considerations might increase (eg, known local outbreak) or decrease (recent travel, attendance at a political event) the number.

Abbreviations: VHFs, viral hemorrhagic fevers; VEE, Venezuelan equine encephalitis; JE, Japanese encephalitis; WNV, West Nile virus.

and intervention to optimize the patient's ABCs, in keeping with ATLS guidelines [4]. This step returns the EHCP's focus to the patient or patients who have aroused suspicion, to find and treat those conditions that present an immediate threat to life or limb. Biologic casualties may also have conventional injuries; therefore, attention should focus at this point on maintaining a patent airway and providing adequate support for breathing and circulation.

The fourth step (following patient stabilization) is D—Decontamination, if appropriate. Decontamination is rarely necessary after a biological attack, however. This is partly because of the inherent incubation periods of biologic agents. Because most victims will not become symptomatic until several days after exposure to an agent, they will likely have bathed and changed clothing (often several times) before presenting for medical care, thus effectively accomplishing "self-decontamination." Rare exceptions might include personnel near ground zero in an observed attack, where common sense might dictate topical disinfection. Even in these situations, bathing with soap and water and conventional laundry measures would likely be adequate, unless concomitant exposure to chemical agents were a concern [10].

At this point, the EHCP will have reconsidered the likelihood of a biologic attack and made a decision whether to initiate appropriate patient, ED, and possible hospital responses. Continuing life support has been provided, and personal protection and decontamination issues considered. Now it is time to proceed to the more specific aspects of the Secondary Survey.

Steps 5–10: diagnosis, treatment, and epidemic control

These more definitive diagnostic, treatment, and public health interventions will focus squarely on victims of a biological attack (Table 4, Steps 5–10). After decontamination, if warranted, the fifth step for the EHCP is to establish a diagnosis. This requires the usual components of a careful but focused history, thorough physical examination, and selected laboratory tests that are routinely available on a "stat" basis. In approaching the focused history, the ATLS "AMPLE" mnemonic (allergies, medications, past medical history/pregnancy, last meal and events/environmental issues) certainly applies to this group of patients also, especially if the *events* category is conceptualized as a focused history of the presenting medical illness. Even the "last meal" construct, intended as a pre-operative surgical consideration, might be expanded to include an inquiry into food and water exposures that could have been potentially targeted by a terrorist attack, resulting in an epidemic of gastrointestinal illness.

Several critical historical features (events) of the presenting illness may be sought, including acuity of disease onset and presence of a febrile prodrome; particular attention should be paid to respiratory, neurologic, or dermatologic symptoms. Most biological agent-induced diseases will have a sub-acute onset over several days from time of exposure, though this may vary. Most will also have a febrile prodrome, though this is not true of botulism, a toxin-mediated disease. Relevant physical examination findings include vital signs and a brief but focused evaluation of the cardiorespiratory, neurologic, and dermatologic status. Specific diagnostic tests might include a chest radiograph in patients with respiratory findings and a complete blood count or coagulation studies in patients manifesting purpura. For convenience, we note that most of the relevant bioagent–induced diseases can be characterized by a predominance of respiratory, neurologic, or dermatologic manifestations (Table 4).

Unfortunately, not all diseases caused by biological agents fit nicely into these three categories. For example, a disease such as viral equine encephalitis could present as an undifferentiated febrile illness or with central neurologic symptoms such as headache, meningismus, and encephalopathy. Many other diseases such as Q fever or brucellosis may lack a significant respiratory or neuromuscular component and present merely as undifferentiated febrile illnesses. Intentional food poisoning, which has already accounted for at least one notorious bioterrorism incident involving Salmonellosis [11], would likely manifest with epidemic numbers of victims with gastrointestinal illness (Table 3). Finally, many of the biological agents considered to have the potential for the most devastating population impact, such as

Table 4
Critical biological agent syndromes[a]

Organ-system specific	
Syndrome	Disease
Respiratory syndrome	
Fever, cough, chest pain, dyspnea, cyanosis	Anthrax, plague, tularemia, melioidosis
Neurologic syndrome	
Fever, encephalopathy, seizures, coma	Venezuelan encephalitis, Japanese encephalitis
Weakness, bulbar palsies, respiratory failure	Botulism
Cutaneous	
Pustulovesicular rash	Smallpox
Hemorrhagic rash	Viral hemorrhagic fevers

Febrile illness—undifferentiated: Suspect in patients especially when presenting in epidemic numbers, after earlier patients in community have been diagnosed or strongly suspected of having these diseases.

Syndrome	Disease
Non-specific febrile prodrome	Anthrax, plague, smallpox, tularemia, brucellosis, Q-fever, viral hemorrhagic fevers, melioidosis
Fever, fulminant progression to shock	Anthrax, plague, tularemia, viral hemorrhagic fevers

[a] Syndromes indicative of diseases that require urgent diagnosis, empiric antibiotic treatment or isolation, and vaccination considerations. Most have delayed onset from known exposure, prodromal phase with fever, and systemic symptoms.

anthrax, tularemia, plague, smallpox, and others, may present as undifferentiated febrile illnesses during their early, prodromal periods.

In many cases the use of a simple algorithm (Fig. 1) along with epidemiologic clues may allow the ECHP to establish a syndromic diagnosis of an advanced bioagent disease, before a specific diagnosis and definitive laboratory confirmation is possible. This could allow early administration of empiric antibiotic therapy for these recognized patients. In addition, in the context of one or two such "index" patients, a cluster of later-arriving casualties with undifferentiated febrile illnesses that do not conform to the categories outlined here may nonetheless require consideration of empiric antimicrobial therapy, particularly if an index patient with a more advanced clinical course has alerted the EHCP to the possibility of one of these diseases.

Although more definitive diagnosis at this point might be beyond the capabilities of a typical ED, especially in the case of biological diseases with nonspecific symptoms, appropriate specimens should nonetheless be collected and forwarded to a public health laboratory. The CDC has set up a laboratory network with four levels of capabilities designated Levels A through D. Level B laboratories capable of "ruling in" putative agents of biological terrorism are available at most state health departments [12]. Blood, sputum, nasal swabs, throat swabs, and urine samples might be obtained from representative patients and sent through hospital laboratory channels to these state health laboratories for analysis [13].

After establishing a syndromic diagnosis, the sixth step of management by the EHCP is to provide prompt therapy. Note that there is some redundancy in the agents assigned to the syndromic categories listed in Table 4. Although definitive diagnosis of clinical cases is of paramount importance in forming a prognosis and determining follow-up care, it is less important in the ED, where saving lives and evacuating casualties are the overwhelming medical concerns. Most of the treatable biological agent-induced diseases can be covered by the empiric administration of ciprofloxacin or doxycycline [14]. Two important exceptions are botulism, a toxin-induced disease, and smallpox, a viral infection, for which no licensed antiviral therapy is currently available. If a diagnosis of botulism is plausible, consideration should be given to the rapid procurement and administration of botulinum antitoxin, which may mitigate disease progression if administered early, and the provision of ventilatory assistance, if needed. If smallpox is suspected, patient isolation and vaccination of exposed persons must be instituted at the earliest possible time. For these scenarios, specialist consultation with the CDC (770-408-7100) or the US Army Medical Research Institute of Infectious Diseases (888-USA-RIID) would be warranted and would facilitate the rapid acquisition of botulinum antitoxin or smallpox vaccine.

As mentioned previously, one important potential group of patients might be the first wave of bioterrorism victims presenting with undifferentiated febrile illnesses. Such illnesses are ubiquitous and often the result of common viral infections and other endemic and epidemic infectious diseases. In most cases of bioagent-induced disease, success of therapy is contingent on its early initiation. The potentially lethal diseases in this category (eg, prodromal plague, anthrax, and tularemia) that require specific treatment are generally the same diseases that progress to delayed-onset respiratory syndromes. We therefore advocate similar therapy, namely the empiric administration of ciprofloxacin or doxycycline, to such patients once a treatable bioagent disease has been diagnosed or strongly suspected in the community. In select situations in which naturally occurring disease seems unlikely or in which a credible terrorism threat exists, such therapy may be life saving.

The seventh step is to ensure that contagious diseases do not spread to health care staff or other patients; therefore, the EHCP must institute proper infection control measures. Current guidelines [15] advocate the use of "standard precautions" in all patient-care encounters. More stringent "transmission-based precautions" are applied to patients with certain infectious diseases. Three subcategories of transmission-based precautions exist; one is appropriate for each of three potential biological warfare diseases [10,16].

Droplet precautions should be used when approaching the pneumonic plague victim, which includes wearing a surgical mask within three feet of a patient [8]. Contact and droplet precautions should be used for certain viral hemorrhagic fever patients. Elevation to higher protection levels may be required if patients have significant cough, vomiting, diarrhea, or profuse bleeding [17]. Airborne and contact precautions, ideally including a HEPA-filter mask and negative pressure isolation, should be used when approaching smallpox victims [9]. Anthrax, tularemia, brucellosis, Q-fever, the toxin-mediated diseases, the equine encephalitides, and most other diseases considered as potential biological terrorism agents may be safely managed by employing standard precautions.

The eighth step is to alert the proper authorities so that the appropriate warnings may be issued and outbreak control measures implemented. In most cases, this entails notifying local or state health department officials. Law-enforcement personnel must be involved also, because they will be important in traffic and crowd control, gathering of evidence, maintenance of a chain-of-custody, and the potential transport of victims.

Because successful bioterrorism attacks are man-made epidemics, public health officials are key to outbreak containment. The ninth step, therefore, is to prepare to assist in an epidemiologic investigation. EHCPs must have a working knowledge of basic epidemiology and of the proper sequence for conducting an outbreak investigation so they can assist their public health colleagues who will likely spearhead the investigation. This sequence of steps, the so-called "epidemiologic sequence," is detailed elsewhere [18], and includes the formulation of a case definition, determination of the number of cases and an approximate attack rate, followed by a careful description of the epidemic with regard to onset of illness, location of victims, illness characteristics, and comparison of demographic and clinical features of unaffected individuals with victims.

The tenth and final step for the EHCP is to "know and spread the gospel." Once trained, they must endeavor to remain proficient in the skills necessary to manage the consequences of a biological attack and must assist others in their departments and institutions in obtaining the requisite training.

Summary

We have purposely expanded on the well-known ATLS paradigm to aid EHCPs in their approach to a potential bioterrorism event. By building on a process that is already familiar, we hope this will aid the EHCP to remember a systematic approach to such an incident. By following this ten-step process, we believe that all EHCPs, and especially those practicing at the first echelons of care in urgent care clinics and EDs, can approach the daunting problem of biological defense with a good deal more confidence. This same model advocated for bioterrorism also may apply to natural infectious disease epidemics, particularly of emerging or re-emerging diseases, that might not be optimally managed by reliance on the conventional public health strategy that requires physician-dependent definitive diagnosis and active reporting mechanisms. The authors hope the acquired knowledge and skills one might gain will rarely be needed, but if the events surrounding the dispersal of anthrax-contaminated mail in the fall of 2001 are any indication of the future, such competencies will be invaluable.

References

[1] Centers for Disease Control and Prevention. Biological and chemical terrorism: strategic plan for preparedness and response. Morb Mortal Wkly Rep 2000;49(RR-4):1–14.

[2] Kortepeter MG, Parker GW. Potential biological weapons threats. Emerg Infect Dis 1999;5:523–7.

[3] Henderson DA. The looming threat of bioterrorism. Science 1999;283:1279–82.

[4] Committee on Trauma. American College of Surgeons. Initial assessment and management. In: Advanced trauma life support student manual. Chicago: American College of Surgeons; 1998. p. 9–46.

[5] Eitzen EM. Education is the key to defense against bioterrorism. Ann Emerg Med 1999;34:221–3.

[6] Henretig FM. Special considerations in the poisoned pediatric patient. Emerg Med Clin North Am 1994;12:549–67.

[7] Pavlin JA. Epidemiology of bioterrorism. Emerg Infect Dis 1999;5:528–30.

[8] Inglesby TV, Dennis DT, Henderson DA, et al. Plague as a biological weapon: medical and public health management [consensus statement]. JAMA 2000;283:2281–90.

[9] Henderson DA, Inglesby TV, Bartlett JG, et al. Smallpox as a biological weapon: medical and public health management [consensus statement]. JAMA 1999;281:2127–37.

[10] Keim M, Kaufmann AF. Principles for emergency response to bioterrorism. Ann Emerg Med 1999;34:177–82.

[11] Torok TJ, Tauxe RV, Wise RP, et al. A large community outbreak of Salmonellosis caused by intentional contamination of restaurant salad bars. JAMA 1997;278:389–95.

[12] Gilchrist MJR. A national laboratory network for bioterrorism: evolution from a prototype network of laboratories performing routine surveillance. Milit Med 2000;165 (Suppl 2):S28–31.

[13] US Army Medical Research Institute of Infectious Diseases. USAMRIID's medical management of biological casualties. 4th edition. Fort Detrick, MD: US Army Medical Research Institute of Infectious Diseases; 2001. Appendix F.

[14] Cieslak TJ, Rowe JR, Kortepeter MG, et al. A field-expedient algorithmic approach to the clinical management of chemical and biological casualties. Milit Med 2000;165:659–62.

[15] Garner JS. Guideline for infection control in hospitals: the hospital infection control practices advisory committee. Infect Control Hosp Epidemiol 1996;17:53–80.

[16] English JF, Cundiff MY, Malone JD, et al. Bioterrorism readiness plan: a template for healthcare facilities. Available at: http://www.apic.org/bioterror/. Accessed March 26, 2001.

[17] Centers for Disease Control and Prevention. Management of patients with suspected viral hemorrhagic fever. Morb Mortal Wkly Rep 1988;37(Suppl 3):S1–16.

[18] Centers for Disease Control and Prevention. Investigating an outbreak. In: Principles of epidemiology: self study course SS 3030. 2nd edition. Atlanta: Centers for Disease Control and Prevention; 1998. p. 347–424.

EMERGENCY
MEDICINE
CLINICS OF
Emerg Med Clin N Am   NORTH AMERICA
20 (2002) 365–392

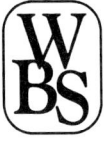

Medical management of vulnerable populations and co-morbid conditions of victims of bioterrorism

Suzanne R. White, MD, FACEP[a],*,
Fred M. Henretig, MD, FACEP[b],
Richard G. Dukes, MD[c]

[a]Children's Hospital of Michigan Regional Poison Control Center,
4160 John R Suite 616, Detroit, MI 48201, USA
[b]Department of Pediatrics and Emergency Medicine, Children's Hospital of Philadelphia,
34th and Civic Center Blvd., Philadelphia, PA 19104, USA
[c]Wayne State University School of Medicine and Detroit Medical Center,
Department of Emergency Medicine, 4201 St. Antoine, Detroit, MI 48201, USA

Medical planning for bioterrorism primarily focuses on the needs of the military or population as a whole. There has been little discussion pertaining to certain vulnerable groups such as children, pregnant women, or immuno-compromised patients, who are likely to comprise a subset of the exposed population. Take the unthinkable scenario involving a major bioterrorism release near a nursery, preschool, nursing home, or even a hospital, in which affected individuals, at higher risk for complications, may pose unique challenges. Identification of these groups is crucial so that specialized care can be arranged. The following discussion focuses primarily on three uniquely susceptible populations: pregnant women, children, and immunocompromised patients, in the context of those bioagents most likely to be used.

Pregnancy

Overview

Susceptibility to infections in pregnancy is altered. Hormonal, biochemical, cellular, and humoral changes suppress the maternal immune response to the fetus [1]. Progesterone-mediated smooth muscle relaxation of the

---

* Corresponding author.
E-mail address: swhite1@dmc.org (S.R. White).

respiratory tract results in stasis of secretions and increased local bacterial growth. High circulating levels of steroids inhibit humoral responses. Despite increased numbers of circulating white blood cells, neutrophil chemotaxis and adherence, cell-mediated immunity, and natural killer cell activity are all decreased. These processes markedly depress defense mechanisms, resulting in a more susceptible host. These factors along with concerns for fetal safety will undoubtedly create clinical challenges.

Variola virus (smallpox)

The possible re-emergence of smallpox as the result of a deliberate release has been raised with the recent discovery of Russia's extensive bioweapons program [2]. Historically, three forms of illness existed: *variola major*, or classic epidemic smallpox, *variola minor*, or alastrim, a much milder form of the disease that was often sporadic, and *varioloid* that occurred in partially immune subjects [3].

After viral entry into the respiratory tract, local multiplication is followed by spread to regional lymph nodes. Viremic phases during the 12-day incubation period occur with the prodromal phase and with onset of eruptions. Variola crosses the placenta and infection of the fetus may occur during either of these viremic stages [4]. Increased susceptibility to variola infection and greater severity of illness are documented during pregnancy [5]. Maternal mortality is approximately 50%, compared with 30% in men and nonpregnant women [3,6,7]. High rates of fetal loss are associated with first trimester variola major, and increased rates of prematurity are described with illness during the latter half of pregnancy [8–10]. Most terminations occur during the pre-eruptive and early eruptive stages [10]. These observations are not consistently noted, because none of four pregnant women in one epidemic miscarried [4] and only two spontaneous abortions occurred during a variola minor outbreak involving hundreds of pregnant women [11]. It is likely that the virulence of the involved strain plays a role in explaining these disparate findings.

Maternal smallpox infection

Pregnant women are more susceptible to hemorrhagic smallpox (purpura variolosa), characterized by fever, backache, a diffuse, coppery-red rash, and rapid decline. The illness classically occurs in unvaccinated or remotely vaccinated individuals, although recent vaccination does not confer full protection [10]. An association with pregnancy was first described by Rao, who noted that 72% of patients with purpura variolosa were female, and of those of childbearing age, 51% were pregnant. Others have corroborated this link [12,13]. Mehta described three patients with fever, backache, abdominal pain, and symptoms of threatened abortion [12]. Within 24 hours of symptom onset, spontaneous ecchymoses, epistaxis, bleeding gums, an intense, erythematous rash, and subconjunctival hemorrhages were noted. Two patients developed vaginal or gastrointestinal bleeding, and all died within 48 hours. Larger series provided similar descriptions and have confirmed the uniform fatality of this form of smallpox [7,10]. Death generally results from a toxic (septic) state. Hematologic derangements in this setting include thrombocytopenia, increased capillary fragility, and depletion of coagulation factors and fibrinogen [12,13].

Fetal smallpox infection

The incidence of congenital variola varied from 9%–60% of deliveries during epidemics [10,11]. Congenital variola is characterized by giant dermal pox and diffuse necrotic lesions of the viscera and placenta [8,14]. Observations from a 1956 Brazil variola minor epidemic illustrate the unpredictable nature of transmission to the fetus [4]. One unvaccinated woman delivered a term infant 13 days later, who manifested prodromal symptoms and then a typical eruption at 6 days of age. The timing of illness was consistent with in utero exposure to variola at the onset of the maternal eruptive phase. Another unvaccinated woman delivered a child 4 days before the onset of variola minor. Sixteen days after delivery, variola occurred in the newborn, consistent with extra-uterine transmission. A third unvaccinated woman acquired variola during the fifth month of pregnancy and delivered a dead fetus at term. In a fourth case, a healthy term infant was delivered 56 days following maternal infection. Despite latter stage exposure and living with other household members with variola, several infants escaped illness. They were born to mothers with a history of (1) childhood smallpox, (2) vaccination within five years, or (3) a mother (infant's grandmother) with variola during the latter stages of pregnancy during a previous epidemic. This suggests maternal immunity may confer some fetal protection. Despite heavy, persistent viremia during hemorrhagic smallpox, none of 21 children born to 84 infected women developed congenital smallpox [10].

In another outbreak, 22 of 36 infants born to women who contracted variola minor late in pregnancy acquired disease. The unaffected infants were born before the mother's illness or at least one week after the onset of maternal rash [3,11]. Delivery of newborns with smallpox to mothers without clinical manifestations is also reported [15], demonstrating the unpredictable nature of transmission. Aside from one report of congenital cataract [16], there is no evidence for teratogenicity of the variola virus.

Vaccination

Treatment of smallpox is primarily supportive. There are currently no approved, effective chemotherapeutics [2]. This has historically rendered preventive and post-exposure smallpox vaccination programs critical to the containment of outbreaks and eradication of the disease.

Depressed immunity during pregnancy creates a dilemma—protection of a more susceptible host versus increased vaccination risk in the setting of an altered immune system. The licensed US smallpox vaccine is a live-virus preparation derived from a related Orthopoxvirus, vaccinia. Live virus vaccination during pregnancy has generally been avoided because of concerns regarding maternal infection and fetal safety.

Maternal complications of smallpox vaccination

Uncomplicated primary vaccinia follows successful vaccination. A vesicle appears within 2–5 days, matures through a pustular phase, crusts, and heals within 3 weeks. Fever and regional adenopathy are common during the first week. Antibodies appear 7–10 days after inoculation and peak at week three. Samples from 422 pregnant smallpox re-vaccinees showed titer development similar to that of nonpregnant patients [17]. Humoral and cell-mediated immunity play roles in containing the primary infection and in limiting post-vaccination complications.

Complications occur in 0.13% of primary and 0.01% of re-vaccinated individuals [18]. Maximal viral shedding from the site occurs 4–14 days post-vaccination and inoculation of other body sites (vaccinia autoinoculata) accounts for half of the complications (530 cases per million vaccinations) [18,19]. Autoinoculation sites include the face, eyelid, nose, mouth, genitalia, and rectum. A re-vaccinee with vaccinia autoinoculata of the eye and genitalia during the fifth month of pregnancy gave birth to a healthy child five weeks later [20]. A woman developed vaccinia blepharoconjunctivitis with unspecified fetal outcome [21]. A recent case of vaccinia autoinoculata during pregnancy resulted from dermal exposure to a recombinant vaccinia-rabies vaccine bait intended for wild animals. The patient delivered a term, healthy child [22].

The most severe vaccination complications are encephalitis and vaccinia necrosum, occurring in 12.3 and 1.5 cases per million primary vaccinees, respectively. Vaccinia necrosum involves extensive necrosis of the vaccination site, often spreading to secondary areas. It occurs primarily in immunocompromised patients. Moderate complications include generalized vaccinia (241.5 cases per million) and eczema vaccinatum. Generalized vaccinia is a vesicular eruption occurring in the first or second week after vaccination and is self-limited in the immunocompetent individual. Eczema vaccinatum occurs in those with a history of eczema or other exfoliative skin conditions and may involve localized or systemic dissemination [19]. Children with eczema are at greatest risk and may acquire this simply from contact with a recently vaccinated household member [3]. Other rare complications include urticaria, Stevens-Johnson syndrome, bacterial superinfection, malignancy at the scar site, and monoarticular arthritis.

Maternal complications from immunization have not been well delineated. Of 101 women vaccinated during the first trimester during the 1972 Yugoslavia smallpox outbreak, one primary vaccinee developed encephalitis, and one primary and seven re-vaccinees experienced significant infections with fever, local swelling, and lymphadenopathy. In an evaluation of 257 first trimester vaccinees, no reactions were reported [23]. The only potential treatment for vaccine complications is vaccinia immune globulin (VIG), effective for eczema vaccinatum, progressive vaccinia, and possibly ocular autoinoculation. VIG supply is extremely limited, the Center for Disease Control and Prevention (CDC) being the only source for civilians. The risks associated with VIG use in pregnancy are unknown, although similar products are Federal Drug Administration (FDA) Pregnancy Category B drugs (see Table 1).

Fetal complications of smallpox vaccination

Viremia may occur with primary vaccination and re-vaccination [24]. Early attempts to isolate vaccinia virus from placentae of vaccinated pregnant women yielded negative or equivocal results [17,25,26]. Subsequent animal and human investigations, however, demonstrated viral seeding of the placenta with transmission to the fetus [17]. In the largest clinical study, vaccinia virus was isolated in 3.2% of the products of conception in 366 women undergoing abortion after recent re-vaccination [24]. Trophoblasts are able to fully support the replicative cycle of the vaccinia virus and, in doing so, undergo cytopathic changes [27]. The virus persists in placental tissues for more than 30 days and causes premature placental senescence. Pathologic changes include abnormal vascularization of villi, diffuse interstitial hemorrhage, inflammatory response, calcifications, and total or partial moles [17,28]. Whether these changes translate to an increased rate of spontaneous abortion, prematurity, or low birth weight following vaccination has been debated. A higher incidence of fetal loss occurred in vaccinated women compared with unvaccinated controls (47% versus 13%) during the Glasgow outbreak of 1950 [29]. Higher rates of spontaneous abortion, low birth weight, and prematurity have been associated with mass vaccination during other outbreaks [17,25,30]. Nevertheless, it seems that the absence

Table 1
Risk categories of antimicrobials in pregnancy

Drug	FDA pregnancy risk category
Aminoglycosides	
Gentamicin, streptomycin	D
Beta lactams	
Penicillins	B
Chloramphenicol	—
Cidofovir	C
Fluoroquinolones	
Ciprofloxacin, ofloxacin, Levofloxacin, moxifloxacin	C
Tetracycline, doxycycline	D
Ribavirin	X

Abbreviations: A, studies in pregnant women show no risk; B, animal studies show no risk but human studies are not adequate or animal toxicity has been shown but human studies show no risk; C, animal studies show toxicity, human studies are inadequate but benefit of use may exceed risk; D, evidence of human risk but benefits may outweigh risks; X, fetal abnormalities in humans, risk outweights benefit.

of detrimental effects of smallpox vaccination on pregnancy outcome is more frequently reported [31–35].

Fetal vaccinia. Fetal vaccinia, a rarely reported complication, is characterized by placental infection, viral dissemination to most fetal organs, and giant pox skin lesions. The first description in 1932 involved a six-month fetus born with large, generalized skin lesions four weeks after maternal vaccination. Approximately 50 other cases have been described [5,18,19,36–40]. Most followed primary vaccination or re-vaccination after a 20-year hiatus, and occurred during second trimester. Of concern are reports of unvaccinated, asymptomatic mothers who delivered infants with vaccinia, presumably contracted from contact with recent vaccinees [41,42]. If mass vaccination programs are implemented in response to bioterrorism, pregnant women must be cautioned against close contact with those recently vaccinated.

The risk for congenital defects caused by maternal vaccination has affected public health decisions. In one outbreak, vaccination was considered grounds for abortion and was contraindicated during pregnancy [5]. Although there are a few reports of associated congenital abnormalities [23,43–45], several studies, including a cumulative review of 8599 vaccinees and 11,104 control subjects, found no evidence of increased rates of malformations, and no cases of fetal vaccinia in the setting of vaccination beyond the twelfth week of pregnancy [5,46]. Vaccination during pregnancy is not considered an indication for therapeutic abortion.

In summary, sporadic reports of fetal vaccinia and limited evidence of increased rates of premature delivery and spontaneous abortion following smallpox vaccination exist, and suggest that the live vaccine should not routinely be administered to pregnant women. Recommendations do promote vaccination of pregnant women during a bioterrorism incident if there has been a definite exposure to the virus (ie, face-to-face, household, or close-proximity contact with a smallpox patient) [19]. Some authorities suggest the simultaneous administration of VIG to prevent maternal complications and to protect the fetus. Although this approach may be considered for primary vaccinees or those not vaccinated within the past three years, others probably don't require VIG and its use could be reserved for higher-risk patients [2,5,47]. Clinical evidence for "prophylactic" VIG administration to pregnant women is lacking.

Yersinia pestis *(plague)*

Clinical features

Yersinia pestis, the bacteria that causes plague, spreads in nature from infected fleas to humans. Despite the occurrence of four major historical pandemics, little is documented regarding the medical aspects of plague acquired during pregnancy.

Fetal wastage attributed to *Yersinia pestis* infection has been proposed to result from severe maternal systemic infection and placental transmission of the agent to the fetus [48,49]. Early descriptions of plague acquired during pregnancy from the pre-antibiotic era reported universal fetal loss [50]. Paré chronicled that one could predict the onset of plague in a region by an increasing number of abortions and stillbirths. Boghurst observed that the illness was especially severe in pregnant women [51]. Early World Health Organization (WHO) reports summarized that "serious attacks of plague in any form usually lead to abortion or miscarriage in pregnant patients, events which exert a most unfavorable influence on the outcome of the illness" (48). During one epidemic, 13 of 14 pregnancies ended in spontaneous abortion or stillbirth. There were only four maternal survivors. The only live neonate, who appeared well at birth, died the next day [50].

More favorable outcomes are found in post-antibiotic era reports, albeit all cases were bubonic. In one instance, bubonic plague occurred during the fifth month of pregnancy [48]. Clinical course was characterized by high fever, leukocytosis, thrombocytopenia, elevated fibrin split products, and an inguinal bubo. Treatment included streptomycin for five days with delivery of a normal neonate. Another case acquired near term was complicated by fever, fetal tachycardia, inguinal buboes, and leukocytosis. Treatment included gentamicin and ampicillin. A healthy child, delivered within 24 hours of presentation, was treated empirically with the same medications [52]. Another second trimester patient exhibited fever, vomiting, prostration, pyuria, and inguinal buboes. After treatment with tetracycline and streptomycin, recovery was uneventful and the infant was not affected [51]. A fourth case, acquired near term, involved fever, lymphadenopathy, and fetal tachycardia Labor was induced and maternal treatment was initiated with streptomycin. The normal infant was treated empirically with streptomycin. Cord blood cultures were negative and the infant did not mount an antibody response. The post-partum course was complicated by disseminated intravascular coagulation. Chloramphenicol and tetracycline were added, and complete maternal recovery occurred [53].

Treatment

Maternal and fetal outcomes associated with modern chemotherapy of bubonic plague are favorable. The major determinant of maternal/fetal outcome is the time to administration of antibiotics. Because the fetus may be exposed to *Yersinia pestis* in utero or through contact with maternal blood during delivery, empiric antibiotic treatment of the newborn should be considered [53]. A killed bacilli *Yersinia pestis* vaccine was discontinued in 1999. It did not prevent or ameliorate primary pneumonic plague.

Recent recommendations for treatment of and prophylaxis against pneumonic plague in pregnancy are based on clinical and evidence-based criteria and do not necessarily correspond to the FDA approved indications [54]. Traditionally avoided in pregnancy, gentamicin is the most efficacious treatment for pregnant patients with pneumonic plague. The recommended dose is 5 mg/kg IM or IV once daily or a 2 mg/kg loading dose followed by 1.7 mg/kg IM or IV three times daily. Alternatives include doxycycline (100 mg twice daily or 200 mg once daily IV) or ciprofloxacin (400 mg IV twice daily) for 10 days. Other fluoroquinolones may be substituted. Conversion to oral therapy depends on clinical status. Chloramphenicol is the treatment of choice for plague meningitis (see Table 2).

Although the tetracycline class of antibiotics has been associated with fetal dental enamel hypoplasia and retarded skeletal growth, extensive use of doxycycline in pregnancy has not demonstrated an increased risk for these or other teratogenic effects. Liver toxicity during pregnancy has been reported, so it is prudent to monitor hepatic transaminases. The marrow toxicity of chloramphenicol is not believed to be enhanced by pregnancy. Although streptomycin appeared to be efficacious in three of the four cases of bubonic plague described above, it has limited availability, and its rare association with vestibular and cochlear toxicity and irreversible deafness in children following maternal administration makes it a second-line agent [54].

Following a bioterrorist attack, prophylaxis of exposed pregnant patients would need to be considered. The preferred agent is doxycycline 100 mg orally twice daily. Tetracycline may be substituted, with consideration of the risks outlined above. Alternatives include ciprofloxacin 500 mg orally twice daily or chloramphenicol 25 mg/kg orally four times daily (this latter formulation is not available in the United States). Sulfonamides such as TMP/SMX are inferior to the previously mentioned antibiotics and are not recommended.

Breastfeeding

Consensus recommendations promote the provision of a single antibiotic to mother and infant based on the most appropriate agent for the infant. Gentamicin is recommended for treatment of plague in breast-feeding mothers. Doxycycline or a fluoroquinolone are advocated for prophylaxis [54].

Bacillus anthracis (anthrax)

Clinical features of illness

A detailed discussion of the manifestations of anthrax can be found elsewhere in this monograph. Anthrax in pregnancy has not been studied.

Treatment

No clinical trials have assessed treatment of inhalational anthrax in humans. Treatment during an outbreak of inhalational anthrax in the former Soviet Union in 1979 entailed use of antibiotics, vaccination, antianthrax immunoglobulin, corticosteroids, and ventilatory support. Still, 68 of 79 patients died. Neither the relative efficacy of these therapies nor the strain susceptibility to the antibiotics used is known [29].

Table 2
Initial antibiotic therapy for principal bacterial agents of bioterrorism in pregnant or breast-feeding patients[a]

Contained casualty setting Agent	Pregnant Antibiotics	Dose and route	Breastfeeding Antibiotic
Anthrax inhalational, oropharyngeal, or GI)	Ciprofloxacin or Doxycycline plus one or two additional antibiotics[b]	400 mg IV q 12 h 100 mg IV q 12 h	Same
Cutaneous[c]	Ciprofloxin or Doxycycline multiple drug IV therapy indicated for those with systemic involvement, extensive edema, or head and neck lesions	500 mg PO bid 100 mg PO q 12 h	
Plague	Gentamicin or Doxycycline Ciprofloxacin	5 mg/kg IM or IV q 24 h or 2 mg/kg loading dose IV then 1.7 mg/kg q 8 h 100 mg IV q 12 h or 200 mg IV q 24 h 400 mg IV q 12 h (other fluoroquinolones may be substituted)	Gentamicin
	Chloramphenicol is treatment of choice for meningitis		
Tularemia	Gentamicin or Streptomycin or Doxycycline or Ciprofloxacin	5 mg/kg IM or IV q 24 h 1 g IM bid 100 mg IV q 12 h 400 mg IV q 12 h	Gentamicin

Mass casualty setting or Prophylaxis Agent	Pregnant Antibiotics	Dose and route	Breastfeeding Antibiotic
Anthrax	Ciprofloxacin If strain is susceptible Doxycycline or Amoxicillin	500 mg PO q 12 h (ofloxacin 400 mg every 12 h or levofloxacin 500 mg q 24 h may be considered) 100 mg PO q 12 h 500 mg PO bid	Ciprofloxacin Doxycycline or Amoxicillin
Plague	Doxycycline or Ciprofloxacin	100 mg PO bid (tetracycline can be substituted if doxycycline is not available) 500 mg PO bid	Doxycycline or Fluoroquinolone

(continued on next page)

Table 2 (continued)

Mass casualty setting or Prophylaxis	Pregnant		Breastfeeding
Agent	Antibiotics	Dose and route	Antibiotic
Tularemia	Ciprofloxacin or Doxycycline	500 mg PO bid 100 mg PO bid	Ciprofloxacin

[a] Compiled and adapted from references 54,55,62.

[b] Such as rifampin, vancomycin, penicillin, ampicillin, chloramphenical, imipenum, clindomycin, or clarithromycin.

[c] Amoxicillin is an option for completion of therapy following clinical improvement and once strain sensitivities are known.

Early antibiotic administration is likely to be the most important determinant of maternal-fetal outcome. Recommendations for treatment and prophylaxis in pregnancy are based on clinical and evidence-based criteria and do not necessarily correspond with FDA drug indications [55]. Preferred antibiotic treatment of pregnant patients with suspected inhalational, otolaryngeal, or GI anthrax is ciprofloxacin 400 mg IV q 12° or doxycycline 100 mg IV q 12° and one or two other antimicrobials (see Table 2). Fluoroquinolones are not recommended during pregnancy, based on a rare association with arthropathy in children, but the risk for infection with an engineered strain resistant to penicillin is high. Because of concerns for inducible Beta lactamases penicillin and ampicillin should not be used alone. If meningitis is suspected, doxycycline is less optimal based on poor CNS penetration, and steroids may be considered as an adjunct to antibiotic therapy. Duration of therapy is 60 days, with oral therapy replacing parenteral as soon as clinical improvement is noted. Preferred antibiotic treatment of the pregnant patient with suspected cutaneous anthrax is ciprofloxacin or doxycycline 100 mg PO bid. 500 mg po bid. (Multiple drug IV therapy is indicated for those with systemic symptoms, extensive edema, or head and neck lesions). Oral amoxicillin in an option for completion of therapy following clinical improvement and once strain sensitivities are know. The duration of therapy is 60 days if the risk of simultaneous aerosol exposure is high.

As discussed in the section on treatment for plague, similar precautions exist concerning use of tetracycline-like drugs in pregnancy. Because antibiotics are not effective against the spore form of B. anthracis, inhaled spores may reside in tissues for prolonged periods. Thus, post-exposure vaccination with Anthrax Vaccine Adsorbed (AVA), the only licensed human anthrax vaccine, is advised [55]. The vaccine has been used widely among military personnel. It is safe and is extremely effective in animal studies, providing protection against high-dose aerosol exposures to virulent anthrax strains. AVA use in pregnancy has not been studied. Accordingly, current vaccination recommendations are somewhat vague [56]. Currently, vaccine supplies are scarce, but if available, potential benefits would likely outweigh potential risks of this inactivated, cell-free product.

Pregnant women with significant inhalational exposure to anthrax spores should be given post-exposure prophylaxis with oral ciprofloxacin 500 mg every 12 hours or doxycycline 100 mg twice daily for 60 days. (In vitro studies also suggest that alternative quinolones such as ofloxacin 400 mg every 12 hours or levofloxacin 500 mg every 24 hours could be substituted orally.) If strain susceptibility testing is favorable, amoxicillin 500 mg by mouth every 8 hours should replace ciprofloxacin [55].

Breast-feeding women should be offered prophylaxis with an antibiotic that is safe and effective for the infant. Recommendations suggest that ciprofloxacin or doxycycline is appropriate in this setting [55]. Both ciprofloxacin and doxycycline are compatible with breast feeding because the amount absorbed by infants is small, but safety with long-term use is not known. Amoxicillin is an option once strain sensitivities are known. Alternatively, breast milk can be pumped and discarded with resuming of breast feeding upon completion of drug therapy. Killed vaccine administration is not medically contraindicated during breast-feeding, and no data suggest increased side effects in breast-feeding women or breast-fed children following administration of AVA [56].

Clostridium botulinum (botulism)

Clinical features

Botulinum toxin, the most potent toxin known, is considered to be a significant bioterrorism threat. A detailed discussion can be found elsewhere in this article.

Botulism during pregnancy is rare, but a few cases deserve mention. In the first instance, third trimester illness was associated with placental abruption, but no evidence of botulism in the infant [57]. In another report, the newborn of a heroin abuser with third trimester wound botulism required several weeks of intensive care after cesarean section delivery at 34 weeks. Details on the infant's course are lacking [58]. More recently, second trimester severe maternal botulism was not associated with ill effects in the fetus [59]. Finally, a full-term, normal fetus was delivered to a woman who acquired severe food-borne botulism during the second trimester [60]. One could speculate that the large 150,000-dalton botulinum toxin would not likely cross the placenta, but too few cases have been reported to fully assess this possibility.

Treatment

Treatment is primarily directed at providing respiratory support. Available antitoxin neutralizes the botulinum toxin. Administration shortens the course of illness and decreases mortality, but probably does not improve existing neurologic symptoms. Any benefit of antitoxin administration after 72 hours from time of exposure is minimal in patients without a declining neurologic status. The CDC licensed antitoxin is a trivalent equine IgG product with attendant risks of anaphylaxis and serum sickness on administration. The USAMRIID product is a heptavalent (effective against toxin types A through G) FAB-fragment with a theoretically lower risk. It is only available for use under an IND protocol, however. The trivalent antitoxin is FDA Pregnancy Category C. Supplies of antitoxin are extremely limited.

Francisella tularensis (tularemia)

Clinical features

Tularemia is a zoonotic illness that most commonly manifests as an ulceroglandular form in humans exposed to diseased animal fluids or bites from infected deerflies, mosquitoes, or ticks. A complete discussion of the clinical manifestations of this illness can be found elsewhere in this article. Tularemia in pregnancy is rare, with the latest case described in 1936 [61].

Treatment

Recommendations for treatment are based on consensus guidelines and not necessarily on FDA recommendations [62]. First-line options include either gentamicin 5 mg/kg once daily or streptomycin 1 g IM twice daily. Alternatives include doxycycline 100 mg IV twice daily or ciprofloxacin 400 mg IV twice daily. Treatment duration is 10 days for streptomycin, gentamicin, or ciprofloxacin, and 14–21 days for doxycycline. Conversion to oral therapy is guided by the patient's clinical status.

Post-exposure prophylaxis for pregnant women is advised. The antibiotics of choice are ciprofloxacin 500 mg orally twice daily or doxycycline 100 mg twice daily for 14 days.

Immunity following tularemia infection is permanent. Person-to-person transmission does not occur, and respiratory isolation is not required. A live, attenuated vaccine has been used in laboratory personnel working with *Francisella tularensis*. Its safety in pregnancy has not been established, however [63], and it has not been universally effective in protecting against inhalational tularemia. Vaccination is not recommended for post-exposure prophylaxis or as part of management of infection [62].

Filoviruses

Ebola

RNA viruses such as Ebola and Marburg are highly infectious by the aerosol route, are associated with high mortality rates, and are easily grown in cell culture. These characteristics make them obvious bioterrorism threats. A detailed discussion of these agents can be found elsewhere in this article.

Illness from Ebola is generally more severe in pregnant women, with more serious hemorrhagic and neurologic complications than in nonpregnant patients [64,111]. The case fatality rate of pregnant women with Ebola Hemorrhagic Fever (EHF) was 95.5% versus 77% in nonpregnant infected persons in one study. The mortality of pregnant women with EHF seems to be equal in all trimesters.

Spontaneous abortion is frequent, with fetal losses reported to be as high as 23%–66% [65,66]. In one outbreak, pregnant women became iatrogenically infected after receiving vitamin injections with contaminated needles and syringes. During this outbreak, factors believed to contribute to the high rate of fetal wastage included pyrexia, intravascular coagulopathy, and infection of the fetus. All infants born to mothers with EHF ultimately died within 19 days of delivery. Whether they became infected during pregnancy or delivery, by breast-feeding, or through contact with other body fluids after delivery is not known [65].

Treatment of EHF in pregnancy involves supportive care and blood product replacement. Neither antiviral agents nor convalescent sera are reported to be effective.

Arena viruses

Lassa fever

The causative agent of Lassa Fever is an RNA virus of the arenavirus group. Illness is transmitted by way of contact with rodent excreta or through person-to-person body-fluid exposure. Early symptoms are nonspecific and include fever, malaise, exudative pharyngitis, conjunctivitis, lymphadenopathy, and rash. Hepatitis is universally seen and prostration out of proportion to pyrexia is characteristic. Late findings include pleural effusions, cardiac and renal failure, encephalopathy, and hemorrhage.

The first reported case of Lassa Fever occurred during pregnancy. Ultimately, 11 residents and workers on the index patient's obstetrics ward died. Lassa Fever now accounts for 25% of maternal deaths in Sierra Leone, a country that has reported vast experiences from many large outbreaks. The case fatality rate among pregnant women varies from 30%–75% as compared with 1%–36% in nonpregnant victims [67,68]. Women in the last trimester of pregnancy have the highest fatality rate.

Clinical trials suggest ribavirin treatment is associated with a decreased case fatality rate as compared with treatment with convalescent serum [67]. It is effective at any point in the illness, but is most beneficial when given early. It has typically been withheld from pregnant women based on concerns of teratogenicity. It is an FDA Pregnancy Risk Category X [69]. Decisions to treat pregnant women with convalescent serum have typically been made based on the degree of SGOT elevation. Risk for death is greatest during the third trimester (odds ratio 5.57). One study found that evacuation of the uterus, regardless of method, or by normal delivery, improved the mother's chance of survival [70].

Children

Overview

> Ring around the rosy,
> A pocket full of posies,
> Ashes, ashes
> We all fall down...

This popular nursery rhyme is believed to date back to The Great Plague of the fourteenth to sixteenth centuries [71]. The verses might depict a child's take on the plague epidemic of that era: the "rosy ring" representing the erythematous band of cervical lymphadenopathy common to plague victims; the posies, presumably sweet-smelling flowers carried to disguise the stench of necrotic tissues; and ashes the ultimate outcome of cremation after death.

Since the anthrax incidents in Florida, Washington DC, and New York City after September 11, 2001, the possibility of pediatric victims of bioterrorism seems more real than ever. Children and bioterrorism—the notion is more heinous than can be imagined. Yet, terrorists have the capacity to consider this "unthinkable" crime. Timothy McVeigh viewed children killed in the bombing of the Murrah Federal Building as "collateral damage." A 1995 plot to release chlorine gas in the Disneyland amusement park was averted by the Federal Bureau of Investigation (FBI) [72]. These examples indicate that motivated terrorists may not alter plans to avoid hurting children, and some groups might target young children to maximize public outcry and horror. An aerosol attack with infectious agents would affect children and adults. For communicable agents, the fallout to children would be inevitable, even if they were not initially targeted [110].

Special pediatric vulnerabilities

Few of the most threatening infectious or toxin-mediated diseases under consideration are common in the Western world, and experience with them in children is particularly rare, with the possible exception of infantile botulism. Virtually no experience exists in the bioterrorism context, with the exception of the children infected with Salmonella in the 1984 incident of intentional contamination of salad bars in The Dalles, Oregon [73] and the one child infected with anthrax in October 2001 [73a]. Thus, a lot of what we posit here is speculative, but we can delineate some general issues that might be relevant in the pediatric context of a bioterrorist incident.

Some physiologic differences between children and adults bear comment. Children have higher minute ventilation rates and live "closer to the ground" than do adults [72,74]. Thus, an increased exposure to many aerosol particles might ensue. Children have thinner and more permeable skin than adults that could enhance susceptibility to many chemical warfare agents, and one agent class, the tricothecene mycotoxins, is believed to be dermally active even on intact skin. Children, with their large body surface area, lose heat quickly and become hypothermic more readily, a factor to consider during gross decontamination. Immunologic immaturity or a more permeable blood–brain barrier might increase susceptibility to, or worsen prognosis for, several diseases, though this is not clear for most. It is clear, however, that several of the recommended antibiotics and other chemotherapeutic agents are not approved for use in children and may have relative contraindications to their use in this population. Finally, vomiting and diarrhea may complicate biowarfare agent-induced diseases, and the smaller fluid reserves in children would predispose them to a more fulminant course of dehydration and potentially to shock.

A second area of distinction is that of developmental and psychologic vulnerability. Infants and young children cannot escape or evade an attack, nor would they likely be able to understand the danger. The usual guardians against these developmental vulnerabilities—the child's parents—may be dead or incapacitated and thus unable to effect this role. The child who witnesses death or severe illness may be less able to cope, and be more at risk subsequently for post-traumatic stress disorders.

Finally, the health care system response to children is unique, and might be further compromised by such an incident. Our Emergency Medical Services systems and emergency departments are often stressed when faced with critically ill infants and children. Experience with and availability of pediatric resuscitation drug doses and equipment and pediatric procedural skills are often less "fine-tuned" than for the critically ill adult. A demand to demonstrate cognitive and procedural skills on numerous children during a mass casualty incident or while garbed in protective gear would stress systems further. Many urban hospitals usually transport critical pediatric patients expeditiously to regional children's hospitals. This would likely disappear in a mass casualty incident, and those hospitals would have to provide resuscitative and definitive care for large numbers of children. Children's hospitals or pediatric services at the regional medical centers would be inundated by patients seeking care, and by frantic calls from neighboring hospitals. Finally, the National Disaster Medical System, a federal plan to expand hospital bed capacity in response to a catastrophic event, does not include provisions for increased pediatric beds.

Specific pediatric considerations in the primary bioagent diseases

The clinical manifestations of the primary bioweapon diseases are similar in children and adults. Because of their importance as potential weapons, a few specific comments are offered here regarding anthrax, plague, smallpox, and botulism in children.

Bacillus anthracis *(anthrax)*

All forms of anthrax may occur in children, though cutaneous infection accounts for 90% [75,76,110]. In the past decade, several pediatric cases were reported from the Middle East and France. In most reports, the source was ingestion of contaminated meat. There were no pediatric cases reported from the anthrax release in Sverdlosk in 1979 [29,74]. Whether this represented some relative resistance in comparison with adults, or more likely, decreased exposure, is unknown. Most recently, one child developed cutaneous anthrax during the October–November 2001 outbreak in the United States related to anthrax-spore contaminated mail (90a).

In 1993, two cases of anthrax meningitis in siblings were reported from Iran [77]. Four members of this family, of which three died, had eaten contaminated sheep meat and became ill. The two-year-old girl presented with fever, coma, right focal seizures, right pupillary dilatation, ptosis, nuchal rigidity, and positive Kernig and Brudzinski signs. Lumbar puncture revealed 1100 WBCs, with 80% neutrophils, CSF protein 200 mg/dL and glucose 20 mg/dL, but no organisms on Gram stain. She was started on penicillin and streptomycin but died three hours after admission. Her six-year-old brother presented with fever, headache, vomiting, nuchal rigidity, and positive Kernig and Brudzinski signs, but normal mental status and without focal neurologic findings. His CSF revealed 1100 WBCs with 67% neutrophils, protein 120 mg/dL, and glucose 30 mg/dL with Gram-positive bacilli. He was similarly started on parenteral antibiotics, was afebrile within five days, and improved gradually over two weeks. He apparently recovered completely.

Another two-year-old Iranian child developed a fulminant case of intestinal anthrax after the ingestion of contaminated lamb meat [78]. This child presented with three days of fever, nausea, vomiting, and diarrhea that had progressed to bloody vomitus and abdominal distention. She was in shock on presentation, with systolic blood pressure of 40 mm Hg and cool, cyanotic extremities. Her abdomen was markedly distended. Peritoneal aspirate yielded turbid ascitic fluid with 4100 neutrophils/mm^3 and Gram-positive bacilli in chains. She was started on intravenous antibiotics but died 12 hours after admission.

An 11-year-old French girl developed anthrax meningitis 16 days after eating contaminated sheep liver [79]. She was ill with fever, headache, and vomiting for four days before presentation, by which time she was comatose. CSF had 10,000 WBCs, with protein 1.2 g/dL, and large Gram-positive rods. She died after two days. Such a case is rare in Western Europe, but this was a Muslim family who had slaughtered the sheep themselves; in review, it was noted that the sheep's lungs and liver were black at the time of slaughter.

A Turkish infant presented in 2000 with fever and erythema surrounding the umbilicus that had been tied with a wool thread at birth. The infant had positive cultures of blood, urine, and from the umbilicus for *B. anthracis*; all the maternal cultures were negative. On investigation of the infant's home, it was found that the wool tie used on the umbilical cord was from an infected wool hide [76].

In October 2001, a seven-month-old boy was admitted to the hospital for treatment of a presumed infected spider bite on his arm in New York City [73a]. The child was treated with ampicillin-sulbactam, and then clindamycin was added. Despite this, he developed progression of the lesion to a depressed black eschar, with marked surrounding edema, and systemic complications including transient disseminated intravascular coagulation and renal insufficiency. After the epidemiologic association to the concurrent anthrax-contaminated mail outbreak was recognized, diagnostic tests confirmed his infection was caused by anthrax. The child was hospitalized approximately 10 days, and was discharged in stable condition, on oral ciprofloxacin therapy after the diagnosis was confirmed. Such systemic effects of cutaneous anthrax infection without overt sepsis are not typically reported, and may suggest some unique pediatric susceptibility.

Yersinia pestis *(plague)*

Most cases of plague in children are of the bubonic type [48,80,112]. Sepsis and meningitis can certainly occur, though undifferentiated septicemia is less common than in adults. Treatment is similar for children as for adults [54]. When it does occur, primary plague sepsis in children has a much higher fatality rate than the bubonic form, 71% versus 3% in one series from the 1970s [112]. Gastrointestinal signs and symptoms can be prominent and at times can mimic an acute abdomen [81]. Two 1980s cases of primary plague septicemia in children highlight some of these observations.

A 14-month-old girl presented with one day of high fever, without lymphadenopathy or localizing signs of infection, and was treated expectantly with antipyretics [80]. Four days later, she suddenly had explosive diarrhea, vomited, and collapsed. On evaluation, she was cyanotic, hypotensive, and minimally responsive, with scattered petechiae noted. She soon went into cardiac arrest and was unable to be resuscitated. Post-mortem blood and spleen cultures grew *Y. pestis*. The child's family had recently moved into housing that was discovered to have been infested with plague-carrying rock squirrels and their fleas.

An eight-year-old boy presented with a three-day history of fever and malaise, and was diagnosed with otitis media and started on erythromycin [81]. Two days later he developed vomiting and severe right lower quadrant tenderness. His white blood count was 29,000/mm^3 with 30% segmented neutrophils and 56% band forms. He underwent exploratory laparoscopy that revealed a normal appendix but marked mesenteric and retroperitoneal lymphadenopathy. Post-operatively he developed higher fever and a sepsis syndrome with shock, respiratory distress requiring ventilatory support, disseminated intravascular coagulation, renal failure, and gastrointestinal hemorrhage. Blood culture was positive for *Y. pestis*. He was treated with chloramphenicol and cefotaxime, and survived with full recovery.

Smallpox

Scant recent literature exists to distinguish pediatric from adult smallpox [2]. Historically, children less than five years of age and adults more than

45 years of age had the highest mortality. Today virtually all children in the United States are unvaccinated, and have no immunity to smallpox; thus their potential susceptibility might actually be greater than in those older Americans who were immunized before 1972. Older textbooks [82] offer noteworthy observations regarding manifestations of smallpox in children. During the prodromal phase, in addition to high fever, head and muscle aches, chills and prostration, a child may develop delirium, coma, and seizures. A viral osteomyelitis was described, occurring between the tenth and twentieth days and involving multiple bones and joints, accompanied by radiographic evidence of bony destruction that might lead to serious sequelae, including deformed bones, stunted growth, and ankylosis.

Clostridia botulinum (botulism)

Clinical manifestations of botulism are similar in adults and children, and even the "infant botulism" syndrome is now described in adults as intestinal botulism [72]. Infants have narrower pharyngeal airways and thus might be expected to experience increased mortality from an equivalent dose per body size in the absence of effective supportive care [83].

Specific pediatric treatment issues

Several issues pertain to the treatment of children in the context of bioterrorism (see Table 3). Foremost, many of the highest threat agents are treated in adults with ciprofloxacin or doxycycline. Fluoroquinolone and tetracycline classes of antibiotics have been considered contraindicated in young children [84]. The fluoroquinolone concern has been based primarily on the theoretic risk for arthropathy and growth abnormality from studies in small mammals. Tetracyclines stain children's teeth, particularly in those children less than eight years of age who are undertaking prolonged or repeated courses of this antibiotic. In each case, however, further evaluation has mitigated much of this concern as it applies to the use of these agents in children potentially at risk for serious diseases such as anthrax, plague, or tularemia.

The past decade has seen a great deal of clinical use of ciprofloxacin in young children with cancer [85] and cystic fibrosis [86] in Western nations. In addition, it has been used considerably for the treatment of other common infections including shigellosis [87], typhoid fever [88], and neonatal sepsis [89], particularly in underdeveloped countries. One study [86] followed 26 children with cystic fibrosis treated with twice-daily ciprofloxacin for 14 days, who were monitored by magnetic resonance imaging (MRI) during or just after drug administration, and at three months after therapy. None showed evidence of arthropathy. Another study [88] examined more than 300 Vietnamese children treated with ciprofloxacin or ofloxacin for seven-day courses in the therapy of multidrug-resistant typhoid fever. The patients were examined daily during therapy, and followed up at 1, 12, and

Table 3
Initial antibiotic therapy for principal bacterial agents of bioterrorism in children

Agent	Antibiotics	Dose and route
Contained casualty setting		
Anthrax Inhalational, GI, or oropharyngeal	Ciprofloxacin or	10–15 mg/kg IV q 12 hr (max 1 g/day)
	doxycycline could be substituted if strain is susceptible. Plus one or two additional antimicrobials such as rifampin, penicillin, ampicillin, clindamycin, vancomycin, chloramphenicol, imipenum, or clarithromycin	
Localized cutaneous anthrax	Ciprofloxin or doxycycline PO (IV therapy with multiple agents is recommended if systemic involvement, extensive edema, lesions of the head or neck, or age less than 2 years)	
Plague	Streptomycin or	15 mg/kg IM q 12 hr (max 2 g/day)
	Gentamicin	2.5 mg/kg IM or IV q 8 hr (q 12 hr in neonates <1 week old)
	or	
	Doxycycline	2.2 mg/kg IV q 12 hr (max 200 mg/day)
	(Ciprofloxacin, chloramphenicol might also be considered, especially chloramphenicol for plague meningitis.)	
Tularemia	Streptomycin or	15 mg/kg IM q 12 hr (max 2 g/day)
	Gentamicin	2.5 mg/kg IM or IV q 8 hr
	(q 12 hr in neonates <1 week old)	
	or	
	Doxycycline	2.2 mg/kg IV q 12 hr (max 200 mg/day) (Chloramphenicol, ciprofloxacin may also be considered.)
Mass casualty setting or prophylaxis		
Anthrax	Ciprofloxacin	10–15 mg/kg PO q 12 hr (max 1 g/day)
	(Amoxicillin or doxycycline could be substituted if strain is susceptible.)	
Plague	Doxycycline or	2.2 mg/kg PO q 12 hr (max 200 mg/day)
	Ciprofloxacin	15–20 mg/kg PO q 12 hr (max 1 g/day)
Tularemia	Doxycycline or	2.2 mg/kg PO q 12 hr (max 200 mg/day)
	Ciprofloxacin	15 mg/kg PO q 12 hr (max 1 g/day)

Compiled and adapted from references 54,55,62.

24 months post-treatment. No evidence of joint toxicity was found. Growth velocity was slightly increased for ciprofloxacin-treated patients at one year, and equivalent at two years.

Several studies have examined ciprofloxacin pharmacokinetics in children [90,91]. The drug is well absorbed with a typical half-life of four to five hours in young children under steady-state conditions. Oral doses of 30–40 mg/kg/day in two divided doses seem to provide area under the concentration time curves comparable to 400 mg three times per day intravenously, or 750 mg orally two times per day in adults [91].

The American Academy of Pediatrics now considers the use of ciprofloxacin justified for several pediatric indications, particularly when its oral route confers an advantage over other drugs that would require parenteral administration, and for multidrug-resistant pathogens [84]. Finally, the FDA approved ciprofloxacin in 2001 for use in a bioterrorist-related anthrax exposure for children and adults [92].

Among the tetracyclines, doxycycline is least likely to cause dental staining. It has now been recognized as the drug of choice for treatment of pediatric life-threatening rickettsial infections [84]. One recent study on a few patients treated with doxycycline for Rocky Mountain Spotted Fever found no significant differences in dental staining between patients and control subjects [93]. Doxycycline seems appropriate as a first- or second-line agent for the treatment of potential bioterrorist infections in children.

Additional considerations include issues related to vaccine efficacy and safety in children and the possible use of botulism antitoxin therapy. Vaccines exist for several of the bioterrorism agents, but aside from vaccination for smallpox, they are generally unavailable and none have been used to any significant degree in children, nor are they approved for pediatric use. Currently, availability of anthrax vaccine is even in question, and antibiotic prophylaxis will play the primary treatment role [54,55,62]. Finally, botulinum antitoxin is available, and could be used in children [72]. There is an investigational human-derived antibody, Botulism Immune Globulin Intravenous (Human), developed by the California Department of Health Services, but its use is limited at present to treatment trials of infant botulism [72].

Immunocompromised patients

Over the past decade, the population considered to be immunocompromised has grown. Increasing numbers of patients are elderly, afflicted with HIV or cancer, or harbor co-morbid conditions. Advances in medical therapy such as hemodialysis and the use of potent immunosuppressive or cytotoxic regimens have resulted in more "compromised hosts" than ever before. A bioterrorist attack involving this segment of the population could result in complication and death rates greater than expected for the general population. Scant information is available on clinical manifestations and the most appropriate treatment for immunocompromised patients following exposure to bioterrorism agents. Consensus guidelines regarding anthrax and plague treatment and post-exposure prophylaxis for immunocompromised persons recommend the same antibiotic regimen as for immunocompetent adults and children [54,55].

Elderly patients

During this century, the rate of growth of the elderly population has greatly exceeded that of the country as a whole. The fastest growing segment of the elderly population is comprised of those aged 85 years and older. The number of persons more than 65 years of age may more than double to 80 million by 2050 [94]. Given that a large percentage of these individuals would have pre-existing disease states, their susceptibility to infections and post-infectious sequelae will be increased in the event of a biological attack. The potential for drug–drug interactions and adverse effects from antibiotics used to treat or prophylax against bioterrorist agent exposure will be greatly increased in this population also.

In anticipation of their special needs, pre-identification of sites such as nursing homes and senior citizen complexes should be carried out to identify pre-existing illness in the residents of these facilities. Health officials also will need to develop a plan for rendering care to those elderly who are unable to access public information alerts, travel to medication points of distribution, follow evacuation or quarantine instructions, or attend to their basic needs following the loss of their spouse or primary caregiver.

Patients with HIV

It is known that the depression of cell-mediated immunity induced by HIV infection is associated with a higher incidence of opportunistic infections [95]. In theory, this places these individuals at an increased risk for infection and post-infectious complications following a bioterrorist attack.

Smallpox

There is little information about how individuals with different types of immune deficiency would respond to smallpox infection. Early investigators reported that hemorrhagic smallpox occurred in eight out of nine persons with immunologic deficiencies who were vaccinated late after contact [96]. Details regarding the specific types of immunosuppression in these patients, however, are not available. Smallpox was eradicated before human immunodeficiency virus (HIV) was identified and before suitable techniques became available for measuring cell-mediated immunity [2]. This fact renders any prediction regarding the clinical course of smallpox in patients with HIV as speculative.

Monkeypox, an illness caused by a related Orthopoxvirus, is similar to smallpox. Although this virus is not a high priority agent, there are concerns over its use for the purposes of bioterrorism. Cross-immunity exists between smallpox and monkeypox. With the global decline in smallpox vaccine-derived immunity, monkeypox has the potential to replace smallpox in unvaccinated populations [97,98]. Estimated attack rates are much lower than for smallpox; however, the presence of depressed immunity has not been accounted for in such modeling. A prolonged outbreak of monkeypox occurred as recently as 1997 in the Congo among a population known to have waning smallpox antibody protection. Although the HIV prevalence in this population was not determined, in comparison to other monkeypox outbreaks, greater rates of human-to-human transmission were noted [97].

The smallpox live virus vaccine has been a source of severe complications when inadvertently administered to recipients with impaired immunologic function. (Complications were discussed in detail earlier in the section on pregnancy.) In one series, for example, vaccinia necrosum developed in a child with hypogammaglobulinemia and in an adult with depressed levels of IgM. Specifically, when used in patients with T-cell deficiency, eczema vaccinatum, generalized vaccinia, progressive vaccinia, and death have been reported. A military recruit with subclinical T-cell deficiency developed disseminated vaccinia after receiving the vaccine [99]. When immunocompromised members of the population require live virus vaccination following a biological attack, one option is to administer vaccinia immune globulin (VIG) concomitantly with the smallpox vaccine in an effort to minimize post-vaccination complications. The recommended dose in this setting is 0.3 ml/kg of body weight. Vaccine efficacy will not be altered by VIG co-administration. Realistically, VIG is in short supply and will likely not be available for mass casualty use. This highlights the potential difficulties in coordinating an effective medical response to a smallpox or monkeypox outbreak in regions with high HIV prevalence. Foregoing vaccination in this segment of the population will make it difficult to contain the outbreak and will pose challenging questions regarding isolation and quarantine. Finally, pre-identification of immunocompromised patients through careful screening will be critical to avoid inadvertent vaccine administration and prevent serious sequelae.

Francisella tularensis *(tularemia)*

Experience regarding tularemia in immunocompromised patients is limited. This agent causes more protracted illnesses in HIV-infected individuals, who then require extended courses of antibiotic therapy and longer convalescence [100]. Relapses and treatment failures following use of bacteriostatic agents should be anticipated, and aminoglycosides are the preferred antibiotics [62].

Coxiella burnetti *(Q fever)*

Coxiella burnetti, which causes Q fever, is a potential biological threat. It has been hypothesized that HIV infection could result in increased severity or reactivation of Q fever [101]. This concern is based on the fact that host defenses against the organism are primarily cell-mediated. In one study of HIV-infected patients exposed to *Coxiella burnetti*, cellular immunosuppression favored the development of symptomatic Q fever [102]. Yet another large investigation found the clinical and radiographic findings to be similar for HIV-positive and HIV-negative individuals [103]. The transmission of Q fever occurs more frequently in HIV-infected persons than in the general population. This is likely explained by the fact that *Coxiella burnetti* is able to reside in a phagolysosome like other microorganisms known to cause opportunistic infection [101]. In the event of a bioterrorist attack, HIV-positive individuals could be at a substantial risk for developing Q fever and transmitting the infection to others.

Patients with cancer or organ transplantation

Recent advances in medical oncology have resulted in improved survival rates for patients with cancer. Similarly, modern immunosuppressive drug therapy has made organ transplantation a highly successful procedure. Corticosteroids, cyclosporine, alkylating agents, antimetabolites, and radiation therapy may each suppress the host's immune response to agents of bioterrorism.

Smallpox

There have been cases of generalized and progressive vaccinia following smallpox vaccination in individuals being treated for malignancy. Examples include a patient with lymphosarcoma and hypogammaglobulinemia taking prednisone [104], a patient with chronic lymphocytic leukemia [105], and two re-vaccinees with CLL. The latter patients survived with VIG, gamma globulin and thiosemicarbazone treatment. There are also reports of malignant tumors occurring in vaccination scar sites. One report delineated several tumor types, including malignant melanoma, basal cell carcinoma, and squamous cell carcinoma. Usually a primary vaccination site was involved [106]. Another malignancy-related complication of the smallpox vaccine is post-vaccinial lymphadenitis, characterized by a reactive change in lymph nodes that histologically mimics malignant lymphoma and results in frequent misdiagnosis [107].

Q fever

Coxiella burnetti infection occurred during immunosuppressive therapy for graft-versus-host disease following bone marrow transplantation [108]. Similarly, Q fever has occurred in individuals with malignancy on chemotherapy. Of five such patients in one case series, four were clearly immunocompromised. The only patient without a history of malignancy or immunosuppressive drug use was suspected to have defective host defense mechanisms based on substandard living conditions and an overall poor state of health [109]. This case introduces the possibility that increased infection and complication rates from a bioterrorist incident may be seen in those individuals with homelessness, alcoholism, and malnutrition.

Summary and recommendations

Many issues surrounding bioterrorism have not been adequately addressed in the context of vulnerable populations. Pregnant women, children, the elderly, and immunocompromised patients have physiologic and sometimes developmental differences affecting their susceptibility to an attack. Some features of illness and treatment require special consideration, but similarities among these populations far outweigh differences. Refinement of our approach could lessen the devastation caused by these agents. Research should include a more critical assessment of the optimal types and dosing of pharmaceuticals used for these populations.

Planning efforts should address early identification of the complex needs of the groups discussed here. Medical conditions such as pregnancy, cancer, HIV, and eczema require rapid identification before the institution of a smallpox vaccination program. Unexposed pregnant women and immuno-compromised patients will require education about avoiding close contact with recent vaccinees. Quarantine of those individuals unable to be vaccinated will need to be addressed. Counseling of children and women who have miscarried should be anticipated. Strategies need to be developed to reach individuals such as homeless people and shut-ins.

The greatest challenges may lie in our ability to respond to multiple pregnant or pediatric biological casualties at a time when the health care system is under extreme duress. Only by careful medical education and planning involving the pre-hospital, pediatric, and obstetric communities can we hope to mitigate such a catastrophe. Pediatricians, pediatric emergency physicians, and obstetricians must have a robust role in disaster preparedness. At the same time, government agencies charged with overall coordination of disaster response must include specific plans for adequate pediatric and obstetric bed capacity, resuscitation and delivery equipment, fetal monitoring devices, and availability of pediatric medications.

References

[1] Yancey MK. Host defenses and bacterial resistance. Obstet Gynecol Clin North Am 1992;19:413–34.

[2] Henderson DA, Inglesby TV, Barlett JG, et al. Smallpox as a biological weapon: medical and public health management. JAMA 1999;281(22):2127–37.

[3] Hanshaw JB, Dudgeon JA. Smallpox and vaccinia. Major Prob Clin Pediatri 1978;17: 209–21.

[4] Megale P, Angulo JJ, Pederneiras CA. Variola minor in Braganca Paulista County, 1956. Bull Soc Pathol Exot Filiales 1979;72:11–20.

[5] Levine MM, Edsall G, Burce-Chwatt LJ. Live-virus vaccines in pregnancy. Risks and recommendations. Lancet 1974;2:34–8.

[6] Paranjothy D, Samuel I. Pregnancy associated with hemorrhagic smallpox. J Obstet Gynaecol Br Commonw 1960;67:309.

[7] Rao AR. Haemorrhagic smallpox: a study of 240 cases. J Indian Med Assoc 1964;43:224–9.

[8] Lynch FW. Dermatologic conditions of the fetus with particular reference to variola and vaccinia. Arch Derm Syph 1932;26:997.

[9] Rao AR, Prahlad T, Swaminathan M, et al. Pregnancy and smallpox. J Ind Med Assoc 1963;40:353–63.

[10] Rao AR, Sukumar S, Mascreen RK, et al. Vaccination and pregnancy: placental transmission of antibodies. Ind J Med Res 1969;57(7):1250–60.

[11] Marsden JP, Greenfield CRM. Inherited smallpox. Arch Dis Child 1934;9:309–14.

[12] Mehta BC, Doctor RG, Purandare NM, et al. Hemorrhagic smallpox. A study of 22 cases to determine the cause of bleeding. Indian J Med Sci 1967;21(8):518–23.

[13] Mitra M, Bhattacharya DK. Some observations on haemorrhagic smallpox (type 1). J Indian Med Assoc 1976;67(11):237–40.

[14] Garcia AGP. Fetal infection with chickenpox and alastrim with histopathological studies of the placenta. Pediatrics 1963;32:895–901.

[15] Bancroft IR. Clinical observations on variola. J Med Res 1904;11:322–44.

[16] Jelliffe DB. Possible teratogenic effects of exotic viruses. Lancet 1973;1(7806):774.

[17] Teodorescu M, Topciu V, Plavosin L, et al. The influence of smallpox revaccination upon the foetus. Virologie 1975;26(2):137–9.

[18] Lane JM, Ruben FL, Neff JM, et al. Complications of smallpox vaccination, 1968: results of ten statewide surveys. J Infect Dis 1970;122(4):303–9.

[19] Advisory Committee on Immunization Practices. Vaccinia (smallpox) vaccine: recommendations of the Advisory Committee on Immunization Practices (ACIP). Morb Mortal Wkly Rep 2001;50(RR10):1–25.

[20] Walter N. Vaccinia autoinoculata during pregnancy. Hautarzt 1979;30(9):501–2.

[21] Kistler G, Gertsch R. Smallpox vaccination and pregnancy. Dtsch Med Wochenschr 1970;95(23):1254–6.

[22] Rupprecht CE, Blass L, Smith K, et al. Human infection due to recombinant vaccinia-rabies glycoprotein virus. N Engl J Med 2001;345(8):582–6.

[23] Rajhvajn B, Krznar B, Stoiljkovic C, et al. Vaccination against smallpox in early pregnancy. Acta Med Iugosl 1973;27(4):351–7.

[24] Mihailescu R, Petrovici M. Effect of smallpox vaccination on the product of conception. Arch Roum Pathol Exp Microbiol 1975;34(1–2):67–74.

[25] Topciu VL, Braga V, Plavosin L, et al. The action of the vaccinia virus upon placenta and fetus in revaccinated pregnants. Zbl Bakt Hyg I Abt Orig B 1976;161:552–6.

[26] Wentworth P. Studies on placentae and infants from women vaccinated for smallpox during pregnancy. J Clin Pathol 1966;19:328–30.

[27] Norskov-Lauritsen N, Zachar V, Petersen PM, et al. In vitro infection of human placental trophoblast by wild-type vaccinia virus and recombinant virus expressing HIV envelope glycoprotein. Res Virol 1992;143:321–8.

[28] Todorovic M, Kulis M. Histological changes of the placenta in women vaccinated with anti-variola vaccine. Srp Arh Celok Lek 1974;102(2):121–7.

[29] Meselson M, Guillemin J, Hugh-Jones M, et al. The Sverdlovsk anthrax outbreak of 1979. Science 1994;266:1202–8.

[30] Bieniarz J, Dabrowski Z. Effect of smallpox vaccination on pregnancy. Pol Tyg Lek 1956;11:2183.

[31] Greenberg M, Yankauer A, Krugman S, et al. The effect of smallpox vaccination during pregnancy on the incidence of congenital malformations. Pediatrics 1949;3:456.

[32] Bellows MT, Hyman ME, Merritt KK. Effect of smallpox vaccination on the outcome of pregnancy. Publ Hlth Rep 1949;64:319.

[33] Bourke GJ, Whitty RJ. Smallpox vaccination and pregnancy. BMJ 1964;4:1544.

[34] Liebeschuet HJ. J Obstet Gynaec Br Commonw 1964;71:132.

[35] Ladnyi ID. Smallpox vaccination during pregnancy. ZH Mikrobiol Epidemiol Immunobiol 1974;7:121–5.

[36] Aitkens GH, Bowman R, Hansman D. A case of foetal vaccinia. Med J Aust 1968;2(4):173–4.

[37] Entwistle DM, Bray PT, Laurence KM. Prenatal infection with vaccinia virus: report of a case. BMJ 1962;2:238.

[38] Green DM, Reid SM, Rhaney K. Generalised vaccinia in the human foetus. Lancet 1966;1(7450):1296–8.

[39] MacDonald AM, MacArthur P. Foetal vaccinia. Arch Dis Child 1953;28:311.

[40] Tucker SM, Sibson DE. Foetal complication of vaccination in pregnancy. BMJ 1962;2:237.

[41] Luisi M. Smallpox vaccination and pregnancy. Am J Obstet Gynecol 1977;128(6):700.

[42] Lycke E, Ahren C, Stenberg R, et al. A case of intrauterine vaccinia. Acta Pathol Microbiol Scand 1963;57:287.

[43] Harley JD, Gillespie AM. A complicated case of congenital vaccinia. Pediatrics 1972; 50:150–3.

[44] Konstantinova B, Iordanov G, Ivanov S. Agenesis of the prosencephalon and mesencephalon due to a contact with the virus of the antivariolar vaccin. Meditsina I Fizkultura 1988;27(2):49–55.

[45] Naderi S. Smallpox vaccination during pregnancy. Obstet Gynecol 1975;46(2):223–6.

[46] Koplan JP, Goldstein J, Foster SO. Congenital vaccinia: some doubts. Pediatrics 1972; 50(6)971–2.

[47] Goldstein JA, Neff JM, Lane JM, et al. Smallpox vaccination reactions, prophylaxis and complications of therapy. Pediatrics 1975;55(3):342–7.

[48] Mann JM, Moskwitz R. Plague and pregnancy: a case report. JAMA 1977;237: 1854–5.

[49] Pollitzer R. Plague. Geneva: World Health Organization monograph series no. 22. 1954. p. 417–18.

[50] Jennings WE. A manual of plague. Vol 90. London: Rebman Ltd.; 1903. p. 150–1.

[51] Coppes JB. Bubonic plague in pregnancy. J Reprod Med 1980;2:91–5.

[52] Wong TW. Plague in a pregnant patient. Trop Doct 1986;16:187–9.

[53] Welty TK, Grabman J, Kompare E, et al. Nineteen cases of plague in Arizona: a spectrum including ecthyma gangrenosum due to plague and plague in pregnancy. West J Med 1985;142(5):641–6.

[54] Inglesby TV, Dennis DT, Henderson DA, et al. Plague as a biological weapon: medical and public health management [consensus statement]. JAMA 2000;283:2281–90.

[55] Inglesby TV, Henderson DA, Bartlett JG, et al. Anthrax as a biological weapon: medical and public health management. JAMA 1999;281:1735–45.

[56] Advisory Committee on Immunization Practices . Use of anthrax vaccine in the United States: recommendations of the Advisory Committee on Immunization Practices. Morb Mortal Wkly Rep 2000;49(RR15):1–20.

[57] St Clair EH, DeLiberti JH, O'Brien ML. Observations of an infant born to a mother with botulism. J Ped 1975;87:658.

[58] Gollober M, Beyer RA, Kwan S, Bates PO, Oster H, Billimek M, et al. Wound botulism—California. Morb Mortal Wkly Rep 1995;44:889–92.

[59] Robin L, Herman D, Redett R. Botulism in a pregnant woman. N Engl J Med 1996;335: 823–4.

[60] Polo JM, Martin J, Berciano J. Botulism and pregnancy. Lancet 1996;348:195.

[61] Bowe DP, Wakeman DC. Tularemia and pregnancy: report of a case. JAMA 1936; 102:577.

[62] Dennis DT, Inglesby TV, Henderson DA. Tularemia as a biological weapon: medical and public health management. JAMA 2001;285:2763–73.

[63] Albrecht RC, Cefalo RC, O'Brien WF. Tularemia immunization in early pregnancy. Am J Obstet Gynecol 1980;138:1226–7.

[64] Bwaka MA, Bonnet MJ, Calain R, et al. Ebola hemorrhagic fever in Kikwit, Democratic Republic of the Congo: clinical observations in 103 patients. J Infect Dis 1999;179:S1–7.

[65] Mupapa K, Mukundu W, Bwaka MA, et al. Ebola hemorrhagic fever and pregnancy. J Infect Dis 1999;179:S11–2.

[66] WHO/International Study Team. Ebola hemorrhagic fever in Zaire, 1976. Bull World Health Org 1978;56:271–93.

[67] McCormick JB. Lassa fever: epidemiology, therapy and vaccine development. J Japanese Assoc Inf Dis 1988;26:353–66.

[68] Zuckerman AJ, Simpson DI. Exotic virus infections of the liver. Progress Liv Dis 1979;6: 425–38.

[69] Walls B. Lassa fever in pregnancy. Midwives Chron 1985;1168:136–8.

[70] Price ME, Fisher-Hoch SP, Crave RB, et al. A prospective study of maternal and fetal outcome in acute Lassa fever infection during pregnancy. BMJ 1988;297:584–7.

[71] Baring-Gould WS, Baring-Gould C. In: The annotated mother goose. NewYork: Bramhall House; 1962. p. 252–3.

[72] Arnon SS, Schecter R, Inglesby TV, et al. Botulinum toxin as a biological weapon: medical and public health management [consensus statement]. JAMA 2001;285:1059–70.

[73] Torok TJ, Tauxe RV, Wise RP, et al. A large community outbreak of Salmonellosis caused by intentional contamination of restaurant salad bars. JAMA 1999;278:389–95.

[73a] Roche KJ, Chang MW, Lazarus H. Cutaneous anthrax infection. N Engl J Med 2001;345:1611.

[74] Henretig FM, Cieslak TJ, Madsen JM, et al. The emergency department response to incidents of biological and chemical terrorism. In: Fleisher GF, Ludwig S, editors. Textbook of pediatric emergency medicine. 4th edition. Philadelphia: Lippincott Williams & Wilkins; 2000. p. 1763–84.

[75] American Academy of Pediatrics. Anthrax. In: Pickering LK, editor. 2000 red book: report of the committee on infectious diseases. 25th edition. Elk Grove Village, IL: American Academy of Pediatrics; 2000. p. 168–70.

[76] Ozcaya E, Kirimi E, Berktas M, et al. *Bacillus anthracis* sepsis in a newborn. Ped Inf Dis 2000;19:487–8.

[77] Tabatabaie P, Syadati A. *Bacillus anthracis* as a cause of bacterial meningitis. Ped Inf Dis 1993;12:1035–6.

[78] Alizad A, Ayoub EM, Makki N. Intestinal anthrax in a two-year-old child. Ped Inf Dis 1995;14:394–5.

[79] Berthier M, Fauchere JL, Perrin J, et al. Fulminant meningitis due to *Bacillus anthracis* in 11-year-old girl during Ramadan. Lancet 1996;347:828–9.

[80] Leopold JC. Septicemic plague in a 14-month-old child. Pediatr Infect Dis 1986;5:108–10.

[81] Humphrey M, McGivney R, Perkins C, et al. *Yersinia pestis*: a case of mistaken identity. Pediatr Infect Dis 1988;7:365–6.

[82] Phillips C. Smallpox (variola). In: Vaughn VC, McKay RJ, Behrman RE, editors. Nelson textbook of pediatrics. 11th edition. Philadelphia: WB Saunders; 1979. p. 876–80.

[83] Thompson JA, Glasgow LA, Warpinski JR, et al. Infant botulism: clinical spectrum and epidemiology. Pediatrics 1980;66:936–42.

[84] American Academy of Pediatrics . Fluoroquinolones, tetracyclines. In: Pickering LK, editor. 2000 red book: report of the committee on infectious diseases. 25th edition. Elk Grove Village, IL: American Academy of Pediatrics; 2000. p. 645–6.

[85] Freifeld A, Pizzo P. Use of fluoroquinolones for empiric management of febrile neutropenia in pediatric cancer patients. Pediatr Infect Dis 1997;16:140–5.

[86] Redmond A, Sweeney L, MacFarland M, et al. Oral ciprofloxacin in the treatment of pseudomonas exacerbations of paediatric cystic fibrosis: clinical efficacy and safety evaluation using magnetic resonance image scanning. J Internat Med Res 1998;26:304–12.

[87] Salam MA, Dhar U, Khan WA, et al. Randomized comparison of ciprofloxacin suspension and pivmecillinam for childhood shigellosis. Lancet 1998;352:522–7.

[88] Bethell DB, Hien TT, Phi LT, et al. Effects on growth of single short courses of fluoroquinolones. Arch Dis Child 1996;74:44–6.

[89] Gurpinar AN, Balkan E, Kilic N, et al. The effects of a fluoroquinolone on the growth and development of infants. J Internat Med Res 1997;25:302–6.

[90] Peltola H, Ukkonen P, Saxen H, Stass H. Single-dose and steady-state pharmacokinetics of a new oral suspension of ciprofloxacin in children. Pediatrics 1998;101:658–62.

[91] Schaefer HG, Stass H, Wedgwood J, et al. Pharmacokinetics of ciprofloxacin in pediatric cystic fibrosis patients. Antimicrob Agents Chemother 1996;40:29–34.

[92] Food and Drug Administration. Approval of ciprofloxacin for use after exposure to inhalational anthrax. FDA talk paper. August 31, 2001. Available at: http://www.fda.gov/bbs/topics/ANSWERS/ANS01030.html.

[93] Lochary ME, Lockhart PB, Williams WT. Doxycycline and staining of permanent teeth. Ped Infect Dis 1998;17:429–31.

[94] Hobbs FB. The elderly population. Washington, DC: US Census Bureau, Population Division and Housing Economic Statistics Division; 2001. p. 1–5.

[95] Masur H. Approach to the patient with human immunodeficiency virus infection: clinical features. In: Gorbach SL, Barkett JG, Blacklow NR, editors. Infectious diseases. Philadelphia: WB Saunders; 1992. p. 897–907.

[96] Kecmanaovc M, Suvakovic V. The effect of vaccination status on the clinical outcome of the disease in smallpox patients. MMW Munch Med Wochenschr 1974;117(3):87–92.

[97] Heymann DL, Szczeniowski M, Esteves K. Re-emergence of monkeypox in Africa: a review of the past six years. Br Med Bull 1998;54(3):693–702.

[98] Georges AJ, Georges-Courbot MC. Biohazards due to orthopoxvirus: should we vaccinate against smallpox? Med Trop (Mars) 1999;59(Suppl 4, part 2):S483–7.

[99] Redfield RR, Wright DC. Disseminated vaccinia in a military recruit with human immunodefiency virus (HIV) disease. N Engl J Med 1987;316:673–6.

[100] Gries DM. Typhoidal tulameria in a human immunodefiency virus-infected adolescent. Ped Inf Dis J 1996;15:838–40.

[101] Raoult D. Host factor in the severity of Q fever. Annal NY Acad Sci 1990;590:33–8.

[102] Belec L, Gresenguet G, Ekala MT, et al. Coxiella burnetti infection among subjects infected with HIV type I in the Central African Republic. Eur J Clin Microbio Inf Dis 1993;12:775–8.

[103] Boschini A, Giovanni DP, et al. Consecutive epidemics of Q fever in a residential facility for drug abusers: impact on persons with human immunodeficiency virus infection. Clin Inf Dis 1999;28:866–72.

[104] Rosenbaum EH, Cohen RA, Glatstein HR. Vaccination of a patient receiving immuno-suppressive therapy for lymphosarcoma. JAMA 1966;198:737–40.

[105] Paradinas FJ, Wiltshaw E. Necropsy findings in a case of progressive vaccinia. J Clin Path 1972;25:233–9.

[106] Marmelzat WL. Malignant tumors in smallpox vaccination scars. Arch Derm 1968;97:400–6.

[107] Hartsock RJ. Postvaccinial lymphadenitis: hyperplasia of lymphoid tissue that simulates malignant lymphomas 1968;21:632–48.

[108] Kanfer E, Farrag N, et al. Q fever following bone marrow transplantation. Bone Marrow Transplant 1988;3:165–6.

[109] Heard SR, Ronalds CJ, Heath RB. Coxiella burnetti infection in immunocompromised patients. J Inf 1985;11:15–8.

[110] American Academy of Pediatrics. Chemical and biological terrorism and its impact on children: a subject review. Pediatrics 2000;105:662–70.

[111] Khan AS, Tshioko FK, Heymann DL, et al. The re-emergence of ebola hemorrhagic fever, Democratic Republic of the Congo, 1995. Commission de lutte contre les epidemies a Kikwit. J Infect Dis 1999;179:S76–86.

[112] Mann JM, Shandler L, Cushing AH. Pediatric plague. Pediatrics 1982;69:762–7.

EMERGENCY
MEDICINE
CLINICS OF
NORTH AMERICA

Emerg Med Clin N Am
20 (2002) 393–407

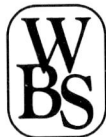

Emergency mental health management in bioterrorism events

David M. Benedek, MD, MAJ, MC[a],*,
Harry C. Holloway, MD[b], Steven M. Becker, PhD[c]

[a]Walter Reed Army Medical Center, Department of Psychiatry,
Forensic Psychiatry Service, Building 6 (Borden Pavilion),
Washington, DC 20307-5001, USA
[b]Department of Psychiatry, Uniformed Services University of the Health Sciences,
4301 Jones Bridge Road, Bethesda, MD 20814, USA
[c]School of Public Health and Center for Disaster Preparedness,
University of Alabama at Birmingham, 317 Ryals Building,
1665 University Boulevard, Birmingham, AL 35294-0022, USA

In addition to producing toxic or infectious sequelae, a bioterrorist attack has the potential to cause widespread psychophysiologic, social, behavioral, and psychiatric morbidity. Psychosocial casualties may appear in large numbers in the emergency department or the doctor's office immediately after an incident, creating major challenges for even the best-prepared healthcare facility. In addition, psychosocial casualties may continue to appear in the months and years following the event. Beyond those directly exposed to biological agents, emergency responders, other caregivers, relatives and friends of casualties, children, and other subpopulations may be at substantial risk for developing emotional and behavioral reactions and disorders. In short, the psychosocial effects of bioterrorism may be profound, and any effort to manage the consequences of a bioterrorism event needs to include a robust and well-developed emergency mental health component [1].

As of this writing the healthcare system in the United States has not yet had to manage mass casualty situations resulting from the large-scale use of biological weapons. The morbidity, mortality, and psychosocial disruption observed following the distribution of anthrax-tainted letters in the fall

---

* Corresponding author.
E-mail address: david.benedek@na.amedd.army.mil (D.M. Benedek).
The ideas and opinions expressed herein are those of the authors and do not necessarily reflect the views of the US Department of Defense, The Uniformed Services University of the Health Sciences, or any of its component services.

of 2001 merely suggest the potential complication that may arise following a larger-scale attack. Thus, principles of emergency mental health management of bioterrorism events must be extrapolated from our knowledge of the social, neuropsychiatric, and behavioral effects of industrial accidents involving toxic exposures, terrorism incidents, natural disasters, and infectious disease outbreaks. These principles can be refined through consideration of the characteristics of biological warfare agents, the means of their dissemination, and emotional and behavioral responses related specifically to these factors. In addition, consideration of other nations' experiences after chemical weapons incidents, knowledge gained during exercises that simulate attacks, and observations of responses to bioterrorism hoaxes can further inform our understanding [2].

This article reviews the mental health effects of bioterrorism and examines the implications for emergency medical response. It begins by addressing principles of primary and secondary prevention of neuropsychiatric and psychosocial sequelae of bioterrorist events and the implications of applying these principles for treatment and triage. The traumatic stress response to bioterrorism is then reviewed. This is followed by a discussion of neuropsychiatric and behavioral syndromes resulting from biological terrorism events and therapeutic interventions aimed at reducing morbidity acutely and during prolonged recovery from such events. The significance of perception, appraisal and attribution of bioterrorist incidents for involved populations, and the role of communication in influencing behavioral and psychiatric effects is outlined. Finally, planning issues related to mental health management in bioterrorism situations are summarized.

Primary and secondary prevention in the emergency setting

The September 11, 2001 terror attacks on the World Trade Center and the Pentagon dramatically and nearly instantaneously taught Americans painful lessons about the effects of international terrorist activity within the United States. These atrocities considerably reduced the state of denial in most US communities regarding the potential for terrorism in general, and alerted Americans to the specific threat of bioterrorism. The attacks also demonstrated that terrorist incidents may have far-reaching social and psychologic effects.

The emotional consequences of an event are strongly affected by the manner in which the event is anticipated. Although widespread denial has been effectively shattered in the aftermath of the September 11 attacks, bioterrorism remains, to many, incomprehensible. The invisibility of biological agents and the insidious nature of bioterrorist events makes them especially frightening, and most people—including medical practitioners—would still prefer not to contemplate the nature and extent of destruction that could be caused by a bioterrorism event. The sense of crisis may be most intensely experienced by community leaders and those who must respond to the emergency.

They must deal simultaneously with the consequences of denial, lack of resources, and a profoundly injured sense of justice. Absent training and preparation, it may be difficult to mobilize flexibility, adaptability, and decision-making skills in an atmosphere dominated by feelings of rage and helplessness. Such emotions can contribute to inadequate appraisal of the realities of the situation with negative impact on subsequent decisions. Mistaken attribution of excessive power to the attackers may be one potential unfortunate consequence: endemic problems may be erroneously interpreted as a consequence of the attack, and overestimates of the probability of subsequent attacks may lead to prolonged additional or intensified emotional symptoms.

Primary prevention

Because a lack of emotional preparedness would make chaos and disorder more likely after a bioterrorist attack [3], primary prevention must begin with a recognition of the need for realistic information regarding the threat, followed by the development of a planned response, the practice of that response, and the provision of appropriate funding and logistic facilities in support of the plan [4]. All of these steps facilitate primary prevention by mitigating a community's sense of helplessness well before an attack ever occurs. Doing so also increases the community's capacity to provide social support to victims. Because poor planning or failed execution would increase the risk for feeling helpless or overwhelmed, there is a pressing need to practice continually and to evaluate the effectiveness of the planned actions and the capacity of the responders to carry out the plans.

Secondary prevention

Bioterrorist attacks are likely to create acute, sub-acute, and chronic mental health effects. Most victims have friends and relatives in the community. An unfortunate outcome for any given patient has consequences for all those with whom the patient is socially joined in the community. When deaths occur, the emotions and psychophysiologic changes associated with bereavement may be added to effects elicited by the attack itself [5].

Secondary prevention of psychosocial consequences begins at the point of initial triage and treatment. First responders, pre-medical care personnel, and mental health treatment providers must be prepared to provide some level of treatment for individuals with acute (and most often transient) emotional and behavioral disorganization or other symptoms [4]. For persons who develop transient symptoms, response managers may facilitate recovery by creating a location or locations where symptoms can be observed and monitored that is sufficiently removed from high-tempo triage activity but close enough to permit return for re-evaluation should symptoms worsen. This "holding environment" favors social and psychologic recovery. The purpose of a terrorist attack is to produce terror and create a sense of chaos. This is accomplished through acute disruption of the social order and cultural assumptions that support community bonding. Any such attack creates an opportunity for governmental and other institutional officials either to make errors and behave in ways that discredit themselves or to demonstrate outstanding capacities as leaders. Creating an environment in which emotionally and behaviorally disorganized individuals are afforded transient protection from chaotic conditions created by the attack is one way to contribute to the psychosocial recovery and health of the community as a whole.

Because of the need for a "holding environment" and the reality of numerous acute, sub-acute, and chronic neuropsychiatric effects, mental health treatment and rehabilitative services (tertiary preventive resources) within the community will be needed to address psychosocial consequences. These services, including Red Cross disaster assistance, community mental health centers, social workers, home nurses, and hospice care providers should be an integral part of bioterrorism response planning and training. The use of these resources can promote adequate care for those suffering psychosocial impacts while emergency and primary care personnel are addressing the life-threatening somatic consequences created by the attack [6]. Combined with the development of an intelligence and information system, a thoroughly rehearsed response plan that provides for effective triage and initial treatment and incorporates community resources beyond the emergency department are measures that decrease community disruption. To the degree that the community can maintain effective social organization and respond to the demands created by the attack, the social supports provided by the community will be increased and the risk for psychiatric stress casualties decreased.

The traumatic stress response as it relates to bioterrorism

The state of autonomic arousal associated with fear will occasion the development of various rapidly evolving somatic symptoms. Although signs and symptoms may result from the direct effects of exposure to specific biological agents (see later discussion), these symptoms and somatic complaints will also occur in individuals neither exposed nor secondarily infected as a consequence of the attack. Some will attribute their rapid heart rate, shivering, muscle aches, and shortness of breath to exposure to toxic agents [7]. They will present to primary care providers requesting (or demanding) post-exposure treatment during and following the incident. In some cases, psychogenic symptoms may mimic the symptoms of exposure to an agent, creating challenges for the triage process. Because these persons may seek emergency treatment, an understanding of the emotional and behavioral responses (termed the traumatic stress response) to disaster or crisis is as critical to appropriate triage as an understanding of the specific effects of biological agents.

It is useful to divide the traumatic stress response into four phases. The first phase during or immediately following a disaster consists of strong emotions including varying feelings of disbelief, numbness, fear, and confusion. There may be high levels of autonomic arousal. These feelings are the normal emotional responses to an abnormal or traumatic event. The second phase usually lasts from a week to several months. Adaptation to environmental changes and intrusive symptoms (unbidden thoughts or recollections of the event) accompanied by symptoms of hyper-arousal, such as an abnormal startle response, frequently occur during the second phase. Somatic symptoms such as dizziness, headache, fatigue, and nausea may also develop. The third phase is notable for feelings of disappointment and resentment when initial hopes for aid and restoration are not met. In this phase the sense of community is weakened as individuals focus on their personal needs. The final phase, reconstruction, may last for years. During this phase, survivors rebuild their lives and re-establish occupational and social identities [2,4,8].

Because individuals progress through these phases at variable rates, medical responders must realize that persons may manifest emotional symptoms over different timelines in response to the same event. Moreover, depending on the severity of the trauma, the capacity of the community to respond and retain its social organization, the resources available during the event, and individual coping skills within members of the community, varying numbers of the affected population will develop persistent symptoms requiring tertiary treatment. Anger and frustration may be manifest toward caregivers including medical responders and outside agencies aiding in consequence management.

Microbial and viral agents are invisible and odorless. Exposure occurs in the absence of a warning signal. Once suspected, the separation of the infected from the non-infected will require the use of expert evaluation and tests. The uncertainty created by the lack of warning, the variability of exposure and incubation period, and the potential use of mixed agents may evoke a more potent stress response. Terrorists, knowing that these agents are colorless, odorless, and variable in the symptoms they produce, may claim to deploy one agent while in reality deploying a different agent or multiple agents. Thus, these characteristics lend themselves to a type of (mis)information warfare that enhances the potential for confusion, uncertainty, and a maladaptive traumatic stress response.

Specific agents may also produce pathologic consequences and lesions that further intensify the stress response. For example, as hemorrhagic fevers and smallpox progress, grotesqueries are produced that generate revulsion and horror. When observed by persons naïve to the physical consequences of these illnesses, lasting mental images are created that may be re-experienced in the form of unwelcome intrusive memories or recollections (flashbacks), or may be generalized to include fantasies of one's own tortured disfigurement or death [9]. The impact of observing such medical grotesqueries has been noted to produce post-traumatic symptoms in children [10] and may generate symptoms in adults. Sick children constitute an especially stressful set of patients in this circumstance. A large influx of such patients to a care facility can be difficult for the treatment staff, particularly if these patients have an unavoidably high mortality rate. Furthermore, a large influx of pediatric patients will require mental health staff to have in place specialized materials and protocols that are appropriate for assisting children.

Neuropsychiatric syndromes in bioterrorism

The clinical emotional and behavioral consequences of trauma are rooted in a combination of social, autonomic, and voluntary mechanisms only now being elaborated at the molecular level. In the immediate phase, the release of Corticotrophin Releasing Factor (CRF), the secretion of Adrenocortico-trophin Hormone (ACTH), the surge of peripheral catecholamines, and the activation of brain areas related to perception of threat accompany extremes of environmental stress. Behavior and cognitive changes correlate with noradrenergic phenomena. The immediate impact of acute stress under most conditions is improved performance. As preparation and capacity to act in response become inadequate to meet continued or increasing demands, however, the risk for performance and cognitive dysfunction increases. Behavior and thinking may become goal-directed and narrowly focused. Unfortunately, this aroused but focused state results in difficulty shifting goals, scanning alternatives, and changing plans of action [16]. Extreme distress may disrupt cognition to the point of creating chaotic thinking, and under certain social circumstances the over-focused response of flight or immobility may occur. When this response is communicated to others in the immediate social environment, social panic results [12]. Factors contributing to the development of mass panic are listed in Table 1.

The development of massive group panic is rare, and pro-social behavior is the norm after most disasters. In the situation created by a bioterrorist attack, however, medical managers must be sensitive to the idea that community leadership will be faced with inadequate resources, inadequate personnel, and inadequate experience—factors that, when combined, could precipitate a grossly maladaptive panic response in this small but critical group. Prevention of group or social panic is accomplished by militating the

Table 1
Mass panic: risk factors

New risk (eg, new weapon, new disease)
Poor/discredited leadership
Perceived risk very high (regardless of whether or not this perception is realistic)
Perceived small chance of escape (no chance of escape decreases risk)
Perceived group isolation
Untrained or mis-trained with distrust of peers
Intra-group breakdown in communications
Critical response element fails
No effective response perceived

impact of these factors; planning and over-training with regard to response algorithms are critical to this endeavor. Absent group panic, more common responses of scapegoating or paranoia may still detract from the overall response effort. It is not uncommon to see community anger displaced and directed toward caregivers or the community leadership [4,13]. Likewise, it is not uncommon for people perceived to have been affected by an invisible agent to be viewed by others with fear or hostility. Stigma and discrimination, for example, have been seen after chemical and radiologic incidents and in the aftermath of disease outbreaks [14,15].

The immediate alarm response is followed by a cascade of neuronal and intercellular events leading to elevated levels of CRH, increased synthesis of cortisol-related receptors, and activation of protein synthesis in subcortical nuclei of the amygdala responsible for the development of emotionally-laden memories (conditioned responses and habits). Hyper-secretion of epinephrine seems to exaggerate and consolidate fear-related memories of events also. One might speculate that this increased neuronal synthetic activity (neuroplasticity) serves an adaptive role in preparing for future threat by establishing memory of the event. These changes may also play a role, however, in the development of an exaggerated startle response, intrusive thoughts, and low thresholds to autonomic arousal observed as clinically significant pathology in disorders such as Acute Stress Disorder (ASD) and Post-traumatic Stress Disorder (PTSD) [16].

It is less clear how this cascade of neuronal events may relate to the social withdrawal also seen in individuals with ASD or PTSD. Social withdrawal is a major contributor to the pathologic consequences of traumatic experience. One factor that seems to mitigate the psychopathologic effects of these changes is the availability of social supports and a supportive healing environment. When social relationships result in increased demands, however, (eg, if a previously supportive individual becomes critical of one's performance) the risk for post-traumatic psychopathology may be increased [13]. The increased neuroplasticity immediately following the recognition of a threat may provide a rationale for rapid intervention after the traumatic event. Unfortunately, the empiric data are not well enough developed to assure the efficacy of such interventions in asymptomatic populations.

Therapeutic interventions

Symptoms ranging from lethargy and depression to disorientation, dissociation, depersonalization, hallucinations, paranoia, and cognitive slowing have been linked to the direct neurotoxic effects and encephalopathies associated with infectious biological agents [17,18] (Table 2). The rapid identification of an agent and the initiation of antimicrobial or other anti-infectious treatment and containment strategies discussed elsewhere in this text serve to minimize the psychiatric sequelae of initial or secondary infections. Early treatment will reduce the incidence of delirium, which is important because

Table 2
Neuropsychiatric syndromes or symptoms in selected biological agents

Biological agent	Syndrome or symptoms	Comment
Anthrax	Meningitis	May be rapidly progressive
Brucellosis	Depression, irritability, headaches	Fatalities associated with CNS involvement
Q fever	Malaise, fatigue	In 1/3 of patients
	Encephalitis, hallucinations	In advanced cases
Botulinum toxin	Depression	Due to lengthy recovery
Viral encephalitides	Depression, cognitive impairment	Other mood changes also
All biological agents	Delirium	Acutely impaired attention, memory, and perceptual disturbances

even small numbers of delirious patients can place exceptional demands on available staff. Persons who recover from direct exposure or secondary infection remain at significant risk for later development of psychologic symptoms; therefore continued surveillance may direct additional psychosocial or psychiatric intervention in this population.

Antipsychotic and anxiolytic medications used in the acute management of delirium brought about by other causes are effective in infectious causes also. Antipsychotic medications metabolized by way of the cytochrome p-450 system may alter antibiotic levels and antibiotics similarly metabolized may likewise affect antipsychotic levels. Dose-related side effects of the antipsychotics (such as agitation or somnolence) may also be mistaken for primary symptoms of an infectious encephalopathy. Use of the phenothiazines as antiemetic or antipsychotic medications may result in pseudo-parkinsonism, akesthisia, or other basal ganglion disturbances that are difficult to interpret and manage in these circumstances. The importance of keeping treatment simple therefore cannot be overemphasized. The possibility that antipsychotic treatment contributes to a higher incidence of PTSD also cannot be ruled out. A conservative approach that minimizes the use of psychotropic medications is indicated, although these medications can be helpful in controlling behavior when such control is clinically critical. It is clear that acute pharmaceutical suppression of anxiety and arousal symptoms will not prevent PTSD.

Within hospitals or other institutions serving as entry points for care, once the need for anti-infectious or other medical treatment measures has been identified and initiated, establishing a location where persons presenting with psychologic symptoms can receive respite is appropriate. Assignment to this location, which is still nearby but separate from the chaos of initial triage and treatment, should be accompanied by the reassurance that stress symptoms are normal, predictable, and generally transient. Such symptoms, it should be pointed out, are not necessarily a harbinger of further somatic symptoms or even a sign of exposure. Many of the initial psychologic symptoms associated with trauma will respond to these measures alone. Symptom-based treatment for persistent symptoms of agitation or insomnia is appropriate, however [7,19]. Even though stores of psychotropic medications are less likely to be depleted than those of vaccines or antibiotics, triage, followed by an opportunity for holding and observation will ensure that available pharmacologic resources are used optimally. This requirement must be balanced against the advantages of rapidly discharging patients from the treatment facility. Caregivers on site—with appropriate guidance from public health and disaster mental health specialists—are best equipped to make decisions about this tradeoff.

Although group debriefing techniques and critical incident debriefings have often been used in the aftermath of natural disasters, school shootings, and terrorist events, there is no convincing evidence that such debriefings reduce the development of psychiatric illness or prevent the development of PTSD. Nonetheless, evidence suggests that ongoing frank and open discussions among care providers and emergency responders (just as with other potential victims) fosters cohesion and group understanding of the unfolding event. This may serve to sustain the performance of persons critical to the management of the event, decrease individual isolation and stigma, and facilitate identification of care team members who may require further mental health attention [11]. Finally, evidence from clinical trials suggests that cognitive behavioral therapy may be valuable. Cognitive behavioral therapy involves education about the nature and universality of symptoms, examination of the precipitants of symptoms (particularly cognitive distortions), and development of reframing and interpretive techniques to minimize further symptoms. Clinical trials for depression, anxiety, and PTSD suggest that even brief therapeutic interventions of this nature may reduce immediate symptoms and diminish the development of long-term morbidity [20,21]. Given that medical resources may be quickly overwhelmed in the aftermath of a bioterrorist attack, non-physicians trained in the delivery of these therapies (eg, social workers, psychiatric nurses, and specifically trained others such as Red Cross volunteers) will allow for more effective delivery of care. In establishing priorities, delay in instituting mental health diagnosis and treatment may increase long-term morbidity.

Problems related to appraisal and attribution in the course of medical management

Although effective recognition, triage, and treatment will be the most important aspects of emergency management, these efforts must be accompanied by measures aimed at mitigating rage, helplessness, and hopelessness associated with the experience of attack or exposure. The appraisal and attribution of harmful significance to a terrorist event depends on the sociocultural milieu of those attacked and on their understanding of the specific incident at hand. Without a warning, the threat of attack and the attack are experienced nearly simultaneously as a crisis. Providing some opportunity for the treatment staff to come to terms with their emotional response to disfigured and dying patients may be done through worksite group work (such as a facilitated discussion of the triage/treatment activity and individuals' thoughts and emotions stemming from this). Providing support for the staffs' families is also an important dimension. It is unrealistic to expect the medical staff to respond with empathy for their patients if their emotional needs are ignored.

Beyond problems encountered within the emergency department, outreach to the public at large is central to managing community attribution and perception of the crisis. A public information plan must include efforts to inform and prepare the public to interpret the nature of the attack and to understand and carry out measures to protect themselves, their loved ones, and others. Such public information campaigns must address the concerns of the public and of the caregivers. In mass casualty situations, loved ones may include pets and children [22]. It is critical that the information provided be truthful even if it is bad news. Information regarding distribution of medications or vaccinations must be delivered in a manner that does not increase panic when inevitable shortages are recognized. If public information programs are discovered to be providing intentionally incorrect information, restoration of credibility for the program is highly unlikely.

The responsibility for developing public information plans does not rest primarily with emergency and medical care professionals. Medical and behavioral health personnel should however participate in development of the plan as they will have a critical role in plan implementation, and public information will influence what the community expects from healthcare providers. Robust systems must be in place for dissemination of information during and following the attack. Resilience of these systems must be well tested in advance. Medical personnel must be prepared to deliver consistent and updated information to and through the media. Information from official and unofficial sources before, during, and after the terrorist event will shape patients' expectations, behaviors and emotional responses [23]. Confounding official public information campaigns, rumors may lead unexposed persons to seek emergency treatment for various somatic symptoms or for vaccinations or medications. If medical responders accept the same unverified rumors, enormous effort and precious resources may be wasted. It is critical that emergency personnel, including physicians, acquire a dedicated and secure communications net that connects providers to agencies managing the overall community response, laboratories supporting the medical/epidemiologic effort, and the logistic structure that provides personnel, equipment, medications, and vaccines. The delivery of consistent, updated information across multiple channels by way of widely recognized and trusted sources will diminish the extent to which misinformation shapes public attribution [24].

Clinical personnel should also plan and train for the appearance of media at triage and treatment sites. The media response at these sites may be critical in letting the public know who needs to be examined and who does not, and which symptoms should prompt urgent attention. Trusted media representatives may fulfill a vital function by delivering simple, salient, and repeated messages regarding matters of concern to the public. These messages could educate the public concerning the nature of the threat and how to act to avoid harm and get help.

Planning for mental health response

By definition, a mass casualty situation occurs at the time there is a mismatch between demand for and availability of resources. A bioterrorist attack has great potential to create such a situation. Internal debates that develop over allocation of scarce resources once an attack is recognized delay response time and decrease the collaborative response process. This may create demoralization, despair, and reduced confidence in care providers that is subsequently transmitted to the community as a whole. Prevention of these consequences is of particular importance in the emergency response to terrorism because community disruption and reduced sense of community support are fundamental goals of terrorist activity.

Realistic plans and exercises must respond to the challenges within the parameters afforded by available resources. Medical responders must be prepared to deal with many people who seek care although not exposed to the infectious pathogens, and to treat such people with respect and care. That unexposed individuals will seek care in great numbers is illustrated by data from the 1995 chemical attack in Tokyo, where the number of individuals presenting to medical authorities with complaints of post-exposure symptoms exceeded the number who required medical treatment caused by exposure by a ratio of 4:1 [17].

Behavioral scientists can aid in the planning of emergency responses at the hospital, community, state, and national levels. Input from behavioral health specialists will be crucial in assuring appropriate triage and initial management of psychologic casualties. It is important that behavioral casualties be identified and that they receive appropriate assistance to reduce psychologic morbidity and to enable healthcare providers to manage those exposed individuals who require more in-depth evaluation, intervention, or supportive care.

In the social domain, specific measures to inform individuals about who should seek medical evaluation and care (discussed earlier) are vital. Successful communication of this message may help reduce the load at the medical triage sites. At emergency triage sites, rapid medical evaluation, treatment, and institution of infection control procedures must be efficiently and effectively implemented. The establishment of holding facilities that provide a recovery environment for those individuals who cannot be sent home immediately is also important. Public health agencies must play a lead role in providing community infectious disease control. Such actions will provide a sense of safety and restoration of health to the community as a whole. This sense is critical to the mobilization of any positive psychologic and supportive social response within the community.

Although any member of the population who experiences the trauma of a biological attack may experience the psychologic symptoms or syndromes described earlier, specific factors influence the development of these phenomena in subgroups within the population. Predisposing factors must be accounted for in planning the response to an attack for any specific population. Modification of protective factors forms an essential component of the prevention strategy [23]. PTSD, other anxiety disorders, and physical syndromes are more frequently diagnosed among females in the aftermath of traumatic stressors. The neurobiological and psychosocial factors accounting for this include that women seek treatment for stress-related symptoms more frequently than do men, and that duration of illnesses such as PTSD may be longer in women. Men are at greater risk for problems related to alcohol and substance use, and antisocial or violent behavior. Gender-specific neurophysiologic properties, life experiences, and cultural expectations are implicated in these differences [25,26].

Level of psychological function in the aftermath of trauma is also directly related to pretrauma functioning. Individuals who demonstrate marginal social or occupational performance before a disaster are at increased risk. Persons who have experienced and overcome past traumatic experiences may be more resilient to future traumatic insults. If past experiences have resulted in the development of PTSD or other significant symptoms of psychiatric distress, however, subsequent traumatic exposure may increase the likelihood and severity of future episodes of illness.

Medical and rescue personnel are at particular risk. They are repeatedly exposed to trauma in the mass casualty situation and they experience the extreme suffering and death of patients they try to help. This is particularly stressful when these patients are children. If these personnel are afforded an inadequate opportunity to rest or deal with their own emotional responses, they become a population at higher risk for the development of ASD and PTSD.

Emergency and primary care physicians will be at potentially greater risk as a consequence of biological attack. They will be required to take on the role of first responders in terms of recognizing the potential problem and also of responding to the needs of the mass causalities. Even if they perform well, they may have to deal with high personal risk and numerous deaths among their patients. It may be difficult for physicians who are success-oriented by training to deal with an unavoidable sense of failure in this situation. Provision of psychosocial supports for this group, including appropriate work/rest scheduling, visible and accessible leadership, support groups, and early therapeutic intervention may permit these persons to recognize that their disturbing emotional responses are normal [27].

The nature of biological weapons (odorless, colorless, and not immediately noxious or painful on contact) reduces the likelihood that primary exposure will be traumatic. Once an attack has been identified, the subsequent anticipation and eventual experience of physical symptoms and grotesqueries (either personally or vicariously) creates an ongoing risk for secondary traumatic injury including feelings of hopelessness and despair. Critical to the population-based reduction of traumatic stress response is the restoration of a sense of autonomy and provision of social support. Another factor distinguishing the overall medical response to a bioterrorist event from either a natural disaster or a conventional terrorist bomb detonation may be the need for quarantine or other infection control measures to prevent further infection once the deployment of a biological agent is confirmed. The establishment of a supportive recovery environment will require that reassurance and understandable information about expected symptoms (physical and emotional), and plans for delivery of care and containment approaches are transmitted through a variety of channels to homes, offices, schools, and hospitals wherever triage, treatment, and containment efforts are occurring.

Summary

The United States has not suffered significant psychosocial or medical consequences from the use of biological weapons within its territories. This has contributed to a "natural" state of denial at the community level. This denial could amplify the sense of crisis, anxiety, fear, chaos, and disorder that would accompany such a bioterrorist event. A key part of primary prevention involves counteracting this possibility before an incident occurs. Doing so will require realistic information regarding the bioterrorism threat followed by the development of a planned response and regular practice of that response.

Unlike in natural disasters or other situations resulting in mass casualties, emergency department physicians or nurses and primary care physicians (working in concert with epidemiologic agencies), rather than police, firemen, or ambulance personnel, will be most likely to first identify the unfolding disaster associated with a biological attack. Like community leaders, this group of medical responders must be aware of its own susceptibility to mental health sequelae and performance decrement as the increasing demands of disaster response outpace the availability of necessary resources.

A bioterrorist attack will necessitate treatment of casualties who experience neuropsychiatric symptoms and syndromes. Although symptoms may result from exposure to infection with specific biological agents, similar symptoms may result from the mere perception of exposure or arousal precipitated by fear of infection, disease, suffering, and death. Conservative use of psychotropic medications may reduce symptoms in exposed and uninfected individuals, as may cognitive-behavioral interventions. Clear, consistent, accessible, reliable, and redundant information (received from trusted sources) will diminish public uncertainty about the cause of symptoms that might otherwise prompt persons to seek unnecessary treatment. Training and preparation for contingencies experienced in an attack have the potential to enhance delivery of care. Initiating supportive social, psychotherapeutic, and psychopharmacologic treatments judiciously for symptoms and syndromes known to accompany the traumatic stress response can aid the efficient treatment of some patients and reduce long-term morbidity in affected individuals. Preventive strategies and planning must take into account the idea that specific groups within the population are at higher risk for psychiatric morbidity. First responders comprise one group at psychologic risk in this situation, and healthcare providers comprise another. These and other high-risk groups will benefit from the same supportive interventions developed for the community as a whole.

References

[1] Becker SM. Are psychosocial aspects of WMD incidents addressed in the federal response plan: summary of an expert panel. Mil Med 2001;166:66–8.
[2] Norwood AE, Ursano RJ, Fullerton CS. Disaster psychiatry: principles and practice. Psychiatric Quarterly 2000;(71)3:207–227.
[3] Lerner M. The belief in a just world: a fundamental delusion. New York: Plenum Press; 1980.
[4] Ursano RJ, Fullerton CS, Norwood AE. Psychiatric dimensions of disaster: patient care, community consultation, and preventive medicine. Harv Rev Psychiatry 1995;3:196–209.
[5] Call JA, Pfefferbaum B. Lessons from the first two years of project heartland, Oklahoma's mental health response to the 1995 bombing. Psychiatr Serv 1999;50:953–5.
[6] Lystad M. Perspectives on human response to mass emergencies. In: Lystad M, editor. Mental health response to mass emergencies. New York: Brunner/Mazel; 1998. p. xvii–xviii.
[7] Carmeli A, Liberman N, Mevorach L. Anxiety-related somatic reactions during missile attacks. Isr J Med Sci 1991;27:677–80.
[8] Norwood AE, Ursano RJ. Psychiatric intervention in post-disaster recovery. Directions In Psychiatry 1997;17:247–62.
[9] Ursano RJ, McCarroll JE. Exposure to traumatic death: the nature of the stressor. In: Ursano RJ, McCaughey BG, Fullerton CS, editors. Individual and community response to trauma and disaster. New York: Cambridge University Press; 1994. p. 46–71.
[10] Shaw JA. Children, adolescents and trauma. Psychiatr Q 2000;(71)3:227–43.
[11] Rafael B. Conclusion: debriefing-science, belief and wisdom. In: Raphael B, Wilson JP, editors. Psychological debriefing: theory, practice and evidence. NewYork: Cambridge University Press; 2000. p. 351–9.
[12] Sime JD. The concept of panic. London: David Fulton Publisher, Ltd.; 1990.
[13] Solomon SD, Smith EM. Social supports and perceived control as moderators of response to dioxin and flood exposure. In: Ursano RJ, McCaughey BG, Fullerton CS, editors. Individual and community response to trauma and disaster. New York: Cambridge University Press; 1994. p. 179–200.
[14] Becker SM. Meeting the threat of weapons of mass destruction terrorism: toward a broader conception of consequence management. Mil Med 2001;166:13–6.
[15] Becker SM. Psychosocial effects of radiation accidents. In: Gusev I, Guskova A, Mettler FA Jr, editors. Medical management of radiation accidents. 2nd edition. Boca Raton: CRC Press; 2001 [chapter 41].
[16] Shalev AY. Biological responses to disasters. Psychiatr Q 2000;(71)3:277–88.
[17] DiGiovanni Jr C. Domestic terrorism with chemical or biological agents: psychiatric aspects. Am J Psychiatry 1999;156(10):1500–5.

[18] Franz DR, Jahrling PB, Friedlander AM, et al. Clinical recognition and management of patients exposed to biological warfare agents. JAMA 1997;278:399–411.

[19] Holloway HC, Benedek DM. The changing face of terrorism and military psychiatry. Psychiatric Annals 1999;29(6):363–74.

[20] Bryant RA, Harvey AG, Dang ST, et al. Treatment of acute stress disorder: a comparison of cognitive-behavioral therapy and supportive counseling. J Consult Clin Psychol 1998;66(5): 862–6.

[21] Foa EB, Hearst-Ikeda D, Perry KJ. Evaluation of a brief cognitive-behavioral program for the prevention of chronic PTSD in recent assault victims. J Consult Clin Psychol 1995;63(6): 948–55.

[22] North CS, Nixon SJ, Shariat S, et al. Psychiatric disorders among survivors of the Oklahoma City bombing. JAMA 1999;(282)8:755–62.

[23] Holloway HC, Norwood AE, Fullerton CS, et al. The threat of biological weapons: prophylaxis and mitigation of psychological and social consequences. JAMA 1997;278: 425–7.

[24] Peters RG, Covello VT, McCallum DB. The determinants of trust and credibility in environmental risk communication: an empirical study. Risk Anal 1997;17:43–54.

[25] Breslau N, Davis GC, Andreski P, et al. Sex differences in posttraumatic stress disorder. Arch Gen Psychiatry 1997;54:1044–8.

[26] Breslau N, Schultz LR, Peterson EL. Sex differences in depression: a role for pre-existing anxiety. Psychiatry Res 1995;58:1–12.

[27] Raphael B. When disaster strikes: how individuals and communities cope with catastrophe. New York: Basic Books; 1986.

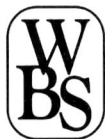

EMERGENCY
MEDICINE
CLINICS OF
NORTH AMERICA

Emerg Med Clin N Am
20 (2002) 409–436

Mass casualty management of a large-scale bioterrorist event: an epidemiological approach that shapes triage decisions

Frederick M. Burkle, Jr., MD, MPH, FAAP, FACEP

The Center for International Emergency, Disaster and Refugee Studies,
Departments of Emergency Medicine, and International Health,
Schools of Medicine and Public Health, The Johns Hopkins Medical Institutions,
1830 East Monument Street, Suite 6-100, Baltimore, MD 21205, USA
Advanced Systems Concept Office, 8725 John Kingman Rd,
Defense Threat Reduction Agency, Fort Belvoir, VA 22060, USA

"No close student of the problems of either military or civilian medicine has ever proposed an alternative to triage"
Garrett Hardin, Promethean Ethics, 1980 [1]

During disasters, health care professionals have an obligation to treat as many victims as possible who have a chance of survival. Clinicians sort, screen, and prioritize victims in a resource-constrained environment, a process referred to as triage. Decision criteria for triage management are the likelihood of medical success and the conservation of scarce resources [2,3].

Triage is common to all disasters, regardless of size. The PICE (Potential Injury/Illness Creating Event) disaster nomenclature (Table 1) attempts to provide a method for consistency in disaster classification, based on the likelihood that outside medical assistance will be needed [4]. Stage 0 means little or no chance, stage I means there is a small chance, stage II means there is a moderate chance, and stage III means local medical resources are clearly overwhelmed.

E-mail address: fburkle@jhsph.edu (F.M. Burkle, Jr.).

The opinions and assertions contained herein are the private views of the author and are not to be construed as official or reflecting the views of the Department of Defense.

Table 1
Potential injury/illness creating event (PICE) nomenclature

A	B	C	PICE stage
Static	Controlled	Local	0
Dynamic	Disruptive	Regional	I
Dynamic	Paralytic	National	II
Dynamic	Paralytic	International	III

Column A describes the potential for additional casualties. Column B describes whether resources are overwhelmed and, if so, whether they must be augmented (disruptive) or first need to be reconstituted (paralytic). Column C describes the extent of geographical involvement. The PICE stage refers to the likelihood that outside medical assistance will be needed.

Adapted from: Koenig KL, Dinerman N, Kuehl AE. Disaster nomenclature—a functional impact approach: the PICE system. Acad Emerg Med 1996;3:723–727.

A bio-terrorist (BT) disaster is an intentional epidemic caused by biological agents or biologically related toxins released on a population with the objective of causing fear, illness, or death. Although of low probability, a large-scale BT disaster would create a public health disaster in which the number of victims would exceed existing health care resources [3,5–8]. Triage will be practiced in a large-scale PICE stage I (dynamic, controlled, regional) to stage III (dynamic, paralytic, international) levels [4]. Stage progression may occur rapidly and uncontrollably: what is first considered a static, well-controlled local event can quickly become a regional or national disaster of paralytic proportions. With stage progression, management and triage inextricably become one.

Historical data suggest that future BT incidents will probably involve hoaxes or small-scale attacks [5,9,10]. There is evidence, however, that the technical barriers to mass-casualty terrorism are eroding [5,11]. Targets of terrorism are also changing. In a sample of 135 terrorist events, two types of targets have increased in frequency: the general civilian population (with the apparent intent of inflicting indiscriminate casualties) and the symbolic federal building or organization [10].

Studies suggest that in most cases the United States will have "some, little, or no capability" for BT mass casualty management and triage at four levels of medical care (local responders, initial treatment facilities, state, and federal) [12]. This study further suggests that existing conventional management and triage protocols for disasters fall short of meeting casualty management needs for a large-scale BT event. Where life-saving resources are either limited or not yet fully developed, management is inescapably connected to a sound epidemiologic approach that will help shape significant triage decisions. Management becomes an exercise in the triage of resources, supply, and distribution, and solutions to this dilemma are best achieved through the application of public health and epidemiologic principles, lateral decision-making processes, and strict adherence to exclusionary criteria, all beginning at the local level.

Conventional triage management

Disaster medicine deals with large populations. Triage is the first of three principles of mass casualty care, followed by standard procedures and evacuation [2]. Modern disaster medicine uses the *utilitarian* approach to triage, in which the greatest good is provided for the greatest number of victims in the shortest time to maximize success with the limited resources available [1–3,13,14]. An example of the utilitarian approach can be seen in International Humanitarian Law, which states that triage must provide the best "opportunity" to survive. This translates to receiving a fair triage process based on available resources, but it does not necessarily guarantee either treatment or survival [3,14–16].

Most of what is known of the triage process comes from treatment of victims of war trauma, in which it is used to determine who can be treated and expeditiously returned to the front line. The rapid treatment and evacuation of more seriously injured individuals is an important but *secondary* objective. Civilian triage protocols have different objectives. Civilian systems treat the most emergent first and attempt, where appropriate, to address broader community public health needs [1,2]. Triage is a dynamic process, constantly changing with victim status and resource availability. Popular triage systems, such as the Simple Triage And Rapid Treatment (START) algorithm, depend on physiologic criteria that are primarily trauma-oriented and are appropriate only for defined circumstances [17].

The management and triage process after a bioterrorism event

Discovery phase

The discovery of a BT incident will most likely occur in an emergency department, doctor's office, or clinic [5,12,18–21]. During the discovery phase, assumptions about the nature of the event will initially guide triage and management. One can assume that the "desired" terrorist bioagent will be an airborne virus or bacterium that is highly stable as an aerosol, highly contagious, has an incubation period of one week or less, a low recovery rate, and a course of at least three weeks duration [5,22]. The Centers for Disease Control and Prevention (CDC) Category A agents would be the most likely pathogens or toxins [23–26]. These agents, however, do not necessarily fit this classic profile: anthrax is not highly contagious, the infection-to-removal/recovery time for inhalational plague is approximately one week, and the incubation period of smallpox is approximately 12 days. Current public health laboratory testing, surveillance, and reporting are not timely enough to detect and then prevent a large, rapidly progressive outbreak. This is especially so if the agent is unusual, not included in state epidemiologic screening batteries, or if identification must be performed by remote laboratories. Initial identification must therefore rely on presenting signs and symptoms and supporting public health information, through a process known as syndromic surveillance [5,27].

Syndromic surveillance

The early clinical manifestations of disease caused by most BT agents may be nonspecific and could appear remarkably similar [20,28]. Immuno-compromised patients or those individuals exposed to higher inoculums may present early in the outbreak, before the event has been discovered. A high level of alertness is therefore required. Schultz challenges the emergency physician and others to "think like an epidemiologist," and to suspect a biological weapon when clusters of syndromes are seen [29].

Certain syndromes would be characteristic of potential BT attacks, and awareness of these syndromes by practitioners may promote early discovery. In anticipation of the 2001 Presidential Inauguration, the Maryland Department of Health asked that physicians maintain a high level of suspicion for any of the following syndromes [30]:

- Gastroenteritis of any apparent infectious etiology
- Pneumonia with the sudden death of a previously healthy adult
- Widened mediastinum in a febrile patient with no other explanation
- Rash of synchronous vesicular/pustular lesions
- Acute neurologic illness with fever
- Advancing cranial nerve impairment with progressive generalized weakness

Similarly, Rega included the following in his list of "covert assault clues" [31]:

- Severe disease manifestations in previously healthy people
- Higher than normal number of patients with fever and respiratory/ gastrointestinal complaints
- Multiple people with similar complaints from a common location
- An endemic disease appearing during an unusual time of year
- Unusual number of rapidly fatal cases
- Greater number of ill or dead animals
- Rapidly rising and falling epidemic curve
- Greater numbers of patients with:
    severe pneumonia
    sepsis
    sepsis with coagulopathy
    fever with rash
    diplopia with progressive weakness

Knowledge of these syndromes by frontline clinicians forms the basis on which to initially confirm or deny the presence of a bioagent. The syndromic events become the target of surveillance. Discovery of an abnormal syndrome or unexpected incidence within the community should lead to the development of a case definition of the infectious disease process in question. At the same time, one must be cognizant of any variation in the case definition that might make one suspect a mixed or genetically altered bioagent. Case definitions may be communicated as "suspect, presumptive, or confirmed" [32–35]. The more refined a case definition, the more realistic triage and management decisions will become.

Epidemiologic analysis phase

The process from discovery to management can be complex. Steps include the active collection of information, rapid verification (early detection devices, rapid laboratory diagnosis), epidemiologic investigation and surveillance, sharing of information, and eventually the implementation of control measures [34,35]. Once an abnormality is discovered, whether it is a single illness, an unexplained cluster of illnesses, or a mass-illness event, an epidemiologic investigation must occur in tandem with case definition development. This epidemiologic function is of paramount importance in the recognition of an epidemic caused by terrorism [5,36]. Epidemiologic assessment, ideally using state-of-the-art epidemiologic resources (ie, computer-assisted–trained epidemiologists, ready links to public health agencies and laboratories) [5,33], may provide objective information about the effects of the bioagent on the population and the projections that may be used to match available resources to a population's emergency needs. It may also increase the efficiency with which finite resources are allocated [32]. Unfortunately the ability to use this information with total objectivity and detachment may be difficult [37]. Additionally, the "working" epidemic models that guide the response may change, especially if the BT event were to escalate to a regional, national, or international crisis.

To assist in rapid data collection and analysis, the CDC has developed the EpiInfo computer software program in which questionnaires can be created, data entered and analyzed, and line listings produced [38,39]. The proposed concept of operations is that this process will be performed on pre-loaded handheld devices that can upload continuous data for dynamic analyses.

Data can be evaluated quantitatively, and graphic representation of this information, known as *epidemic curves* (epi-curves), may prove especially useful in this endeavor. These visual representations depict case frequency over time, and are initially used to obtain tentative answers to questions concerning origin, propagation, incidence, prevalence, and likely modes of transmission. The nature of the epidemic curve varies with the pathogen but allows an estimate of incubation time of the infection, which then assists in the identification of the pathogen itself [39–43]. The frequency curve for most infectious diseases resembles a logarithmic normal curve. Each infectious agent has its characteristic range of incubation periods in a particular host species that can help identify the pathogen during the discovery phase

[40,43,44]. Epi-curve analysis is simple and uses the median incubation period as a measure of central tendency and the dispersion factor as a measure of variability [40,43,45–48]. This process helps in estimating the date of common exposure and a timeframe on which the epidemiologic team should focus further investigations. This methodology has proved instrumental in the eradication of infectious diseases (eg, smallpox) [49].

Simple epidemic models are available to explore the impact of disease variables on healthy and infected populations [39,41,50]. For example, a point source curve (Fig. 1) would be produced by release of *Bacillus anthracis* spores and analysis may allow an estimate of the rate of release. This estimate may then provide valuable guidance in searching for a location common to those individuals exposed during that time period [39,40].

Propagative curves (Fig. 2) would be more characteristic of highly infectious agents such as smallpox and inhalational plague. Early in an outbreak of a progressive BT epidemic, epi-curves may also assist in refining resource allocation that will be tentative at best at this point. Management teams will undoubtedly be struggling to ensure initial and future resource requirements.

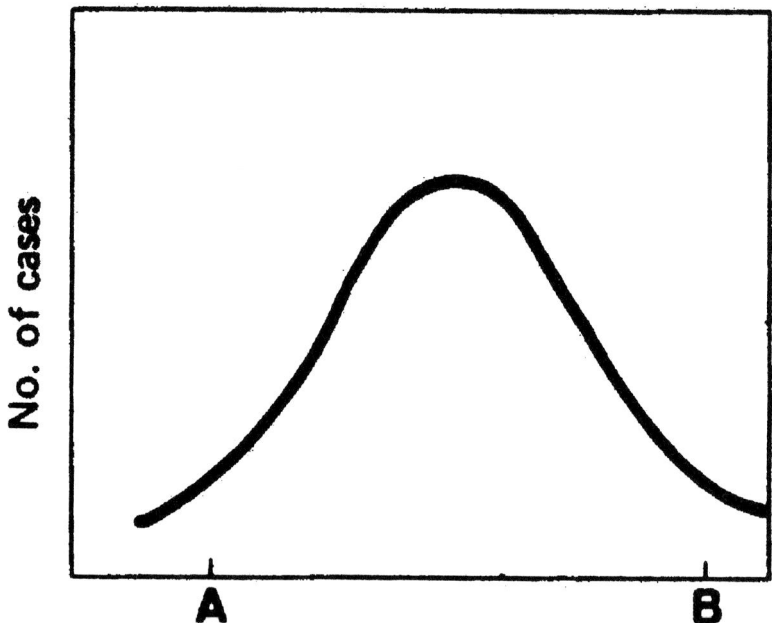

Fig. 1. In a common source epidemic, the population at risk was exposed at one point in time to, for example, botulin (the neurotoxin responsible for botulism). Cases occur suddenly after the minimum incubation time and continue for a brief period, depending on the variability in incubation time of infected individuals. If the interval between A and B is consistent with a known incubation period, then all exposures occurred on the same day. Without a secondary spread of the toxin or pathogen to others, the epidemic ends.

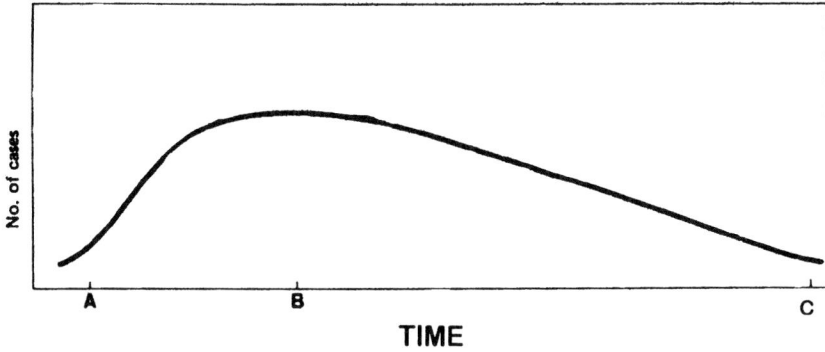

Fig. 2. Propagative or progressive curves give evidence of an epidemic involving the spread of a pathogen by uncontrolled person-to-person transmission from a common source or the presence of a common source over a long time, as would occur with smallpox and inhalational plague. Secondary cases are illustrated by B and C. Irregular peaks occur frequently in propagative epidemics, reflecting the number of infected sources and the numbers of susceptible and exposed persons.

Epi-curves may provide clues that an epidemic involving a naturally occurring pathogen is actually caused by a bioterrorist event, because typical epidemics such as influenza have distinctly different patterns of initiation and spread (Fig. 3). Epi-curves may also be used to update and follow the effectiveness of certain control measures such as vaccination and quarantine (Fig. 4).

Curve analysis may also provide details on unique characteristics of the BT agent. Studies suggest that large (unnatural) inhalational doses of Ebola

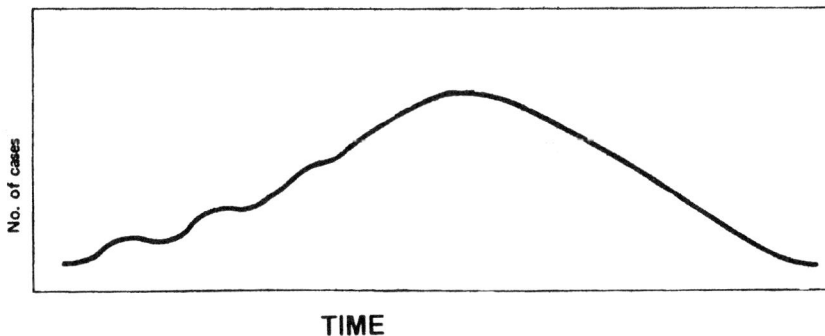

Fig. 3. A slower, gradual buildup of cases in an epidemic that does not originate from a common source of exposure causes a wave-like pattern in the early part of the epidemic. This pattern represents generations of transmission, with the interval between the two crests being the average incubation period. This pattern may be found with a human reservoir aerosol-borne disease [41,50].

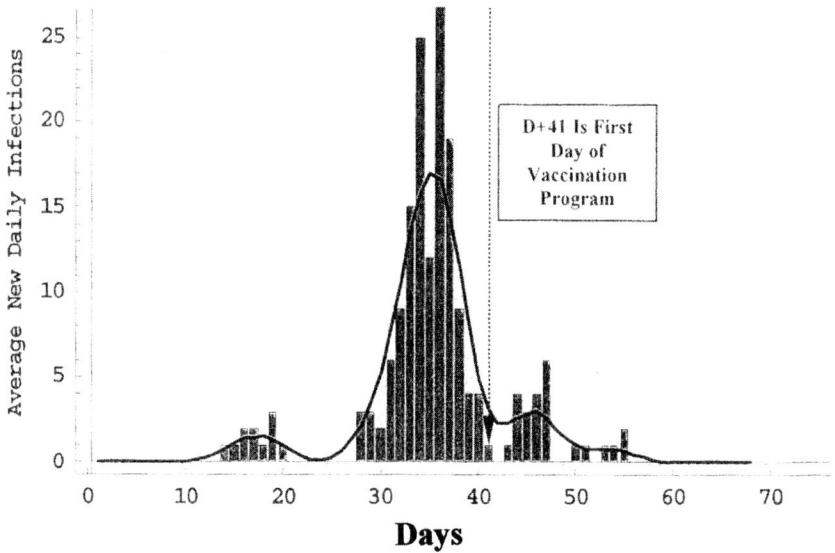

Fig. 4. 1972 smallpox outbreak depicting case distribution, epidemic curve, and onset of vaccination control measure. *Based on*: Bombardt JN Jr. Smallpox transmission and BW casualty assessments. Institute for Defense Analyses document P-3550. 2001.

do appear to substantially shorten the onset-to-death period, a characteristic that might occur in other bioagents [51].

Mathematical modeling

Mathematical modeling (MM) is an analysis tool especially applicable to the understanding of large population dynamics, disease transmission, casualty estimates, and extrapolation of the impact of major control measures such as national or international immunization programs [39,52–55]. MM facilitates understanding of the interplay between variables affecting the course of the epidemic and variables that control the pattern of infection and the disease within the population. MM has already been used to control or eliminate a disease that is usually endemic. Research is currently facilitating new insights into the nature of potential bioagents, the impact of primary and secondary infections, and the effectiveness of disease control measures on such known virulent infections as Ebola, smallpox, and inhalational plague [52,54,56–59].

Such analyses have led to important epidemiologic insights that directly affect emergency medical and triage management, such as decisions to implement quarantine, forced isolation, population evacuation, or control zones [39]. Epidemics cannot be spread in a population of susceptible individuals whose density is low. Without this density threshold, infection cannot be sustained and therefore dies out [60]. The eradication of an epidemic by mass immunization can be understood in reducing the density of susceptible individuals below a threshold required for the spread of infection. Called *herd immunity*, it is critical to the triage management of limited vaccine resources to know the infection can be eradicated with less than 100% effective immunization [39]. Given that there will be limited vaccine and resources, by raising the immunity above a certain population threshold with the vaccine that is available, the remaining non-immune individuals can be protected.

Whether the modeling data can assist the urgent policy decisions required in a bioterrorism event remains unknown. The importance of MM was recognized during the recent Foot and Mouth disease epidemic in Great Britain. Epidemiologists anticipated a "very large epidemic" requiring "drastic measures" to reduce transmission. Data, backed by MM, supported a rapidly expanding epidemic despite existing control measures. Initially these views were considered politically unacceptable, and the epidemic worsened. Once the modeling data were allowed to drive policy decisions the epidemic was brought under control [61].

Lateral decision-making and triage management phase

Triage authority

Early in the Persian Gulf War, triage officers recognized that they might confront multiple weaponry options, including biological, chemical, mixed biological-chemical, or some combination with explosives [62]. During the 1996 Olympics in Atlanta, the CDC enlisted assistance from multiple agencies and laboratories to ensure a robust capacity to identify and manage the consequences of a variety of potential weaponry, including single known, unknown, and mixed pathogens, and multiple chemical and nuclear devices. In both instances, the decision-making responsibilities were more complex than one person or agency could realistically manage [63].

"Environmental resources" have been defined as those resources not internal to the individual making demands for those resources [1]. Normally a community controls environmental resources. The right-of-allocation of these resources may be reserved for the community, acting through its legitimate authorities. It has been argued that triage management should be built on equal concern for each person, regardless of demands on environmental resources; this is referred to as parity policy [1]. Triage policy, however, specifically recognizes the inequality of demands on these resources, and would place the right-of-allocation in the hands of those authorities who have the intent of maximizing the saving of lives (assumed to apply to a triage team given such empowerment). Analyses of both approaches have shown that the efficiency of the triage policy in saving lives consistently increases with the total cohort sample size (variable n) [1,14]. BT events bring new demands and responsibilities in triage, because of the adversarial implications that such an intentional act carries and the potential that available resources are not medically helpful because the bioagents are either genetically altered, mixed pathogens, or antibiotic-resistant [9]. These results make a strong case for communities' responsibility to ensure the preparedness of a pre-selected triage team.

A PICE stage 0 or local disaster assumes that the outbreak will be controlled by local resources without an immediate need for outside aid. In a BT event, however, that assumption may not be entirely valid. Variability in incubation periods may create a situation in which initial victims are given full medical attention with resources available, because a definitive event that hallmarks a mass casualty incident is lacking. It is unlikely that a BT event will have the conventional trigger or threshold point that defines the time at which triage procedures must be initiated, and initial cases might actually be harbingers of a propagative event in which index cases have already widely spread. It is a management responsibility to alert potential assets and open lines of communication for rapid consultation and early lateral decision-making [9,61,64,65]. The CDC phrase "think BT, call this telephone number" is essential to mature triage management [19,31–33,66]. It is expected that any health care provider in charge of triage management will ensure that early notification of the CDC, Public Health agencies, the Federal Bureau of Investigation (FBI), and the Federal Emergency Management Agency (FEMA), by local and state public health officials, has occurred. The CDC has direct links to the World Health Organization (WHO) Outbreak Verification Team that is positioned to coordinate infectious disease surveillance and response on a global level, and has set up a process for timely outbreak verification with capacity to convert large amounts of data into accurate information for suitable action [34]. Although some diseases are almost always regarded as important for international public health (eg, smallpox, plague, Ebola hemorrhagic fever), others may not be [34].

In a suspected or actual BT event, emergency medical management and triage decisions must be, at the minimum, a *team effort*. At the community level, emergency managers (local and FEMA), the Department of Justice (FBI), the political authorities (mayor, governor), and technical experts ("tactical scientists" with expertise in epidemiology and infectious diseases, for example) will make up the *lateral decision-making process* that is necessary for managing these events (as opposed to vertical decision-making in which one agency or individual makes all the decisions) [63,67,68]. Even at the hospital level the triage officer will have pharmacists, infectious disease specialists, administrators, pulmonary care technicians, and others as team members, all of who must think beyond the case at hand and into the future. Emergency medical management and triage decisions will be based on rapidly assessing (Table 2) the evolving epidemiology to forecast a nononsense approach to resource allocation.

Table 2
Questions addressed simultaneously by triage

1. What are the goals and objectives of triage for the hospital? For the community?
2. What is the ranking (priorities) of the goals and objectives?
3. What are the causes of mortality and morbidity associated with the bioagent?
4. What are the causes of mortality and morbidity indirectly associated with the bioagent?
5. What are the consequent public health problems of most concern to the hospital? To the community?
6. What nonhealth problems exist because of the bioagent?
7. What are the biomedical or public health consequences of these problems?
8. What is the ranking (priorities) of these problems?
9. What resources are needed to address these problems?
10. What resources are available now?
11. What are the existing barriers to addressing the above questions?
12. How and for how long can the healthcare infrastructure sustain the demands placed on it from the BT event?
13. What other organizations and agencies can be drawn on for support?
14. What triage behaviors relate to treatment and which relate to prevention?
15. What triage behaviors should be priorities?
16. Does triage address health indicators (water, sanitation, food, shelter) and quality of life issues?

Some will argue that these events can be handled with local coordination of existing resources, as usually happens in other epidemics. As the BT event escalates from PICE stage I to III, however, a more lateral decision-making process, one that mixes managers and technical experts, will be necessary. No one single agency or organization yet possesses the surge capacity required for such an event [44,67,68].

Coordination across multiple agencies presents problems in and of itself. For example, the Hospital Emergency Incident Command system (HEIC) is designed to facilitate decision-making involving such things as staffing, evacuation, and coordination with law enforcement during large-scale disasters. Yet, during the Northridge, California earthquake some hospitals broke from HEIC protocol, re-routing ambulances and refusing to evacuate as ordered. Major decisions were made inefficiently, requiring marathon conference calls with up to 100 people where "...roles, authorities and even identities of those participating were unclear" [44]. In the New York City West Nile Virus outbreak, it was unclear who was in charge, with up to 18 agencies jockeying for authority [44]. It is said that triage is dangerously naïve about political consequences. In the last analysis, triage and management decisions must be enacted in a timely manner despite political challenges to do otherwise.

Triage goals in a BT event

Triage in a BT event is victim- and community-oriented. These events may be ongoing and have the potential for long-lasting effects. With secondary infections, there will be marked increase in intensity and duration. All of this can contribute to an increased consumption of resources.

Triage goals for those bioagents that only produce primary infections should be to rapidly treat those patients with likelihood of success with available resources. There will probably be few opportunities to prevent primary infections or successfully treat many patients with advanced symptoms. EMS management will be directed toward identifying and transporting victims to treatment facilities.

For those bioagents that transmit infection easily (eg, smallpox, Ebola), triage is directed to *prevent secondary infections* [39,56,58]. Traditional prehospital EMS management will be limited or contraindicated. Transport without strict barrier protection will place responders and equipment at great risk for contamination and will compromise EMS early in a contagious epidemic before implementation of these controls. The best method to prevent secondary infections is to reduce Ro (basic reproduction rate) of the bioagent by lowering the effective contact rate between individuals. This can be accomplished by treating infections (eg, prophylactic antibiotics, vaccinations), changing behaviors (eg, preventing religious rites and viewing of the infectious dead), sanitation (proper barrier precautions and handling of corpses), and quarantine (eg, reverse quarantine, forced isolation) [39,69]. If this process is performed using epidemiologic principles, the epidemic will die out.

Another goal of triage is to ensure adequate resources. This includes availability of consumable supplies and maintenance of an organizational structure that provide functional capability and capacity overtime. Resources include hospital and outpatient professional and administrative personnel, detection devices, barrier devices, laboratory resources, pharmaceuticals, ventilators, emergency department and hospitals beds, ICU beds, morgue storage capacity, augmentation facilities and personnel, and volunteers. Analyses of epidemic curves in theoretical BT events reveal that bed days and outpatient visits per patient influence triage systems and decisions. A CDC analysis of three biowarfare agents predicts the resource requirements presented in Table 3 [44].

Table 3
Theorized resource requirements following release of bioterrorist agents in a population of 100,000

Bioagent	Percent hospitalized	No. of in-hospital days	No. of post-hospitalization outpatient visits	No. of outpatient visits	No. of relapse days in 1 year
Anthrax	95%	7	2	28	None
Tularemia	95%	10	2	12	12
Brucellosis	50%	7	7	14	14

Based on: Kaufmann AF, Meltzer MI, Schmid GP. The economic impact of a bioterrorist attack: are prevention and postattack intervention programs justifiable? Emerg Infect Dis. Available at: 3(2): http://www.cdc.gov/ncidod/EID/vol3no2/kaufman.htm. Accessed April–June, 1997.

To anticipate demand for antibiotics, days of treatment (inpatient and outpatient) and efficacy of the treatment course need to be known for each bioagent. For example, in research modeling, intervention strategies for anthrax, tularemia, and brucellosis varied from 14 to 28 days of oral and parenteral antibiotics (efficacy range 80%–90%), plus human anthrax vaccine for an additional 3 doses. This research also suggests that compliance would be 90% for patients exposed in target areas studied [44].

A third triage goal will be to ensure that the "susceptible worried well" subgroup does not overwhelm health facilities dealing with "infective" cohorts. Pre-designated neighborhood collecting, clearing, and information centers for triage, isolation, and education may be needed. A critical measure of effectiveness for triage management in a BT event will be how rapidly a robust system of health information can be mobilized. Once this is established, the subgroup of worried well should decline in number.

Finally, if a goal of the terrorist is to compromise the government by revealing its vulnerability in defending its citizens, a secondary goal of triage is to maintain the continuity of government. A BT event will negatively affect a government's capacity, and may create political, economic, and social instability. Price-Smith defines state capacity (SC) as a country's capacity to maximize its stability in exerting de facto control and protecting its population from infectious agents [70]. The initial SC will determine the scale of adaptive resources that may be mobilized to deal with the disease process. The United States prides itself on its SC, but the only means by which countries with lower SC can ameliorate the overwhelming effects of a BT event is through exogenous resources and mobilization of advanced technical and tactical knowledge.

Triage categories

To be effective, triage requires appropriate categorization of victims. In conventional triage, disposition of a patient at each phase of response and treatment level is determined by the assigned triage category. Usually based on anatomic or physiologic alterations caused by trauma, these categories are not relevant in large-scale BT unless, by chance, the bioagent was combined with an explosive device. In a PICE stage 0 BT event, multiple triage categories may not even be necessary. The triage process would be directed at distinguishing between those patients requiring treatment and those patients not, or those with a lethal infection and those with non-lethal infections [64].

Triage categorization during a large-scale BT event is essential. Categories will not only determine individual victim disposition, but also will serve as markers in the evolving epidemic, such as the distribution of infectious contacts within the population and the rate of spread. They also may be of predictive value in anticipating the ultimate outcome of the disease. Because the ultimate magnitude of the BT epidemic will determine required resources, this information is essential to ensure proper resource allocation. The conventional epidemiologic approach during epidemics is to divide a closed population into susceptible individuals, infective individuals, and removed (by successful immunization, recovery, or death) individuals, and is referred to as the SIR Model (Fig. 5).

The author suggests that an expanded version of SIR analytic framework, referred to as SEIRV (Fig. 6), provides the basis for a triage tool to identify potential steps and avoid missteps in the course of management of a potential bioagent [39,71].

SEIRV uses five categories

1. Susceptible individuals (includes those with incomplete or unsuccessful vaccination)
2. Exposed individuals (those who are infected, incubating, and noncontagious)
3. Infectious individuals (those who are symptomatic and contagious)
4. Removed individuals (those who are no longer sources of infection; they either survive or die from the illness, with the remains no longer contagious)
5. Vaccinated successfully (those with confirmed "take" or who completed course for immunity)

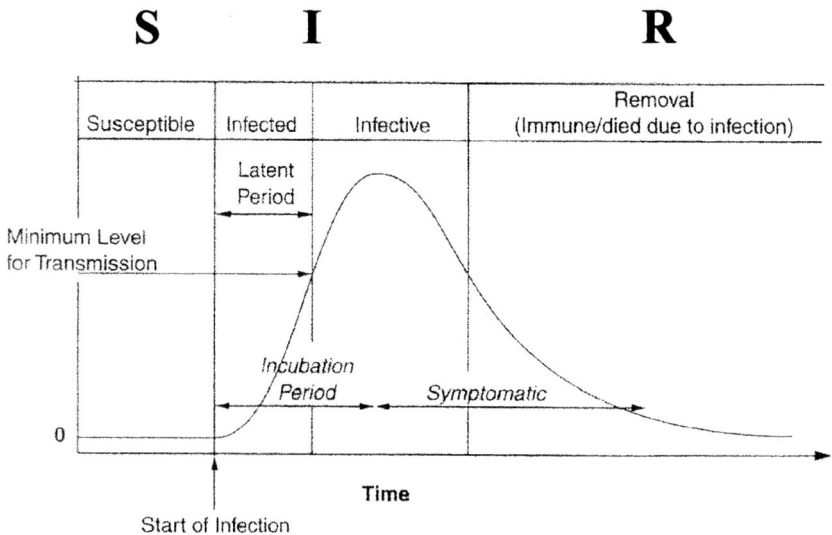

Fig. 5. SIR cohort classification depicting level of bioagent in the host population. *Adapted with permission from.* Aron JL. Mathematical modeling. the dynamics of infection. In: Nelson KE, Williams CM, Graham NMH, editors. Infectious disease epidemiology: theory and practice. Gaithersburg, MD: Aspen Publishers; 2001. p. 151 (used with permission).

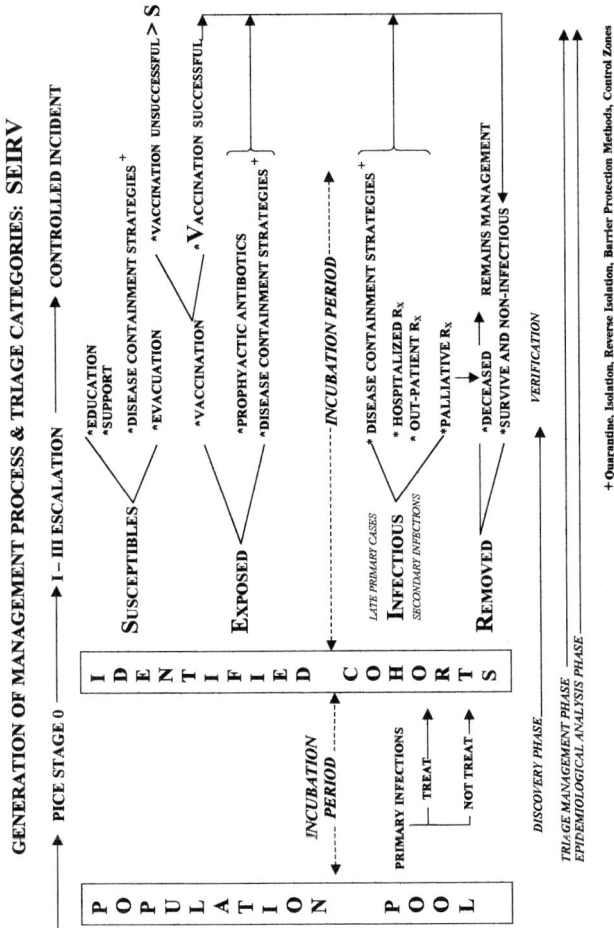

Fig. 6. Depicts PICE stage-related generation of management and triage options for a large-scale population cohort of potential SEIRV categories.

These categories may be further refined to better guide definitive management decisions. For example, the 'infectious' cohort could be subgrouped as follows:

- Those patients so seriously ill that they either cannot survive or require an unreasonably large allotment of medical resources. Victims would receive palliative treatment and appropriate emotional and religious support, unless victims or remains were infective (eg, Ebola, smallpox, or inhalational plague patients and remains).
- Those patients who can be saved by a reasonable amount of care but would die without it, and ultimately require hospitalization.
- Those patients who will survive with a preselected treatment program, best served in a less intensive or outpatient setting, and discharged to home or to observation units with designated outpatient follow-up (eg, oral and parenteral antibiotics for early symptoms and prophylactic antibiotics for those patients in the "exposed" category).

The SEIRV analytic model has identified specific triage priorities (patient isolation, barrier nursing techniques, and strict disinfection procedures of biohazardous materials, including corpses) in Ebola, and monitored the effectiveness of control zones, especially in PICE stage II and III events [39,71].

Even using this approach, difficulties with triage accuracy will arise. If neither the biological agents nor the clinical course of exposed individuals are known, there may be little opportunity for preventive or prophylactic measures and health care providers must "catch up" with the disease as it unfolds. Bombardt suggests that this latter course of action is "perilous, especially in the case of a highly infectious agent like smallpox" [58].

Perhaps most difficulty will come in distinguishing those individuals actually exposed from those individuals potentially exposed, psychologically impaired casualties, individuals with multiple unexplained physical symptoms (MUPS), and those simply susceptible but concerned that they might have been exposed [66,72,73]. This subgroup may well make up most of those seeking care [47,48,68]. Triage personnel not accustomed to managing people with anxiety may under-triage these victims as "worried well." System planning must provide predesignated programs for evaluation, education, and reassurance; emotional support can occur separate from but close to any health facility, to ensure ready access, availability, and compliance.

Overtriage may also occur, especially in those cases with histories of exposure or potential exposure (close contact or family member). There may be a rush to treat all children, the elderly, handicapped people, and individuals with immune compromise with outpatient antibiotics. Triage accuracy should improve with experience or when geographic, plume, and other data (confirmatory tests or demographic data) become known, but there will be a tendency to overtriage in favor of treatment. Overtriage is known in blast injuries, in which initially there may be a total lack of physical findings other than history of being close to a blast (ie, landmine) that resulted in the severe injury or death of another person [74–76]. Because of the risk for delayed adult respiratory distress syndrome or bowel perforation the overtriage rate may be 50% or more. In a BT event, research suggests that an additional 5% to15% of nonexposed but susceptible persons will receive treatment [44]. This percentage may be conservative. These will be difficult decisions and might not even be considered if resources are lacking.

Triage tags aid in identifying victims and their injuries and in determining priorities for treatment and evacuation, and further serve as a rudimentary but essential medical record that follows victims through the treatment process. Tags functionally must reflect identified cohorts within the population requiring intervention, and therefore would be widely distributed to facilities with different health care missions (eg, vaccination centers, collecting, clearing, and information centers, outpatient clinics, and emergency departments) To be effective they must be simple, easily understood, and allow for brief documentation of decisions within categories (Fig. 7). They must be useful to the management process and provide clarification not confusion. If resources improve or deteriorate, warranting a new category, a new tag is added (on top) with time and date, with the new management decisions recorded [2]. Triage tagging is an imperfect science and is often not used for a variety of reasons, including lack of availability or provider unfamiliarity. Research into other means of providing medical records and patient tracking, such as personal archival data sources in the form of "smartcards," is being done, and may provide other options in the future.

Triage efficiency

Triage, and thus resource allocation, efficiency can be measured as "life saved" (L) per unit "effort" (E) or resources required. Hopelessly ill or injured patients have a low L/E value because E is so great. Patients who can be saved by a reasonable amount of care but who would die without it have high L/E values [1]. Most efficient is the use of preventive or prophylactic medications or vaccines to ensure the performance of critical personnel (eg, medical, essential leadership). Each designated triage category should be tested against disaster-specific (ie, bioagent-specific) requirements to ensure resource allocation efficiency and to prospectively set thresholds for initiating care.

Inclusion and exclusion criteria

Conventional triage training and assumptions for care in developed countries are based on *inclusion* criteria [14]. These criteria assume that personnel have been trained in a resource-adequate environment, that they are well versed in basic and advanced standards of care, and that appropriate

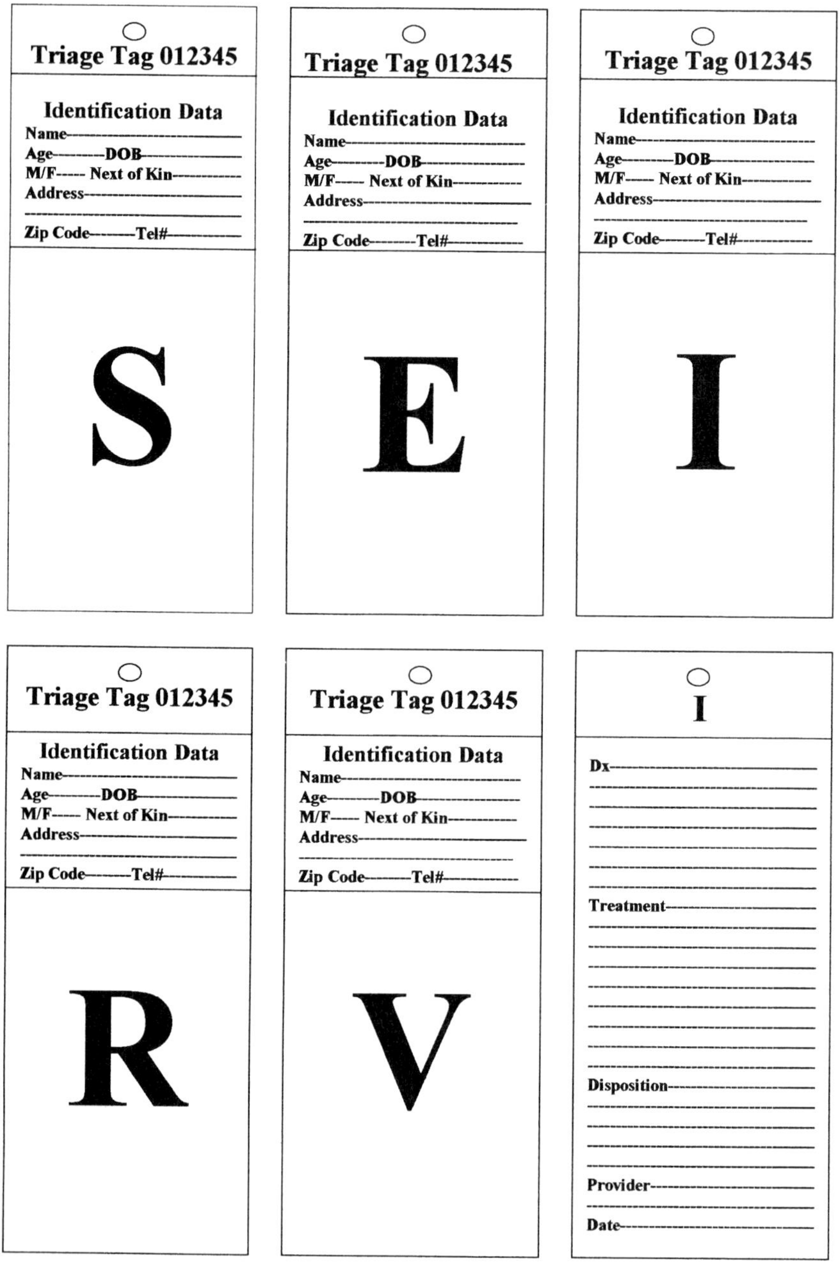

Fig. 7. Example of SEIRV-cohort population triage tags. Tags in a large-scale disaster serve as medical records and may be the only medical documentation available. Large population triage and treatments will occur over a vast geographic area (eg, vaccination centers, outpatient clinics, emergency departments, hospitals, and private offices).

resources will be available without compromise at every level. Few health care providers have experience or practice in large-scale triage or case management in an austere or resource-constrained environment in which, inevitably, some degree of *exclusion* criteria must be practiced [2,13,14]. In such situations, resources are scarce and standards of care may be either limited in scope or not possible at all, making triage totally resource-driven. Although at first glance triage during these large-scale events seems illogical, further exploration usually reveals that strategies were based on exclusion criteria calculated to conserve resources for those individuals with illnesses or injuries who had the greatest likelihood of success (see section on Triage lessons learned from large-scale disasters). In these environments, expectations are that health care providers will discuss resource availability and determine (sometimes on a daily or hourly basis) what supplies can be used and in what amounts (eg, intravenous antibiotics, early intubation and ventilatory support, and intensive care) [77–80].

Minimal qualification for survival

In a resource-constrained environment, exclusionary criteria and other factors, such as ability of the existing health care system to recover and rehabilitate the victim, must be collated to determine which illness or injuries are not amenable to treatment [14]. Health care providers must determine, as soon as possible, the minimal qualifications for survival (MQS), recognizing that these will change with resource availability. As a general rule, anyone requiring major resuscitation (demanding numerous pharmaceuticals and personnel resources) would be immediately excluded. Further MQS criteria will vary depending on factors such as nursing care expertise, security, health infrastructure, and re-supply. This aspect of the triage process is seemingly abhorrent and unthinkable [1,14,81]. MQS, however, remains a necessary tenet of the triage decision-making process that defines its credibility over time.

Triage lessons learned from large-scale disasters

It is rare for the United States to suffer a large-scale disaster requiring triage for a prolonged period of time. Most disasters result in limited numbers of casualties that are easily managed with high physician-to-victim ratios. If resources are a problem, it is usually one of time-limited distribution and not a lack of actual resources. Personnel, equipment, and evacuation are rarely compromised. Documentation of the planning or events during the Cold War, the Persian Gulf War, and complex emergencies of the past decade, however, highlights the potential problems that a large-scale, non-conventional disaster might cause. In all events, resource driven exclusion criteria were required in the triage process.

Triage resulting from weapons of mass destruction

During the Cold War, the British government studied the medical consequences of potential low- and high-yield nuclear explosion scenarios based
on computer-generated estimates of casualties [81,82]. The National Health
Service (NHS) defined a "mass casualty situation" as "one in which the total
medical resources of an area are already overwhelmed or are about to be
overwhelmed, with no prospect of early outside assistance" [81]. The principles of the NHS policy were considered "harsh" when simple rescue and
comfort were abandoned in health planning [81]; yet they were grounded
in reality, meaning that realistic and uncomfortable triage decisions would
need to be made. In some high-yield scenarios that specifically targeted
larger conurbations, the government came close to writing off entire cities
as an act of policy [82].

Health care providers and medical supplies were to be treated as national
commodities of particular value, to be dispersed and stockpiled for the
future. The casualty policy in 1977 repeatedly warned about not wasting
medical staff on "organized life saving operations" [71,81]. The NHS
assumed that deaths and injury in hospital medical personnel (and those
potentially available personnel) occurred in the same proportion as for the
general population, and that health care provider availability would be further compromised as some providers might consider it their duty to stay
with their families in the immediate aftermath of the attack [71,81,82]. In
Hiroshima, physician-victims who were unable to function as health care
providers simply looked after themselves [83–85].

The survival ratio in hospitals was 1 in 14, with 150 candidates for each
surviving bed in a population of 1.1 million. The health departments did not
envisage a general evacuation of patients to other hospitals, believing that
despite national plans to the contrary, this would not realistically occur.
It was impossible to predetermine the proportion of beds that could be freed
quickly [82].

The aim of medical care would be to save the maximum number of lives.
This could only be achieved by refusing medical assistance to those unlikely
to recover, and a NHS system of triage to address these issues was developed [45,71,81]. They defined a 3-tiered system of casualty control consisting
of First Aid Posts (FAPs), Casualty Collecting Centers (CCCs), and hospitals, to limit medical treatment to prevent resources from being overwhelmed. At any treatment facility, victims might or might not receive
treatment. FAP personnel were concerned primarily with reaching the
injured and getting them to the FAPs, sorting out the patients, taking care
of emergency cases, sending suitable patients to hospitals, evacuating others
to community care, and disposing of hundreds of thousands of corpses.
General life-saving procedures might not be possible. CCCs (1 for every
10,000 population) would be set up in each neighborhood between the FAPs
and the hospitals, to treat, sort, and hold casualties until they could be
accepted by a hospital. In some scenarios, CCCs would see more than

1000 victims [71,81,82]. "Triage would be done by a physician (if available), sorting would be necessary on arrival at the CCC...sorting (must) be repeated and continuous, it must be ruthless if it is to be effective; it would often be necessary to give priority to the less severely injured casualties and have regard to the nation's need in the phase of recovery" [82]. Triage teams had four to six practitioners with similar numbers of nurses, volunteers, and local authorities. Casualties were to be sorted into three categories [81]:

1. Those patients who will survive without further attention, who are sent home or to rest centers
2. Those patients who would need major medical attention to survive, who are triaged into a holding unit to die
3. Those patients who might go to a hospital for treatment if, after limited medical treatment, they would be likely to be alive after seven days, with a fair chance of eventual recovery

Each surviving physician would have between 400 and 900 casualties to contend with [82]. Exclusion criteria included those patients requiring major surgery, because of the likelihood that they would need blood products, and those patients requiring intravenous fluids or medication assumed contaminated with radiation.

Quick assessment was essential, because loss of time would result in movement of casualties from the "survival possible" to the "survival improbable" category [82]. Casualty numbers were expected to greatly exceed surviving hospital resources, and directors were to impose strict admission priorities. Triage would inevitably result in the retention at the CCCs of people so badly ill that treatment with limited resources would be wasted on them. Although lower-yield scenarios assumed that there would be enough providers to staff all the areas, under the larger-yield scenarios, "triage would be largely symbolic" [82].

Guidance on mass casualty care included the statement that "there is no objective of offering hope of medical treatment to anyone." It is easy to envisage the state of the holding units in which the "dead and the dying would lie together after a few days" [82]. Consideration was given to preselected triage criteria and government-trained triage officers with authority over a triage process that was designed to save a culture and stabilize a fragile government [82].

Triage resulting from complex humanitarian emergencies

Complex emergencies (CEs) of the last decade resulted in unprecedented numbers of civilian casualties [86]. Epidemiologic studies were integral to the understanding and response to CEs that were caused by major epidemics and migration of large populations [87]. Like BT events, CEs are a threat to safety and security, and often prevent adequate conventional epidemiologic studies from taking place. Rather, to make timely logistic and operational decisions, "quick and dirty" assessments were routinely performed [87].

Coupland has described the CE environment as one in which "few receive adequate medical care and the plight of the rest is appalling" [88]. Personnel, equipment, and evacuation are often compromised, first aid and transport are haphazard, hospital facilities are overwhelmed, inaccessible, or threatening, and water and electricity are non-existent [88]. Despite the warring, a military approach to triage with echelons of care has little relevance. Coupland's studies concluded that patients with life-threatening injuries died from lack of resources, nursing staff, re-supply, a working hospital infrastructure, and evacuation capacity. His investigations found, however, that operative management of some injuries (eg, soft-tissue low velocity wounds) could be delayed with the judicious use of antibiotics, tetanus prophylaxis, splints, and dressings alone until resources arrived [88]. This underscores the need for creative improvisation of care and the optimization of first aid, pain relief, preventive care, and education, especially if there are severe limitations on resources.

In Rwanda, the former Yugoslavia, and Cambodia, selective "cleansing" and genocide were directed at certain populations. In 1994, in Kigali, Rwanda, non-governmental organizations (NGOs) with few resources were confronted with more than 20,000 trauma casualties. With limited personnel and scant basic surgical equipment, the triage decision was to treat only those left standing [89]. By recognizing the limits of their trade, the triage process was appropriately redirected to preventing secondary morbidity and mortality in those individuals who had an opportunity to survive.

During CEs, hastily built refugee camps become overcrowded and lack basic public health infrastructure for the population served [90]. Exclusion criteria strongly influence the camp triage process. Triage decisions must be sensitive and specific enough to seek out severe treatable cases and those cases who present a risk to the refugee camp, such as measles (the most common cause of death in malnourished children), and to exclude chronic non-risk patients who sap limited resources. Case definitions and laboratory confirmation are routine to outbreak investigations necessary to prevent or control epidemics of cholera, dysentery, malaria, tuberculosis, and meningitis. In Rwandan refugee camps on the border with neighboring Zaire, NGOs were faced with an escalating epidemic of cholera and dysentery. Because of poor coordination of limited rehydration resources, lack of personnel expertise, and no minimal qualifications for survival, an initially flawed triage and decision-making process ensued. In these situations, medical care often takes second place to non-medical resources for water, sanitation, shelter, and fuel [86].

Triage from the Persian Gulf War

The threat of biological or chemical weaponry from Iraqi forces led to extensive preparation for contaminated casualties and vaccine and antibiotic prophylaxis programs for allied forces. Medical forces were equipped with detection devices (with high false positive rates), antidotes, and broad-spectrum antibiotics. If such weaponry had been used it would have produced a triage-driven event of large-scale proportions. Expectations were that forward medical facilities would receive between 1500 and 3000 casualties in the first 12 to 24 hours [62]. Multi-specialty triage teams were set up to "lateralize" the decision-making process [74]. Triage plans included rapid evacuation of the dead or nearly dead immediately out of theatre. It was anticipated that the conflict would also produce a large number of psychologically affected patients. Because of this, psychiatrists, psychologists, and chaplains were placed in forward medical facilities and assigned to the triage and expectant areas [62,74,91].

Summary

The threat of a BT event has catalyzed serious reflection on the troublesome issues that come with event management and triage. Such reflection has had the effect of multiplying the efforts to find solutions to what could become a catastrophic public health disaster. Management options are becoming more robust, as are reliable detection devices and rapid access to stockpiled antibiotics and vaccines. There is much to be done, however, especially in the organizing, warehousing, and granting/exercising authority for resource allocations. The introduction of these new options should encourage one to believe that, in time, evolving standards of care will make it possible to rethink the currently unthinkable consequences.

Unfortunately the cost of such preparedness is high and out of reach of most governments. Most of the developing world has neither the will nor the means to plan for BT events and remains overwhelmed with basic public health concerns (ie, water, food, sanitation, shelter) that must take priority. Therefore, developed countries will be expected to respond using international exogenous resources to mitigate the effects of such a disaster. As a result, the state capacity of the effected government will be severely compromised. If triage and management of casualties is further compromised, terrorists will have met their goals.

One could argue that health sciences will continue for decades to play catch up with the advanced technology driving potential bioagent weaponry. If one lesson was learned from the review of the former Soviet Union's biological weapons program, it is that the unthinkable remains an option to terrorists who have comparable expertise. It is crucial to develop realistic strategies for a BT event. Triage planning (the process of establishing criteria for health care prioritization) permits society to see cases in the context of diverse moral perspectives, limited resources, and compelling health care demands. This includes a competent and compassionate management and triage system and an in-depth and accurate health information system that appropriately addresses every level of threat or consequence.

In a PICE stage I to III BT event resources will be compromised. Triage and management will be one process requiring multiple levels of cooperation, coordination, and decision-making. An immediate challenge to existing emergency medical services systems (EMSS) is the recognition that locally there will be a shift of emphasis and decision-making from prehospital first responders to community public health authorities. The author suggests that a working relationship, in most areas, between EMSS and the public health system is lacking.

As priorities shift in a BT event to hospitals and public health care systems, they need to:

1. Improve their capabilities and capacities in surveillance, discovery, and in the consequences of different triage and management decisions and interventions in a BT environment, starting at the local level.
2. Develop triage and management systems (with clear lines of authority) based on public health and epidemiologic requirements, capability, and capacity (triage teams, categories, tags, rapid response, established operational priorities, resource-driven responsible management process), and link local level surveillance systems with those at the national or regional level.
3. Use a triage and management system that reflects the population (cohort) at risk, such as the epidemiologic based SEIRV triage framework.
4. Develop an organizational capacity that uses lateral decision-making skills, pre-hospital outpatient centers for triage-specific treatments, health information systems, and resource-driven hospital level pre-designated protocols appropriate for a surge of unprecedented proportions.

Such standards of care, it is recommended, should be set at the local to federal levels and spelled out in existing incident-management system protocols.

Acknowledgments

The author gratefully acknowledges the review of this document by Peter Merkle, PhD, of the Defense Threat Reduction Agency, Fort Belvoir, Virginia; John N. Bombardt, PhD, of the Institute for Defense Analysis, Alexandria, Virginia; and Denis Mollison, PhD, of Heriot-Watt University, Edinburgh, Scotland.

References

[1] Hardin G. Promethean ethics: living with death, competition, and triage. Seattle: University of Washington Press; 1980. p. 56–71.
[2] Burkle FM. Triage. In: Burkle FM, Sanner PH, Wolcott BW, editors. Disaster medicine. New York: McGraw-Hill (originally published under Medical Examination Publishing Co., Inc, New York); 1984. p. 45–80.

[3] Smith GP. Triage: endgame realities. J Contemp Health Law Policy 1985;1:143–51.

[4] Koenig KL, Dinerman N, Kuehl AE. Disaster nomenclature—a functional impact approach: the PICE system. Acad Emerg Med 1996;3:723–7.

[5] Franz DR, Jahrling PB, Friedlander AM, et al. Clinical recognition and management of patients exposed to biological warfare agents. JAMA 1997;278(5):399–411.

[6] Moore WL. Bioterrorism: a public health issue. Tenn Med Apr 2000;93(4):142–3.

[7] National Health Policy Forum. Biological terrorism: is the healthcare community prepared? Issue brief no. 731. Washington, DC: George Washington University; February 11, 1999. p. 2–7.

[8] Vastag B. Experts urge bioterrorism readiness. JAMA 2001;285(1):30–1.

[9] Centers for Disease Control and Prevention. Strategic Planning Workgroup: Biological and chemical terrorism: plan for preparedness and response. Morbid Mortal Wkly Rep 2000;49(rr04):1–4.

[10] Tucker JB. Historical trends related to bioterrorism: an empirical analysis. Emerging Inf Dis 1999;5(4):1–5.

[11] Seymour J. Terrorist attacks on a city's essential supplies. Available at: http://www.globalideasbank.org/socinv/SIC-79.HTML. Accessed 11 Nov 2001.

[12] Committee on Research and Development for Improving Civilian Medical Response to Chemical and Biological Terrorism Incidents. Chemical and biological terrorism: research and development to improve civilian medical response. Washington, DC: National Academy Press; 1999. p. 97–109.

[13] Pledger HG. Triage of casualties after nuclear attack. Lancet 1986;2(8508):678–9.

[14] Winslow GR. Triage and justice. Berkeley, California: University of California Press; 1982. p. 1–23.

[15] Benedeck EP. The child's rights in times of disaster. Psychiatry Ann 1979;9(11):58–64.

[16] Burkle FM, Rice MM, Madden W. Triage: ethical, operational and legal dilemmas [abstract]. In: Programs and abstracts of the 6th World Congress for Emergency and Disaster Medicine. Hong Kong, September 10, 1989; p. 71–2.

[17] Benson M, Koenig KL, Schultz CH. Disaster triage: START, then SAVE—a new method of dynamic triage for victims of a catastrophic earthquake. Prehospital Disaster Med 1996;11(2):117–24.

[18] Association for Professionals in Infection Control and Epidemiology Inc., and Centers for Disease Control and Prevention. Bioterrorism readiness plan—a template for healthcare facilities. ED Manag 1999;11(Suppl 11):S1–6.

[19] English JF. Overview of bioterrorism readiness plan: a template for healthcare facilities. Am J Infect Control 1999;27(6):468–9.

[20] Scheck A. Threat of bioterrorism out of proportion? Think again, say experts. Emerg Med News 2000;June:3–5.

[21] United Press International. CDC report urges planning for bioterrorism. DIALOG(R)File 261:upi News (c) 2000 United Press International, April 21, 2000.

[22] Centers for Disease Control and Prevention. Preparedness and response initiative: a strategy for public health [briefing report]. Presented at the National Emergency Management Association's 2001 Mid-year Conference. Washington, DC, February 12, 2001.

[23] Armon SC, Schechter R, Inglesby TV, Henderson DA, Bartlett JG, Ascher MS, et al. Botulism toxin as a biological weapon: medical and public health management. JAMA 2001;285(8):1059–70.

[24] Henderson DA, Inglesby TV, Bartlett JG, Ascher MS, Eitzen E, Jahrling PB, et al. Smallpox as a biological weapon: medical and public health management. JAMA 1999;281:2127–37.

[25] Inglesby TV, Dennis DT, Henderson DA, Bartlett JG, Ascher MS, Eitzen E, et al. Plague as a biological weapon: medical and public health management. JAMA 2000;283:2281–90.

[26] Inglesby TV, Henderson DA, Bartlett JG, Ascher MS, Eitzen E, Friedlander AM, et al. Anthrax as a biological weapon: medical and public health management. JAMA 1999;281:1735–45.

[27] Rosen P. Coping with bioterrorism is difficult, but may help us respond to new epidemics. BMJ 2000;320(7227):71–2.

[28] Page D. Epidemic outbreak or biological attack? Emerg Med News 2000;July:41–2.

[29] Schultz CH. Biologic terrorism–diagnose or die [briefing report]. New York: Disaster Preparedness International. Emergency Medicine Connection. April 3, 2000. p. 1–5.

[30] Casani JAP. Medical Coordinator for Emergency Preparedness and Response, State of Maryland Department of Health and Mental Hygiene, Baltimore, MD. Letter to practicing physicians, January 17, 2001.

[31] Rega P. Bio-terry: a stat manual to identify and treat diseases of biological terrorism. Maumee, Ohio: Mascap, Inc.; 2000. p. 1–4.

[32] Epidemiology Program Office. Case definitions for infectious conditions under public health surveillance: definition of terms used in case definitions. Available at: http://www.cdc.gov/epo/dphs/casedef/define97.ht. Accessed April 5, 2001.

[33] Fonesca MGP, Armenian HK. Use of the case-control method in outbreak investigations. Am J Epidemiol 1991;133(7):748–52.

[34] Grein TW, Kamara KO, Rodier G, et al. Rumors of disease in the global village:outbreak verification. Geneva: World Health Organization. Emerging infectious diseases. Available at: http://www.cdc.gov/ncidod/eid/vol6no2/grein.htm. Accessed October 28, 2000.

[35] Klauke DN, Buehler JW, Thacker SB, et al. Guidelines for evaluating surveillance systems. Surveillance Coordination Group. File:///C/windows/TEMP/00001769.htm. January 22, 2001.

[36] Noji EK. Disaster epidemiology: challenges for public health action. J Public Health Policy 1992;13:332–40.

[37] Armenian HK. In wartime: options for epidemiology. Am J Epidemiol 1986;124(1):28–32.

[38] Epiinfo 2000/EpiMap. Centers for Disease Control and Prevention. Available at: www.cdc.gov/epiinfo. Accessed July 2001.

[39] Nelson KE, Williams CM, Graham NMH. Infectious disease epidemiology: theory and practice. Gaithersburg, MD: Aspen Publishers; 2001. p. 119–69.

[40] Armenian HK, Lilienfield AM. Incubation period of disease. Epidemiol Rev 1983;5:1–15.

[41] Bres P. Public health action in emergencies caused by epidemics. Geneva: World Health Organization; 1986. p. 143–57.

[42] Kelsey JL, Whittemore AS, Evans AS, et al. Methods in observational epidemiology. 2nd edition. New York: Oxford University Press; 1996. p. 268–92.

[43] Sartwell PE. The incubation period and the dynamics of infectious disease. Am J Epidemiol 1966;83(2):204–16.

[44] Kaufmann AF, Meltzer MI, Schmid GP. The economic impact of a bioterrorist attack: are prevention and postattack intervention programs justifiable? Emerging infectious diseases. Available at: http://www.cdc.gov/ncidod/EID/vol3no2/kaufman.htm. Accessed June 2000.

[45] Grasman J. Stochastic epidemics: the expected duration of the endemic period in higher dimensional models. Math Biosci 1998;152(1):13–27.

[46] Hill BM. The three-parameter lognormal distribution and Bayesian analysis of a point-source epidemic. J Am Statistical Assoc 1963;58(301):72–84.

[47] Philippe P. Nonlinearity in the epidemiology of complex health and disease processes. Theor Med Bioeth 1998;19:591–607.

[48] Philippe P. Sartwell's incubation period model revisited in the light of dynamic modeling. J Clin Epidemiol 1994;47(1):419–33.

[49] Henderson DA. Eradication: lessons from the past. Bull World Health Organ 1998; 76(Suppl 2):S17–21.

[50] Eickhoff TC. Airborne disease. Am J Epidemiol 1996;144(Suppl):S39–46.

[51] Johnson E, Jaax NK, White J, Jahrling PB. Lethal experimental infections of rhesus monkeys by aerosolized Ebola virus. Int J Exp Pathol 1995;76:227–36.

[52] Bombardt JN, Grotte JH, Schultz DP. CB threats to the corps. Alexandria, VA: Institute for Defense Analysis paper P-3481. November 1999. p. 1–53.

[53] Lefevre C, Picard P. Collective epidemic processes: a general modeling approach to the final outcome of SIR infectious diseases. In: Mollison D, editor. Epidemic models. Cambridge, United Kingdom: Cambridge University Press; 2000. p. 53–68.

[54] Mollison D. The structure of epidemic models. In: Mollison D, editor. Epidemic models: their structure and relation to data. Cambridge, United Kingdom: Cambridge University Press; 1995. p. 17–31.

[55] Rickmeier G, McClellan GE, Anno G, et al. Knowledge acquisition matrix instrument to support bioagent casualty modeling. Presented at the 67th MORS Symposium, Working Group 23. June 1999. p. 1–23.

[56] Bombardt JN. Contagious disease dynamics for biological warfare and bioterrorism casualty assessments. West Point, NY: Institute for Defense Analysis paper P-3488. February 2000. p. 3–33.

[57] Bombardt JN. Pneumonic plague transmission and BW casualty assessments: subtask update for Army OTSG. Alexandria, VA: Institute for Defense Analysis briefing report. June, 2000. p. 6.

[58] Bombardt JN. Smallpox transmission and BW casualty assessments. Alexandria, VA: Institute for Defense Analysis paper P-3550. October 2000. p. 1–57.

[59] Bombardt JN. Summary of smallpox and pneumonic plague casualty estimates. Alexandria, VA: Institute for Defense Analysis briefing report. July 10, 2000. p. 1–35.

[60] deJong MCM, Diekmann O, Heesterbeek H. How does transmission of infection depend on population size? In: Mollison D, editor. Epidemic models. Cambridge, United Kingdom: Cambridge University Press; 2000. p. 84–94.

[61] News Release MAFF. Foot and mouth disease 2001—epidemiological forecasts [note for technical briefing]. Available at: http://www.maff.gov.uk/inf/newsrel/2001/010323a.htm. Accessed March 23, 2001.

[62] Burkle Jr FM, Orebaugh S, Barendse BR. Emergency medicine in the Persian Gulf War, part 1: preparations for triage and combat casualty care. Ann Emerg Med 1994;23(4): 742–7.

[63] Burkle FM, Hayden R. The concept of assisted management of large-scale disasters by horizontal organizations. Prehospital Disaster Med 2001;16:128–37.

[64] Macintyre AG, Christopher GW, Eitzen E, et al. Weapons of mass destruction events with contaminated casualties: effective planning for healthcare facilities. JAMA 2000;283(2): 242–8.

[65] Centers for Disease Control and Prevention, Public Health Practice Program Office. Interim recommended notification procedures for local and state public health department leaders in the event of a bioterrorist incident. Available at: http://www.bt.cdc.gov/protocols.asp. Accessed May 9, 2000.

[66] Human behavior and WMD crisis/risk communication workshop. Defense Threat Reduction Agency [final report]. March 2001; p. 34.

[67] Cole TB. When a bioweapon strikes, who will be in charge? JAMA 2000;284(8):944–5.

[68] Page JO. A dumb way to die. JEMS 1998;2:9–10.

[69] Wilson ML. Ecology and infectious diseases. In: Aron JL, Patz JA, editors. Ecosystem change and public health. Baltimore, Maryland: Johns Hopkins University Press; 2000. p. 311–3.

[70] Price-Smith AT. Wilson's bridge: a consilient methodology for analysis of complex biological-political relationships. Program on Health and Global Affairs (PHEGA), University of Toronto: Center for International Studies working paper 1998 8. November 1998. p. 2–43.

[71] The Royal United Services Institute for Defence Studies. Nuclear attack: civil defence. Aspects of civil defence in the nuclear age. Oxford, United Kingdom: Brassey's Publishers Ltd.; 1982. p. 82–153.

[72] Burkle FM. Triage of disaster-related neuropsychiatric casualties. Emerg Med Clin North Am 1991;9(1):87–105.

[73] Taylor AJ. A taxonomy of disasters and their victims. J Psychosom Res 1987;31(5):536–44.

[74] Burkle Jr FM, Newland C, Meister SJ, Blood CG. Emergency medicine in the Persian Gulf War, part 3: battlefied casualties. Ann Emerg Med 1994;23:755–60.

[75] Stapczynski JS. Blast injuries. Ann Emerg Med 1982;11:687–94.

[76] Wightman JM, Gladish SL. Explosions and blast injuries. Ann Emerg Med 2001;37: 664–78.

[77] Gatter RA, Mostop JC. From futility to triage. J Med Phil 1995;20(2):191–205.

[78] Marco CA, Larkin GL, Mostop JC, et al. Determination of "futility" in emergency medicine. Ann Emerg Med 2000;35:604–12.

[79] Pesik N, Keim MK, Iserson KV. Terrorism and the ethics of emergency medical care. Ann Emerg Med 2001;37:642–6.

[80] Veatch PM, Spicer CM. Medically futile care: the role of the physician in setting limits. Am J Law Med 1992;18(1,2):15–36.

[81] British Medical Association. The medical effects of nuclear war. Report of the British Medical Association's Board of Science and Education. Chichester, United Kingdom: John Wiley & Sons; 1983. p. 36–41.

[82] Campbell D. War plan UK: the truth about civil defence in Britain. London: Burnett Books; 1982. p. 112–413.

[83] Burkle FM. Coping with stress under conditions of disaster and refugee care. Mil Med 1983;148:800–3.

[84] Domres B, Koch M, Manger A, Becker HD. Ethics and triage. Prehospital Disaster Med 2001;16(1):53–8.

[85] Lown B. Sounding board: the nuclear arms race and the physician. N Engl J Med 1981; 304:726–9.

[86] Burkle FM. Lessons learnt and future expectations of complex emergencies. BMJ 1999; 319:422–6.

[87] Centers for Disease Control and Prevention. Famine-affected refugee and displaced populations: recommendations for public health issues. Morbid Mortal Wkly Rep 1992; 41:RR-13.

[88] Coupland RM. Epidemiological approach to surgical management of the casualties of war. BMJ 1994;308:1693–7.

[89] Picard A. World accused by its own silence. Toronto Globe and Mail; July 25, 1994. p. A1.

[90] McGred C. Balladur pleads with UN to speed up plan for Rwanda. The Guardian, July 12, 1994; p. 2.

[91] Burkle Jr FM, Newland C, Orebaugh S, Blood CG. Emergency medicine in the Persian Gulf War, part 2: triage methodology and lessons learned. Ann Emerg Med 1994;23(4): 748–54.

EMERGENCY
MEDICINE
CLINICS OF
NORTH AMERICA

Emerg Med Clin N Am
20 (2002) 437–455

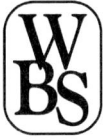

Bioterrorism preparedness I:
the emergency department and hospital

Carl H. Schultz, MD, FACEP[a],
Jerry L. Mothershead, MD, FACEP[b],
Morris Field, DO[c]

[a]Emergency Department, University of California–Irvine (UCI) Medical Center,
#128 Route, 101 City Drive, Orange, CA 92668, USA
[b]United States Navy, Navy Environmental Health Center,
Emergency Medical Services and Prehospital Care,
2510 Walmer Avenue, Norfolk, VA 23513, USA
[c]US Army Medical Research Institute of Infectious Diseases,
Operational Medicine Division, Route 3, Box 227a, Charles Town, WV 25414, USA

As is true for most disasters, hospitals bear the brunt of accepting and treating victims from a bioterrorism event, and the emergency department (ED) is the primary portal of entry. Facility requirements depend on several factors: type and amount of agent used, virulence and persistence in the environment, method of release, population density, demographics, and co-morbidity among those affected. An overt attack using biological toxins will present with an explosive increase in patient load. A covert attack using infective organisms will likely produce demands at a rate parallel to the epidemiologic curve of the ensuing epidemic. In either situation, the emergency physician and the ED play a central role in the early recognition and subsequent medical management of the event. The ability to effectively respond to such an occurrence will therefore depend on the state of preparedness of the practitioner and staff, the department, and the hospital [1,2].

Nature of the problem

No agency or organization is singularly responsible for preparedness and response to disasters. Historically, most disasters result in major property damage but few casualties. As a result, hospitals have typically considered

---

* Corresponding author.
E-mail address: schultzc@msx.ndc.mc.uci.edu (C. Schultz).

0733-8627/02/$ - see front matter © 2002, Elsevier Science (USA). All rights reserved.
PII: S 0 7 3 3 - 8 6 2 7 (0 2) 0 0 0 0 3 - 2

themselves prepared for most events. Hospitals have increasingly implemented "just-in-time" practices for supplies, and little surge capacity is available for potential catastrophes [3]. Excesses in staff have been eliminated commensurately in an effort to reduce overhead, and maintaining back-up capabilities has become especially difficult [4]. In some professions, however, there is a shortage unrelated to hospital staff reductions—this is seen most critically in the current nursing shortage [5]. Finally, the past decade has seen a reduction in total hospital beds nationally, and there is a wide variation in the functional availability of hospital bed space. There were 759,292 acute care hospital beds in the United States in 1996, an average of 2.8 beds per 1000 residents. This represented a 9% decline since 1993. The numbers of hospital beds per 1000 persons varied regionally by a factor of 3.4, from 1.5 to 5.1 beds per 1000 residents [6].

Recent studies suggest that few hospitals in the United States are prepared to manage a disaster with a significant number of casualties, and fewer still are capable of addressing the surge of patients who would be seen in the event of a chemical or biological terrorist attack. One study concluded that sampled hospitals were ill prepared, especially in areas such as mass decontamination, mass medical response, awareness among health care professionals, health communications, and facility security [7]. Another study of surveyed Level I trauma centers revealed that only 6% had all necessary equipment required for safe decontamination [8]. A third study concluded that a significant proportion of hospitals lack a written plan and equipment to allow the ED to safely and effectively manage chemically contaminated patients [9]. Finally, a fourth study stated that fewer than 20% of respondent hospitals had plans for biological or chemical weapons incidents [10]. Although other response organizations may require improvements, most experts believe that America's healthcare system, including its hospitals, are the weakest link.

Basic axioms of hospital disaster planning

This article addresses hospital preparedness for response to a bioterrorism incident. Several points must be kept in mind, however, concerning preparation and planning in general. First, although a large-scale bioterrorism event involving a highly contagious pathogen would certainly task the American healthcare system more than at any time in history, at the local or even regional level, terrorist events or natural or technologic disasters might be equally devastating. A bioterrorism event would have some unique challenges, but in planning, such an event should be viewed as a specific, extreme example of such disasters, and should, to the greatest extent possible, be incorporated into existing response plans under the "all-hazards" approach.

Next, emergency response procedures should be integrated into existing internal organizational structures and operations. During a crisis, individuals are more prone to correctly perform required actions if similar to those performed routinely. Creating different procedures and structures for specific threats complicates planning, training, and response. By incorporating emergency procedures into daily activities, some added value may be gained, or the "costs" of these preparedness actions may be reduced. Another option may be to modify routine procedures to better parallel emergency procedures. Fire departments practice the Incident Command System even for small-scale calamities, to ensure that these procedures are well ingrained in habit patterns before they are needed.

Finally, an individual healthcare facility represents but one node in a three-dimensional functional response "latticework." Response to a major catastrophe requires that links in all axes be firmly established. On one axis are sequentially interdependent response functions, from event discovery to recovery operations, and may involve law enforcement, hazardous materials (HAZMAT) teams, prehospital care services, and hospitals. The second axis, frequently overlooked in planning initiatives, involves parallel networks of organizations with similar responsibilities. These include other regional hospitals but could also include other fixed-site outpatient or rehabilitation facilities if used adjunctively. The third axis represents the time-dependent layering of outside resources that might be remotely located (requiring evacuation to complete the link) or that may be transported into that area in augmentation, such as was seen in the World Trade Center destruction with the use of the Navy hospital ship, *USNS Comfort*. Optimal preparedness occurs when there is full and open communication and collaboration among the disparate organizations during the planning process.

Establishing a baseline: JCAHO standards

An initial level of preparedness for all disasters is a prerequisite to enhance preparation for dealing with major calamities such as a terrorist event. This baseline is most likely compliance with standards established by the Joint Commission on the Accreditation of Healthcare Organizations (JCAHO). Most healthcare organizations in the United States comply with standards set by JCAHO. The Joint Commission evaluates more than 18,000 healthcare organizations in the United States, including 5240 hospitals [11].

The Joint Commission relies on standards that address the hospital's level of performance in specific areas affecting quality of patient care. Standards also specify requirements to ensure a safe environment. Requirements for disaster preparedness fall under Environment of Care (EC) standards that address four areas—the design of the environment, the implementation of safety plans, the monitoring of those plans, and the social environment. Three standards are germane to hospital preparedness for disasters—EC 1.4, 2.4, and 2.91. These standards require that healthcare organizations develop, implement, and exercise emergency operations plans. In past years, these standards focused mainly on the internal safety of the facility. Revised standards effective January 1, 2001 represent a significant effort on the part of JCAHO to task healthcare facilities to prepare and educate their staff for response to "all hazards" events, and to integrate with the emergency management community in ensuring a successful community response [12].

The most significant changes involve EC 1.4, which requires the development of a comprehensive hospital emergency management plan that is integrated with similar efforts in the community. Hospital plans must address the four classic phases of a disaster: mitigation, preparedness, response, and recovery. These terms are given specific definitions that are in concordance with those used throughout the emergency management field [13]. EC 1.4 further describes the anticipated planning process, including performance of a detailed vulnerability and risk assessment of the facility and the supported community and establishing priorities and developing procedures to mitigate and respond to potential disasters. Plans must include procedures for activation, notification, and personnel identification and use in disasters, and must address such diverse issues as patient care, staff support, supplies and logistics, security, communications, and media relations. EC 1.4 requires plans to address facility evacuation and establishment of alternate care sites, patient transportation and tracking, and interfacility communications. It requires plans to ensure alternative means of meeting essential utility needs, backup internal and external communication systems, facilities for radioactive or chemical isolation and decontamination, and alternate roles and responsibilities of personnel during emergencies, including who they report to within a command structure that is consistent with that used by the local community. The plan must also establish orientation and education programs for personnel who participate in response operations that address roles and responsibilities, information and skills required, monitoring of staff knowledge, skills, competencies, and participation, incident reporting, and program evaluation.

EC 2.9.1 requires testing of emergency operations plans. New standards require inclusion of ambulatory care organizations under certain circumstances, integration with community exercises, and full participation through all phases of the exercises. Plans are to be exercised twice yearly, either in response to an actual emergency or as part of a planned drill.

Assessing risks, capabilities, and capacity

Compliance with JCAHO standards is an excellent starting point, but by no means does this ensure the capability of adequately responding to any disaster, much less one of overwhelming proportions. JCAHO standards should be viewed as providing a framework on which to build such ability. Other key areas of interest during initial planning or review of existing plans include assessment of vulnerabilities and threats, determining facility capability and capacity, and identifying staff competencies to respond to disasters.

Risk assessment

Risk assessments include evaluation of hazards or potential threats and the vulnerabilities to those threats. Community and facility vulnerabilities should be addressed, and the threat assessment should include the entire service area of the hospital. Certain community vulnerabilities should be anticipated. Community medical preparedness was a vulnerability of great concern to emergency planners in a survey of all Federal Emergency Management Agency (FEMA) regions in preparation for the new millennium [14]. Several tools are available to assist planners in assessments [15,16]. Assistance in community risk assessments may be available through Local Emergency Planning Committees (LEPC), or the State Emergency Response Commission, mandated by the Emergency Planning and Community Right-to-Know Act (EPCRA) of 1986 [17]. Although EPCRA was enacted to deal with risks involved with toxic industrial chemical spills and exposure, LEPC personnel are usually adept in assessment processes. Many of the subsequent planning factors for response to a bioterrorism event are similar to those for a chemical event. A major difficulty in performing risk assessments for potential terrorism attacks is that any community could be at risk. Certain sites, however, could be especially appealing to terrorists. The Department of Justice, Office of Justice Programs has produced a particularly useful tool to assess community vulnerabilities and threats involving terrorism [18]. Local law enforcement officials may also be a source of identification of potential terrorist threats and targets within the community.

Capabilities and capacity evaluation

Another planning ingredient is a detailed assessment of the hospital's capabilities and capacity. This includes material resources such as medical equipment, antibiotics and other consumable supplies, and human resources. The American Hospital Association (AHA) released a discussion paper that estimated an urban hospital in the United States would require an additional $3 million to accommodate a patient surge of 1000 victims of a chemical or biological attack during the first 24–48 hours; rural hospitals would require approximately half that amount to manage an additional 200 such patients [19]. This is at a time when the fiscal outlook of hospitals is not good. A survey performed by the AHA showed that approximately one third of the nation's community hospitals had negative total margins in 2000, whereas nearly 60% had negative Medicare margins and almost two thirds lost money on patient care services [20].

Equally important is a determination of the capability of the facility to respond to disasters. This goes beyond the mere possession of physical resources or an ample supply of supplemental staff. Capability also includes those policies, procedures, and guidelines that direct the overall response, and the command and control capabilities to oversee this response and interface with other agencies and the public. Tools are available to assist in performing this assessment. One recently developed template is modeled after FEMA's Capability Assessment for Readiness (CAR) [16]. Another one allows more detail for overall community healthcare resource planning [21].

A basic bioterrorism incident management plan

Creating an institutional response plan for a bioterrorism event can be a daunting task. One must insure the plan is comprehensive and flexible enough to cover a variety of scenarios while detailed enough to meet JCA-HO requirements. It must satisfy the needs of the facility and also integrate well with the community. Although no plan can account for every conceivable possibility, a blueprint containing specific elements can provide the flexibility to handle most situations without becoming too cumbersome. Additional detailed procedures, protocols, and algorithms can and should be developed, usually at the department level. Elements unique to a bioterrorism response, or requiring additional emphasis, are listed in Table 1 and will be discussed in detail.

Plan activation and notification

The authority and method for plan activation are significant but frequently overlooked issues. If civil authorities report an attack, activation is simple and usually involves a directive from hospital administration. Release of a biological weapon, however, will probably be a covert event evolving over days, unaccompanied by a warning from the perpetrators [22]. Initial suspicion may arise among emergency or primary care physicians, laboratory personnel, or pathologists. Thus, hospital employees should know whom to contact and how and under what circumstances to activate the plan. It is prudent to identify within the document the circumstances that trigger plan activation. At a minimum this process should include specific notification of the following departments: administration, security, laboratory/pathology, respiratory therapy, pharmacy, infection control, facilities management, and the ED.

Procedures for the notification of agencies and organizations outside the hospital should also be addressed, because timely notification of community public health, law enforcement, and elected officials or other government

Table 1
Components of a bioterrorism response plan

Activation and notification	Supplies and logistics
Facility protection	Staff education and training
Decontamination	Command and control
Expansion of services and alternative care sites	Coordination and communication
	Recovery issues

representatives will improve the responsiveness of resources and assistance that will in turn translate into decreased community morbidity and mortality.

Facility protection

After activation of the bioterrorism response plan, protecting the hospital environment becomes an immediate priority. Depending on the biological agent used, unprotected personnel are at risk for falling victim to the attack secondarily, through contamination (in the event of a toxin) or transmission of infection. Thus, the goal of hospital protection is to prevent infected or contaminated individuals from entering the hospital until the threat they represent is clarified to the extent that appropriate actions can occur, be they decontamination or institution of enhanced infection control measures. Crowd control must also be exercised to prevent paralysis of patient flow.

Several actions should occur simultaneously. Security personnel will be needed to control access points to the facility. This usually involves locking most doors and permitting entrance to the facility through supervised checkpoints. Although controversial, some suggest limiting or eliminating visits by relatives and friends. Under these circumstances, only individuals whose needs are critical, such as parents or guardians of small children, should be given access, and only if they too are adequately protected.

Sequestration of potentially infected individuals from the general hospital population may be required, either because of the risk for transmission if the pathogen is known, or initially while such determinations are being made. External triage to separate access points for unaffected and potentially infected populations may be one option in this endeavor. Alternatively, a second site on the hospital grounds could be opened specifically for exposed patients. Regardless of the option chosen, hospital security must prevent unauthorized access to these areas. Distribution of masks to all patients reduces their exposure or infectious potential. If indicated, decontamination should be performed before permitting entrance to the facility.

Although not a security issue per se, sequestration of infected patients may be necessary once they are admitted. Certain biological agents such as the causative pathogens of smallpox, pneumonic plague, and many of the viral hemorrhagic fevers, can spread in the hospital environment by patient-to-patient transmission, and hospital employees must implement protective isolation strategies. Ideally these include the precautions listed in Table 2 [23]. All patients are treated using standard precautions. Transmission-based precautions are used with certain biological threat diseases. smallpox (airborne), pneumonic plague (droplet), and the VHFs (contact) [23]. Given that the number of isolation rooms is limited, alternatives include creating separate floors for exposed patients, treating them in separate buildings, or transferring them to facilities specifically designated to receive such casualties.

A terrorist attack is not just a medical emergency, it is also a crime. Contaminated personal property removed from victims during decontamination

Table 2
Isolation procedures to reduce secondary transmission

Standard precautions (used in the care of ALL patients)
  Wash hands after patient contact.
  Wear gloves when touching blood, body fluids, secretions, excretions, and contaminated items.
  Wear a mask and eye protection or a face shield during procedures likely to generate splashes or sprays of blood, body fluids, secretions, or excretions.
  Handle used patient-care equipment and linen in a manner that prevents the transfer of microorganisms to people or equipment.
  Use care when handling sharps and use a mouthpiece or other ventilation device as an alternative to mouth-to-mouth resuscitation when practical.

Airborne precautions (in addition to standard precautions)
  Place the patient in a private room that has monitored negative air pressure, a minimum of six air changes/hour, and appropriate filtration of air before it is discharged from the room.
  Wear respiratory protection when entering the room.
  Limit movement and transport of the patient. Place a mask on the patient if they need to be moved.
Diseases requiring airborne precautions: measles, varicella, pulmonary tuberculosis, and smallpox.

Droplet precautions (in addition to standard precautions)
  Place the patient in a private room or cohort them with others with the same infection. If not feasible, maintain at least 3 feet between patients.
  Wear a mask when working within 3 feet of the patient.
  Limit movement and transport of the patient. Place a mask on the patient if they need to be moved.
Diseases requiring droplet precautions: invasive *Haemophilus influenzae* and meningococcal disease, drug-resistant pneumococcal disease, diphtheria, pertussis, mycoplasma, GABHS, influenza, mumps, rubella, parvovirus, and pneumonic plague.

Contact precautions (in addition to standard precautions)
  Place the patient in a private room or cohort them with others with the same infection.
  Wear gloves when entering the room. Change gloves after contact with infective material.
  Wear a gown when entering the room if contact with patient is anticipated or if the patient has diarrhea, a colostomy, or wound drainage not covered by a dressing.
  Limit the movement or transport of the patient from the room.
  Ensure patient-care items, bedside equipment, and frequently touched surfaces receive daily cleaning.
  Dedicate use of noncritical patient-care equipment to a single patient or cohort of patients with the same pathogen. If not feasible, adequate disinfection between patients is necessary.
Conventional diseases requiring contact precautions: MRSA, VRE, *Clostridium difficile*, RSV, parainfluenza, enteroviruses, enteric infections in the incontinent host, skin infections (SSSS, HSV, impetigo, lice, scabies), hemorrhagic conjunctivitis, Viral Hemorrhagic Fevers.

For more information, see: Garner JS. Guideline for infection control practices in hospitals. Infect Control Hosp Epidemiol 1996;17:53–80.

represents evidence of the crime. Security personnel are therefore responsible for identifying and sequestering contaminated clothing and belongings. This not only protects the chain of evidence but also prevents possible inadvertent infection of hospital workers. Hospital security can relinquish this responsibility to law enforcement officers when they arrive and take charge of the evidence, or to infection control if evidence collection is no longer necessary.

Decontamination

Most authorities believe terrorists will not announce the release of a biological weapon. It is likely that days will pass between the time of initial exposure and the time symptomatic patients begin presenting to local EDs. During this time, people will probably have changed clothes and showered. The probability that external contamination remains is small. Under these circumstances, formal decontamination with showers using soap and water is not indicated. Removal of clothing and use of masks should be sufficient.

In the event of an announced or overt release of a biological pathogen, or the release of a fast-acting toxin (such as Staphylococcus B Enterotoxins or T2 Mycotoxins) decontamination will play a role in patient management [24]. Patients who have not been decontaminated at the scene may arrive at facilities still contaminated. In this situation, the theoretical possibility of reaerosolizing the organism or of secondary contamination with the toxin exists, and clothing removal and showering is indicated. Recommendations include the use of preconstructed external decontamination facilities that can be activated quickly, barriers to provide patient privacy, and the use of warm water and soap, which is sufficient to remove most biological agents. Separation of the sexes and discrete decontamination paths for patients requiring assistance and for patients capable of performing self-decontamination is recommended.

The hospital can select either internal or external facilities for decontamination. Internal units protect against inclement weather but have the theoretical disadvantage of permitting contaminated individuals to enter the hospital. They also tend to accommodate fewer patients. External units can handle a large patient volume and keep contaminated patients away from the ED, but hospital personnel must resolve issues of privacy and inclement weather, especially extremes of temperature [25]. An option is to use a nearby parking structure fitted with multiple showerheads. In a situation in which hospital facilities for decontamination are inadequate or nonexistent, improvisation is necessary. A parking lot with several fire trucks spraying high-volume, low-pressure water may be a solution [26].

The issue of how to manage contaminated effluent is vexing. Most hospitals have minimal storage capacity for contaminated wastewater, and drainage of these fluids into sewer systems will likely occur. Although the Inspector General of the Environmental Protection Agency (EPA) has issued an opinion letter to the effect that EPA would not legally pursue response organizations that technically violate the Comprehensive Environmental Response, Compensation, and Liability Act (CERCLA) by performing such acts during operations involving imminent threats to life and health, this letter admonishes response organizations to take all practical steps to avoid such situations, and to preplan for such contingencies [27]. This would seem to indicate that hospitals anticipating receipt of contaminated patients might not qualify for these "Good Samaritan" exemptions. Further, protection from CERCLA provisions does not necessarily translate to insulation from state hazardous materials statutes, even under emergency situations.

Expansion of services and alternative care sites

The large number of victims requiring medical care will soon overwhelm hospital facilities. Plans to expand hospital capacity, internally and then to alternate care sites, can help mitigate the impact. Expansion requirements will include personnel, material resources, and space. Areas that may need early expansion include the ED, inpatient units, the morgue, and possibly decontamination facilities in the case of an announced bioweapon release. This is difficult to accomplish at the time of a crisis unless prior planning has occurred. Creation of a second area for initial evaluation and treatment of patients (a back-up ED) has advantages. A terrorist event will not produce a moratorium on the usual illnesses and injuries occurring on a daily basis. The hospital must therefore continue providing care to the general population and to victims of the attack. Opening a second ED in another area of the hospital or adjacent to primary spaces permits temporary expansion of hospital capacity (providing enough personnel are available to staff two sites). This second site may serve as a work center for outside assistance such as disaster medical assistance teams. During planning for such additional initial services, attention should be given to potential choke points that may now be faced with a surge of requirements from this additional patient population. The surge in laboratory and radiographic testing, without a commensurate increase in staff to perform these tests and the equipment with which to do so, will only serve to move the choke point from outside the hospital (at initial triage) to inside the hospital.

These actions may be of limited value, however, unless there are adequate inpatient beds to accommodate patients requiring admission. Additional internal bed capacity can be accomplished by several actions. Elective cases may be cancelled or rescheduled, and these sites with their attendant equipment and staff can serve as overflow points within the hospital. Expedient discharge of patients may free more beds for anticipated admissions. If spare hospital beds or gurneys are available, some patients' rooms may accommodate these additions. Finding additional staff for these patients may prove problematic. In addition to the chronic shortage of qualified nursing personnel, some staff members may themselves be victims of the bioterrorism attack or may fail to come to work for a variety of reasons. Stretching the hospital staff to meet the burgeoning demand for services in the aftermath of a bioterrorism event may be one of the most challenging aspects of response. Possible sources of additional personnel could include staff from closed clinics or outpatient surgery departments, community healthcare retirees, medical, nursing, and allied healthcare students, and volunteers from within or outside the community. If the event is of a large enough scale, the governor of the affected state may suspend certain licensure and certification requirements during the initial phases of the response effort, or may exercise agreements under Emergency Management Assistance Compacts (EMAC) with neighboring states for volunteers. Plans for integration of these personnel must obviously be made in advance. These individuals will require expedient orientation and may be asked to perform below their levels of competency under supervision. Of some concern is the possibility that imposters may seek to volunteer. Thus, some evidence of training should be required.

Augmentation facility sites on or off the hospital campus must be selected in advance. Using schools or sports stadiums for mass decontamination of stable patients is one way to supplement hospital capacity. Ice rinks may serve as temporary morgues. Arriving medical support teams can convert open land or parking lots into temporary field hospitals, and medical facilities can transfer patients there. Although it may take several days for these assets to arrive, an attack using biological weapons will create a disaster lasting for weeks. Hospitals need to plan conjointly with local government and public health authorities to implement a strategy for using these sites.

A template for domestic preparedness that uses the concept of alternate sites has been formulated by the Department of Defense (DOD) [28]. This model, the Modular Emergency Medical System (MEMS), prepared in response to the Nunn-Luger-Domenici Domestic Preparedness Program legislation [29], is an organizational mechanism for coordinating and expanding community medical capacities when overwhelmed by a noncontagious bioterrorism (BT) event. At this writing, development of a similar mechanism to address contagious pathogens is in progress. MEMS is also applicable to natural, chemical, or radiologic disasters. The system is comprised of four modules, all managed under a unified command system: the Acute Care Center (ACC), the Neighborhood Emergency Help Center (NEHC), the Community Outreach (CO) module, and the Casualty Transportation System (CTS). A goal of MEMS is to shift the entry point of patient flow and the bulk of treatment away from the area hospital.

The initial entry point for patients into the system is the NEHC, which serves to direct noncritical casualties and asymptomatic potentially exposed patients away from the ED, supply basic evaluation and triage, and provide limited treatment including stabilization and antibiotic treatment. Patients arriving by their own means would be directed to an initial sorting area. Critical patients would be transported to the treatment and stabilization area. After any required first aid, patients only in need of prophylaxis are directed to out-processing where they are given medications and instructions and are discharged. The discharge process allows collection of patient records while providing referral for psychologic counseling and social services. Patients identified as requiring more than first aid are referred to the treatment and stabilization area. Once treated within the capabilities of the NEHC they are either transferred to an observation area or, if requiring inpatient care, are transported to either a hospital or ACC.

The ACC is designed to treat patients requiring inpatient treatment but not assisted ventilation or those triaged as expectant. The ACC will concentrate on providing agent-specific and ongoing supportive care. Interventions such as IV antibiotic therapy, hydration, bronchodilator therapy, and pain management are appropriate management at this level. The ACC model was based on a 1000 patient bed capacity, with initial staffing provided by local resources and supplemented through mutual aid, state, and federal resources. This could be scalable.

The CO effort has a broad role in dispensing information related to the incident, assessing the affected area, conducting mass prophylaxis, and assisting patients who are unable to reach higher levels of care. Analysis of epidemiologic information will dictate the mobilization and use of resources. Perhaps key to ameliorating the impact of the event will be the mass prophylaxis effort conducted at this level. Such assets as the National Pharmaceutical Stockpile could be distributed through this system.

The intention of the CTS is to address casualty transportation issues within the construct of MEMS. The CTS has two essential duties: to provide coordinated transportation between the components and to transport non-critical patients not suspected of being BT victims from local medical facilities to distant hospitals outside the affected area. The removal of unaffected patients from local facilities will free resources, and coordinated transportation within the alternative system allows for more efficient patient flow.

Supplies and logistics

The adequacy of existing medical caches and equipment may be problematic. Regardless of the quality of response design, the system will grind to a halt when supplies of antibiotics, vaccines, personal protective equipment (PPE), ventilators, and other materials are exhausted. In the era of managed care and just-in-time inventories, it is impractical to expect hospitals to carry significant additional stockpiles of materials in excess of anticipated demand [3]. The National Pharmaceutical Stockpile program is designed to provide "push packs" of supplies and antibiotics within 12 hours of release by the Director of the Department of Health and Human Services (DHHS). Offloading, transporting, and distributing these supplies are time consuming, however. Thus, hospitals must pursue other possible sources of equipment, including neighboring medical facilities, pharmacies, medical suppliers, and veterinarians. Supplies include appropriate antibiotics and vaccines (if available), required equipment to provide standard precautions, disposable clothing for decontaminated patients, biohazard bags, masks (HEPA filter or N-100), ventilators, and supplies routinely required for all patients (eg, bed pans, linens). It is crucial in determining availability of additional resources during the planning phase that these resources are not "double counted," wherein agreements are made by several facilities for the same supplies from the same vendor.

PPE requirements for most medical personnel treating victims of a biological weapon are fairly straightforward and inexpensive. Standard precautions (Occupational and Safety Health Administration (OSHA) Level D) consisting of gloves, gowns, caps, eye protection, shoe covers, and N-100 or HEPA filter masks may be all that are necessary. The use of such equipment is credited with stopping the nosocomial spread of the Ebola virus in a Zaire hospital in 1995 [30]. Healthcare workers who are designated as part of initial triage teams or who are involved with decontamination of patients should wear appropriate levels of hazardous materials protective garments and respiratory protection appropriate for their roles that are OSHA and NIOSH approved.

Staff education and training

Hospital personnel cannot be expected to perform adequately without specific education and training. Minimum requirements for staff education are listed in Table 3. The local fire department, HAZMAT team, emergency medical services (EMS) agency, the CDC, and the Domestic Preparedness Program can offer assistance in training healthcare workers.

Staff preparedness requirements will depend on the level and type of event and the staff member's role in response. Hospitals typically are not overwhelmed by community disasters—staff shortages rarely occur and supplies are usually ample for the task at hand. In the event of a bioterrorism event of any magnitude this will most likely not be the case, and all available staff will need to know exactly how to respond. Minimum levels of general disaster response education and training must be provided to all staff in a targeted fashion. More detailed education should be provided to those personnel in supervisory or management positions.

One of the critical functions of primary and ED clinicians will be early recognition of a bioweapon release. Although pathogen detection and identification technologies are improving and eventually may be widely available in hospitals, an individual clinician will still need sufficient suspicion that a potential terrorist attack has occurred to use these technologies. Maintaining a high index of suspicion and recognizing important epidemiologic clues are important to differentiating a biological attack from naturally occurring disease. In many cases an initial diagnosis based on patterns of clinical

Table 3
Minimum recommended bioterrorism response staff education

Hospital disaster response procedures, including hospital incident management system
Mass casualty triage protocols
Bioagent and terrorism awareness
Use of personal protective equipment
Decontamination procedures and protocols
Isolation techniques

findings will lead to a syndromic versus a specific diagnosis. All clinicians should have a level of awareness of the typical presentations of potential bioagents and some appreciation of the epidemiologic patterns by which these will appear. Syndromic surveillance coupled with regular epidemiologic data collection and analysis will provide for earlier warning in the face of a covert bioterrorism event. These healthcare personnel should possess knowledge regarding the signs, symptoms, patterns of presentation, diagnostic evaluation, and initial treatment of likely biological agents. Because early manifestations of diseases produced by bioterrorism agents may mimic those of common, benign maladies, such knowledge, if continuously or periodically refreshed, may provide an elevated level of suspicion [31,32]. The CDC has grouped potential biological weapons into three categories, discussed elsewhere in this article. Personnel should be familiar with at least those posing the greatest threats.

Other hospital personnel may benefit from awareness education and training also. Microbiology laboratories may be key in early presumptive diagnosis of these pathogens, provided that laboratory officers and technicians are aware of these possibilities [33]. Unfortunately many laboratory personnel are not trained in the specifics of collection and handling of specimens containing such agents. This lack of knowledge may not only render those specimens unusable, but collection itself may place those personnel at risk. The CDC publishes guidelines for laboratories in collection, handling, and packaging of biological pathogens [34,35]. Furthermore, the CDC has developed a Laboratory Response Network (LRN) that has been designed to facilitate the rapid and safe identification of potential bioterrorism agents through a series of increasingly sophisticated and linked laboratories. The LRN is discussed in greater detail elsewhere in this article. Pathologists and medical examiners might be first to identify diseases caused by these agents, and awareness training and enhanced educational opportunities should also target these professionals [36].

All staff also should be educated in personal protection appropriate for their roles. With the exception of biological toxin release that directly affects the facility, there should be little need for training in expedient collective protection, because the release of bacterial or viral agents would precede clinical manifestations by several days. For most biological pathogens, personal protection will entail universal precautions that should be routinely used during normal operations. In the event of an unknown or highly contagious pathogen, however, additional requirements such as respiratory and droplet protection may be needed. Protocols and algorithms for institution of these precautions should be developed, and all staff educated on them. Personnel performing functions with an increased risk for exposure, such as decontamination, and requiring higher levels of personal protection, should be trained in the appropriate use of this additional equipment.

Periodic assessment of performance is necessary. Otherwise, knowledge and skills will atrophy over time. Several methods including written self-assessment can measure performance. The best test, however, is participation in disaster drills. This permits evaluation of staff knowledge and skills, including appropriate use of PPE, correct decontamination techniques, and overall disaster management. Exercises should emphasize caring for many casualties, using volunteers as victims. Testing performance with simulated (paper) patients is not as effective and is to be discouraged. As painful as these exercises may be to coordinate and implement, there is no better method to test and evaluate performance of a task as complicated as responding to the release of a biological weapon.

Command and control

Events unfold quickly once victims begin presenting in large numbers. An event of the magnitude of a major bioterrorism event will require an established incident management system to integrate the various response functions. It will also be extremely helpful if the various organizations' internal response structures are aligned to the overall management system, allowing a seamless interface between them. The Nunn-Lugar-Domenici Act requires the use of a unified command system, a modification of the Incident Command System (ICS) developed in the 1970s after a series of wild land fires highlighted difficulties in scene command and control. Basic ICS principles include (1) common terminology, (2) a modular organization with a manageable span of control and unity of command, (3) integrated communications and consolidated incident action plans, and (4) comprehensive resource management, including designation of incident facilities [37,38].

Although several hospital models exist, an increasingly popular configuration is the Hospital Emergency Incident Command System (HEICS), developed in California and currently mandated for use by hospitals in that state that are part of disaster response systems [39]. HEICS imposes structure and understandable lines of authority within the hospital system. A single incident commander is responsible for overall guidance and direction. Authority is delegated through a chain of command composed of several functional divisions, typically grouped as operations, finance, logistics, and planning. This incident management system does not instruct how individuals and departments respond, however. Each department is responsible for creating its own plan that specifies how it will respond to the biological threat. In the ED, the functions of triage, decontamination, and initial treatment are frequently assigned to personnel grouped into teams. A single individual should have overall responsibility to coordinate all such team activities.

Coordination and communication

The hospital must coordinate its bioterrorism response with the surrounding community. Successful interdependence with the fire department, EMS, law enforcement, public health, regional government, and other area medical facilities is critical. Agency leaders should regularly communicate and meet in an effort to get to know one another well before the onset of a catastrophic community-wide emergency. Such personal familiarity fosters smoother cooperation among agencies that work together during any disaster response. The fire department should be aware of a potential need for assistance with hospital emergency decontamination. The availability of fire department resources and potential decontamination areas should be identified prospectively. The EMS system may need to modify transport procedures to avoid conflicts with hospital protocols for receiving exposed patients. Contaminated patients must not be taken directly into the ED—a separate entrance or another location on the hospital campus may be designated to receive these patients. Law enforcement may be able to assist with evidence collection and providing additional security. Public health personnel and regional government authorities may provide guidance with such difficult issues as the management of wastewater, distribution of vaccines and antibiotics, and global patient management, such as the treatment of smallpox patients at home versus in a hospital. Finally, assistance may be needed from surrounding hospitals and medical supply vendors to supply such items as ventilators and other critical care equipment. Mutual aid agreements between institutions can facilitate the transfer of such equipment.

Internal and external communications are vital. Phone numbers for the CDC, Federal Bureau of Investigation (FBI), and the local public health department should be kept in the ED and laboratory [40]. Contact with these agencies is useful for reporting a possible bioterrorism attack, activating epidemiologic surveillance, obtaining patient management information, and requesting antibiotics and other supplies. Integration of the hospital laboratory with the local public health agency and National Laboratory Response Network will facilitate identification of unusual microbes. In addition, assets such as Metropolitan Medical Strike Teams, Disaster Medical Assistance Teams, and National Guard Weapons of Mass Destruction—Civil Support Teams may be available.

Local media personnel responsible for reporting health issues can assist in accurate communication with the public. The media can be a valuable asset (or your worst nightmare) in educating the public about what to do during a bioterrorism event. Members of the media should be invited to observe and even "play" in disaster drills and to network with organizational leaders who will lead the response to a bioterrorism event. If ignored, they will likely seek out other less reliable "experts," resulting in the dissemination of inaccurate information that will further confuse an already frightened public and undermine government leaders' efforts to control the message they wish the public to receive.

Information management is important. Requirements provided by affected hospitals can contribute to the optimal deployment of regional, state, and federal resources. With a significant number of victims, many deaths, and transfers between facilities or even out of the area, patient tracking will be difficult. The local American Red Cross has capabilities and experience with tracking, patient information, and social services that should be sought during planning for and responding to these overwhelming events.

Recovery issues

Eventually the outbreak will subside and recovery will begin. Inspectors must examine the entire hospital to confirm no residual biological hazard remains. Contaminated equipment and material can either be disinfected or removed. This will likely be no easy task. For example, in mid-October 2001, the Hart Senate Office Building in Washington, DC was closed after an office worker opened mail containing viable anthrax spores that quickly spread throughout the structure, contaminating several offices and the ventilation system. Multiple fumigation episodes over several weeks were necessary to clear the building of viable spores. Some type of declaration certifying that the facility is hazard-free may be necessary to restore public confidence.

Hospitals should seek financial reimbursement from FEMA or other government agencies for the unrecoverable costs associated with providing care under these disaster conditions. A program for disease surveillance of hospital staff will be needed until the risk for developing infection is determined. It is equally important to offer psychologic support. Hospital personnel will experience high levels of sustained stress while responding to the needs of victims. Post-incident stress management should be offered to anyone involved in responding to or participating in the event. Such intervention can assist in the functional recovery of staff from horrific events of this nature. The psychologic support provided to the staff of Granada Hills Hospital by a psychiatric disaster medical assistance team after the Northridge earthquake was important in maintaining staff morale and performance [41].

Summary

Fundamental precepts in hospital-based planning for bioterrorist events include having a comprehensive well-rehearsed disaster plan that is based on a threat and vulnerability analysis. JCAHO Environment of Care Standards and an "all-hazards" approach to disaster planning and management form the basis for a solid bioterrorism response plan. During preparation, education and training are imperative. Clinicians must maintain a high index of suspicion for use of bioterrorism agents, be able to make a rapid diagnosis, and promptly initiate empiric treatment. Other personnel from administration, security, public relations, laboratory, pharmacy, and facilities management should be familiar with the plan, know when and how to activate it, and understand their roles in the response. A recognized incident command system should be used. Hospital leadership must be aware of the facility's capabilities and capacities, and should have plans for expansion of services to meet the surge in demand. The command center should coordinate emergency personnel teams, decontamination, security, acquisition of supplies, and notification of public health and other authorities and the media. If the plan is ever implemented, stress management with psychologic support will play an important role in recovery.

References

[1] American Hospital Association. Hospital preparedness for mass casualties [summary]. Presented at an invitational forum convened March 8 and 9, 2000. Final report August 2000.

[2] English JF. Overview of bioterrorism readiness plan: a template for health care facilities. Am J Infect Control 1999;27(6):468–9.

[3] Barbera JA, Macintyre AG, DeAtley CA. Ambulance to nowhere: America's critical shortfall in medical preparedness for catastrophic terrorism [discussion paper]. BSCIA 2001.15, ESDP ESDP-2001–07, John F. Kennedy School of Government, Cambridge MA: Harvard University. October 2001.

[4] Johnson LA, Taylor TB, Lev R. The emergency department on-call back-up crisis: finding remedies for a serious public health problem. Ann Emerg Med 2001;37:495–9.

[5] Lynn G. The nursing shortage: causes, impact and innovative remedies Testimony of the American Hospital Association before the United State's House of Representatives Committee on Education and the Workforce. Washington, DC; September 25, 2001.

[6] Center for the Evaluative Clinical Sciences, Dartmouth Atlas Project. Dartmouth Medical School. Acute care hospital beds [chapter 2].

[7] Treat KN, Williams JM, Furbee PM, Manley WG, Russell FK, Stamper CD Jr. Hospital preparedness for weapons of mass destruction incidents: an initial assessment. Ann Emerg Med 2001;38(5):562–5.

[8] Ghilarducci DP, Pirrallo RG, Hegmann KT. Hazardous materials readiness of United States level 1 trauma centers. J Occup Environ Med 2000;42(7):683–92.

[9] Cone DC, Davidson SJ. Hazardous materials preparedness in the emergency department. Prehosp Emerg Care 1997;1(2):85–90.

[10] Wetter DC, Daniell WE, Treser CD. Hospital preparedness for victims of chemical or biological terrorism. Am J Public Health 2001;91(5):724–6.

[11] Healthfinder. Organization resource details. Joint Commission on Accreditation of Healthcare Organizations.

[12] Joint Commission on Accreditation of Healthcare Organizations. Standards Revisions for 2001.

[13] Koenig KL, Dinerman N, Kuehl AE. Disaster nomenclature—a functional impact approach: the PICE system. Acad Emerg Med 1996;3:723–7.

[14] Regional Y2K workshop [summary report]. Washington, DC: Federal Emergency Management Agency, April 1999. Available at: http://www.fema.gov/y2k/wkshp/analysis/intro.htm.

[15] American Society of Healthcare Engineering. Hazard Vulnerability Analysis Tool. 2000.

[16] Healthcare Association of Hawaii Public Library Resources. December 2000 Available at: https://www.hah-emergency.net./

[17] Title 42 USC 116 et. seq.

[18] US Department of Justice, Office of Justice Programs. Fiscal year 1999 State and Local Domestic Preparedness Support Program: assessment and strategy development toolkit. 1999.

[19] American Hospital Association. Survey.

[20] American Hospital Association. Survey.

[21] American Hospital Association Chemical and Biological Checklist.

[22] Eitzen EM. Use of biological weapons. In: Bellamy RF, Azjtchuk MC, editors. Textbook of military medicine, part I: warfare, weaponry, and the casualty (medical aspects of chemical and biological warfare). Washington, DC: Office of the Surgeon General, US Department of the Army; 1997. p. 437–5.

[23] Garner JS. Guidelines for infection control practices in hospitals. Infect Control Hosp Epidemiol 1996;17:53–80.

[24] Macintyre AG, Christopher GW, Eitzen EM, et al. Weapons of mass destruction events with contaminated casualties: effective planning for health care facilities. JAMA 2000;83(2):242–8.

[25] Cole LA. Bioterrorism threats: learning from inappropriate responses. J Pub Health Manage Pract 2000;6(4):8–18.

[26] US Army Soldier Biological and Chemical Command. Guidelines for mass casualty decontamination during a terrorist chemical agent incident. January 2000.

[27] Environmental Protection Agency Alert Bulletin EPA 550-F-00–009. First responders' environmental liability due to mass decontamination runoff. Washington, DC: Chemical Emergency Preparedness and Prevention Office, Office of Solid Waste and Emergency Response, Environmental Protection Agency; July 2000.

[28] US Army Soldier Biological Chemical Command. Expanding local healthcare structure in a mass casualty terrorism event [draft]. October 2001;30:2–38.

[29] Public Law 104–207, Title XIV. The defense against weapons of mass destruction act of 1996.

[30] Outbreak of Ebola Viral Hemorrhagic Fever—Zaire, 1995 [update]. Morbid Mortal Wkly Rep 1995;44(25):468–75.

[31] Richards CF, Burnstein JL, Wackerle JF, et al. Emergency physicians and biological terrorism. Ann Emerg Med 1999;34:185–90.

[32] Keim ME, Kaufmann AF. Principles of emergency response to bioterrorism. Ann Emerg Med 1999;34:177.

[33] Klietmann WF, Ruoff KL. Bioterrorism: implications for the clinical microbiologist. Clin Microbiol Rev. 2001;2:364–81.

[34] Centers for Disease Control and Prevention Public Health Emergency Preparedness and Response. Packaging Critical Biological Agents.

[35] Richmond JY, McKinney RW, editors. Biosafety in microbiological and biomedical laboratories. 4th edition. US Department of Health and Human Services, Centers for Disease Control and Prevention, and National Institutes of Health. Washington, DC: US Government Printing Office; 1999.

[36] Nolte KB. Medical examiners and bioterrorism. Am J Forensic Med Pathol. 2000;4:419–20.

[37] Emergency Management Institute. Incident command system independent study guide (IS-195). Washington, DC: Federal Emergency Management Agency; January 1998.

[38] Irwin RL. The incident command system (ICS). In: Auf der Heide E, editor. Disaster response principle of preparation and coordination. St. Louis: Mosby; 1989.

[39] California Emergency Medical Services Authority. Disaster Medical Services Division. Hospital Emergency Incident Command System III Project.

[40] Kortepeter M. USAMRIID's medical management of biological casualties handbook. 4th edition. Washington, DC: US Army; 2001. p. k14–k27.

[41] Olson RA, Schultz CH, Koenig KL, Auf der Heide E. Critical decisions: evacuating hospitals after the 1994 Northridge earthquake. Natl Sci Found 1998;January:25.

Emerg Med Clin N Am
20 (2002) 457–476

EMERGENCY
MEDICINE
CLINICS OF
NORTH AMERICA

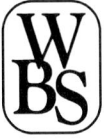

Bioterrorism preparedness II: the community and emergency medical services systems

Lynn K. Flowers, MD, MHA, FACEP[a],*,
Jerry L. Mothershead, MD, FACEP[b],
Thomas H. Blackwell, MD, FACEP[a]

[a]The Center for Prehospital Medicine, Department of Emergency Medicine,
Carolinas Medical Center, 1000 Blythe Boulevard, Charlotte, NC 28232, USA
[b]Plans and Operations Directorate, Navy Environmental Health Center,
620 John Paul Jones Circle, Suite 1100, Portsmouth, VA 23708, USA

Response to any disaster is a local problem first—the local community will be the first affected, and the first responders to the incident will be members of that community. Most communities in the United States have disaster response systems and plans, usually developed in response to specific catastrophes that have befallen those communities, or based on risk analysis of identified hazards. Experts in disaster management emphasize the importance of an "all-hazards" approach to planning and response [1]. Planning for response to a bioterrorism event should be built upon this all-hazards approach; however, because such an event more closely parallels that which would be seen in a rapidly progressing, overwhelming epidemic, specific modifications or additions to such plans must be made. Planning and preparedness for a bioterrorism event are based on many assumptions and possibilities, because there are, fortunately, no historical experience from which to draw. Insight can be gained from examining such events as the 1918–1919 influenza pandemic, the anthrax release in Sverdlovsk, Russia in 1979, and more recently the West Nile viral encephalitis outbreak in 1999 [2,3]. This article discusses the unique aspects of planning for a biological disaster. These catastrophes are primarily public health and medical crises. In contrast to conventional disasters, they also have the potential for larger numbers of casualties ranging in the tens of thousands [4]. Law enforcement

---

* Corresponding author.
 E-mail address: Lflowers@Carolinas.org (L.K. Flowers).

and forensic issues are also discussed, as they may have an impact on the delivery of health care.

Preparation must focus on mitigating the chain of events resulting from such an attack. These include recognizing that a public health crisis is occurring, confirming that it is caused by an intentional act, and responding to and recovering from the consequences of the event. This article discusses the unique aspects of preparedness planning for bioterrorism events, which are primarily public health, public safety, and medical crises. Effective preparedness requires knowledge of the likely events that would unfold, identification and mitigation of potential threats and risks, an initial assessment and subsequent enhancement of system capabilities and capacities, and a program of planning, training, exercising, and incorporating lessons learned into continuous system improvements.

Bioterrorism: a community perspective

Surveillance and event discovery

Timely recognition of an abnormal event is crucial to contain the spread of disease and reduce morbidity and mortality [5]. This requires a pre-existing awareness of what constitutes "normal" that is sufficiently sensitive to identify the aberrancy, but specific enough that episodic deviations do not trigger responses unnecessarily. Information sharing between the law enforcement and medical communities may be valuable in early warning of the potential for a bioterrorist attack. In the case of a covert bioattack, information may come from the environment, population information, or individual patients. Local public health preparedness, then, is crucial [6]. Surveillance systems must be in continuous operation to be effective [7].

Environmental surveillance

Environmental surveillance would theoretically be the best method of discovery, allowing time, albeit minimal, to take actions to lessen the impact of the event. Unfortunately, environmental detection of biological agents is difficult. A number of federal and commercial organizations have developed or are developing air, soil, and water analysis technologies to improve the speed, sensitivity, and accuracy of detection [8–10,42]. Current technologies pose significant obstacles to community use. Most of these items are restricted to the military. Procurement and maintenance costs of those available place them out of reach for most localities. Finally, their accuracy depends on trained and experienced operators, and it is unlikely that a community would have the personnel to dedicate to this function. Hence, use of this method of detection remains for the present time limited.

Epidemiologic surveillance

Current efforts focus on improving epidemiologic surveillance capabilities already in use. Difficulties with current systems limiting usefulness for bioattack discovery include (1) reliance on confirmed diagnoses, (2) enforcement of mandatory reporting, and (3) inadequacies in the timeliness of submission and analysis. Two epidemiologic surveillance tools being aggressively investigated are syndromic surveillance and data mining.

Syndromic surveillance. A syndrome is a set of signs, symptoms, or series of events that often points to a single disease or condition as the cause. Syndromes may be pathognomonic but usually focus attention on several possible diseases. Syndromic surveillance is an enhancement of standard epidemiologic data collection and analysis in which a clinical syndrome (rather than a specific disease) is the target of the surveillance system. By continuously monitoring the prevalence of syndromes associated with potential agents or pathogens of terrorism, changes may be identified that may trigger further investigation to ascertain the cause.

Obstacles exist in the use of syndromic surveillance. Most potential bioagents produce nonspecific syndromes more likely to be attributable to common maladies. Patients seek care from disparate locations, and a single facility or practitioner is afforded limited exposure to a population sample sufficient to rapidly appreciate changes in the prevalence of a particular disease. Thus, a broad spectrum of portals of entry to the healthcare system must be monitored by a common entity. Syndromes must be rigidly defined and clearly understood to ensure inclusion of only those who might have been exposed. Data collection and reporting is labor-intensive and must be near real time to be effective. Patient privacy must be protected. Finally, because enforcement will continue to be problematic, reporting facilities and providers must be convinced that syndromic surveillance has value. If these obstacles are overcome, syndromic surveillance may trigger expedient epidemiologic investigations to clarify the abnormal prevalence and determine the cause. Research in this area has shown promise. The CDC is working with state and local health departments to develop real-time syndromic surveillance methods [39].

Data mining. Data mining is directed at other potential markers of disease. One potential marker is the prevalence of animal diseases—certain bioagents affect animals, frequently sooner than in humans. Clues to the presence of West Nile Virus were present within the bird population before correct diagnosis in humans [2]. Anthrax, certain viral encephalitides, and plague may appear in animals before humans. Other markers relate to the anticipated early behavior of symptomatic individuals before they seek traditional healthcare, such as increased work or school absenteeism or use of over-the-counter medications [11]. An increased incidence of requests for, or demographic alterations in the use of, Emergency Medical Services (EMS) or urgent care, emergency department, or other primary care facility visits for non-traumatic complaints may also provide significant clues [5]. Analysis of this disparate information may hallmark the early phases of a bioterrorism epidemic.

Specific features should alert epidemiologists to a potential bioterrorism event [12]:

1. Rapidly increasing disease incidence in a healthy population
2. Epidemic curve that rises and falls over a short period of time
3. Uncharacteristic timing of an endemic disease
4. Clusters of patients from a single locale
5. Large numbers of rapidly fatal cases
6. Uncommon disease presentation or a disease that has bioterrorism potential (anthrax, tularemia, plague, smallpox)

Syndromic surveillance and data mining may show promise in early discovery of exposure at the community, state, or national level [6]. Improvements in local health surveillance may have value-added effects that enhance ongoing activities that support public health [13]. These efforts may also improve the capability to respond to natural infectious disease outbreaks, such as the influenza pandemic or the West Nile Virus outbreak [2]. The Defense Advanced Research Programs Agency (DARPA) and the Agency for Healthcare Research and Quality (AHRQ) have provided grants to further study data mining and syndromic surveillance.

Event discovery

Discovery may result from a sentinel case—a patient in whom a diagnosis has been entertained consistent with a disease caused by a biological agent. Progression from initial symptoms to debilitating disease or death may be so rapid that unless surveillance systems as described above are instituted, sentinel case recognition may be the primary method of early discovery. Such recognition would likely occur in one of two ways.

Clinical suspicion. Clinical recognition during the initial phases of a bioterrorism-induced epidemic will be extremely difficult because of the non-specific symptoms that most bioagents produce. At some point, patient findings may prompt a presumptive diagnosis consistent with a bioattack. For example, plague is endemic, albeit rare, in the southwestern United States, but not in other locations. A classic bubo in a patient outside these areas should at least raise one's suspicion. Even a single case of pneumonic plague should raise the specter of bioterrorism. Woolsorter's Disease (naturally occurring inhalational anthrax) has been reported in individuals handling hides from infected herbivores, but is virtually unheard of in modern America. There have only been 18 cases of naturally acquired inhalational anthrax reported in the United States from 1900 to 1978 [14]. Smallpox lesions are pathognomonic but may be confused with the lesions of other diseases until the patient is extremely ill. Pathologists may be the first to consider bioterrorism at necropsy. Unfortunately many pathogens produce nearly identical findings, and further tests would still be required. There are exceptions, however—few pathogens produce the extensive necrotizing hemorrhagic mediastinitis found in a patient who has succumbed to inhalational anthrax.

Education is key to the success of this method. Few physicians have treated patients with the diseases of bioterrorism. Education on these diseases falls more into the realm of historical medicine. These diseases, even when attributable to natural causes, are so rare that they might not even enter into a differential diagnosis. Only through education are clinicians likely to consider them. A recent report outlines essential Weapons of Mass Destruction (WMD)-related education and training for emergency medicine physicians, nurses, and EMS personnel [15]. Such training is not currently mandated in medical school or postgraduate training programs, although a number of specialties offer short courses and lectures as part of national educational symposia. A recent survey suggests that, specifically, emergency medicine residencies provide little training on these subjects [16].

Diagnostic studies. Diagnostic studies during early phases of disease produced by bioterrorism would also be nonspecific. Few laboratories are equipped to provide the sophisticated testing required to identify the specific pathogens. A patient presenting with findings consistent with early Venezuelan Equine Encephalitis looks remarkably similar to any other patient with aseptic meningitis, and routine testing of cerebrospinal fluid does not alter this picture. This exact problem occurred during the initial outbreak of West Nile Virus encephalitis in New York City in the summer of 1999. Several months passed before the actual causative agent was identified [2].

Many viral pathogens require sophisticated testing such as enzyme-linked immunosorbent assay or polymerase chain reaction, neither of which is widely available. Even pathogens not requiring sophisticated testing or extreme safety precautions require time for culture growth. Some pathogens can be identified in local laboratories, at least to the degree to justify empiric treatment and healthcare network alert. *Yersinia pestis* is a bipolar Gram-negative rod that can be identified through Gram stain. The identification of *Bacillus* species in a patient with a suggestive clinical picture may trigger a presumptive diagnosis of anthrax. Only anthrax produces the nearly pathognomonic radiographic findings of an unexplained widened mediastinum on chest radiograph in a previously healthy patient with rapidly progressive sepsis.

Laboratories attempting to isolate certain pathogens require appropriate safety precautions. Smallpox and the various viral hemorrhagic fever viruses require laboratories with Biosafety Level IV capabilities. Currently only two facilities in the United States have such capabilities, the Centers for Disease Control and Prevention (CDC) and the US Army Medical Research Institute of Infectious Diseases (USAMRIID). Other organisms such as *Y. pestis* require Biosafety Level II capabilities.

Expedient epidemiologic investigations

A full discussion is beyond the scope of this article, but the same general principles of epidemiologic investigation apply to an attack with a biological agent as would apply to any other disease [7]. Once a sentinel event has occurred or surveillance systems have detected an abnormality, a detailed but expedient epidemiologic investigation will have to be performed, to (1) clarify the causes of the abnormality, (2) determine if the abnormality represents a true emerging epidemic, (3) ascertain if that epidemic is the result of intentional actions, and (4) profile characteristics of the anticipated progression. Such investigations will be laborintensive and may need to occur simultaneously with response activities. They are, however, crucial to ensuing public health and individual patient treatment actions.

Response

Response begins with activation and notification and progresses through emergency response operations, affecting all facets of the medical community—public health, EMS, and fixed site healthcare operations. Healthcare response will include containment of the disease, protecting the healthcare system, mass prophylaxis, mass care, and, unfortunately, mass fatality management. Outside assistance (regional, state, interstate, and federal) must be seamlessly integrated into on-going relief efforts.

Activation

Activation of offices and organizations (law enforcement, hazardous materials, EMS, public health, and political authorities), horizontally and vertically, must occur expeditiously according to prospectively defined agreements or triggered by surveillance systems [17]. Designated local agencies should be identified to interface with state and federal counterparts to streamline communications and reduce redundancy and conflicts in communicated information [18]. The CDC has established an Internet-based rapid reporting system, One Health Alert Network [40].

Notification

The timing, method, and content of information to the public can help or hinder response. During initial public notification, specific but simple instructions need to be provided. Information provided should be accurate but not provoke panic. Many disasters allow sufficient forewarning for area evacuation. If evacuation is not possible, precautions and shelter-in-place actions may be taken to lessen the impact. Terrorists are unlikely to afford that luxury, and it is equally doubtful that local governments will order evacuation based on threats, given the increasing frequency of hoaxes that have plagued communities in recent years.

Related to public notification is general public information and education on issues of bioterrorism well before an incident. Increased public awareness will be of value in reducing anxiety or panic after an attack, and may improve discovery and response—the average citizen will be the true first responder who provides first aid and care to their families and neighbors [26].

The media may play a crucial role in initial notification. Once an attack is public, communications systems may be overwhelmed, and the media may be the primary method for public communications. This was seen in the aftermath of the World Trade Center attacks, during which telephone exchanges in affected areas were essentially locked out and even internet access was difficult for several hours.

Emergency response

Emergency response extends from activation until the event is stabilized. The principle functions of emergency response to a bioterrorist attack include containment of the catastrophe, protection of critical community personnel and response organizations, and management of the health consequences of the event.

Containment. The most important goal of emergency response is to contain the spread of the disaster to unaffected populations. One or more specific measures may accomplish this.

Exposure avoidance is unlikely to be a realistic goal for covert bioagent releases. Subsequent clinical infection may appear days to weeks later. Determining the area of exposure and population at risk will be difficult and will require the expeditious concerted efforts of public health investigators supported by state and federal agencies. Agent characteristics may be helpful, because certain pathogens are exquisitely fragile outside a host. Analysis of activities of initial victims during prodromal or incubation periods is necessary to estimate time and location of release. As more epidemiologic information becomes available, these determinations may be refined.

Isolation and quarantine may reduce spread to secondary contacts. Isolation is the process of separating persons known or suspected of being infectious from others, to prevent the spread of disease, and would occur primarily at hospitals. Quarantine is the compulsory limitation on freedom of movement or sequestration of possibly uninfected persons, to prevent the spread of a disease, and may be applied to individuals or the entire community. A recent study suggests that, for highly contagious diseases, early quarantine might be required to eradicate the epidemic [19]. Most states have quarantine laws, but these may be archaic and not practical in institution or enforcement. Governors also have extraordinary powers to take all necessary measures in the event of a state-declared emergency.

Environmental controls may also be important. Certain contagious diseases affect animals or are carried by insect vectors that might harbor and spread the infection to humans. Water and food may also transmit the disease. Transmission through water supplies is unlikely, because routine water purification systems kill most pathogens, and those that survive are not in concentrations sufficient to cause disease. There are, however, notable exceptions such as *Cryptosporidium parvum*, which is resistant to chlorine and can cause infection in small doses.

Protection of critical community personnel and response organizations. Enormous cost obviates the application of widespread community protection principles. Prospective planning and selective use, targeted at organizations, facilities, and personnel critical to response efforts, are worth consideration. These include traditional first responders (fire services, hazardous materials teams, ambulance and other prehospital care organizations, public health departments, fixed site medical treatment facilities, law enforcement, and critical members of the local government). Methods include collective protection and individual protection, and may be especially important in cases of attacks using toxins or highly contagious pathogens.

Collective protection allows those contained therein to continue operations without cumbersome individual protective equipment. It includes positive-pressure ventilation systems and high-efficiency particulate air filtration. Both require major cost-prohibitive modifications in existing facilities, but may be considered for new construction. To be effective, these must be in continuous operation before release of bioagents or toxins. Unless a facility is downwind from the release site, virtually no risk is present for airborne contamination. Expedient collective protection may include shutting off ventilation systems, sealing all exterior doors and windows, and moving inhabitants to central, upper locations. These actions could be beneficial in overt releases.

Individual protection may be physical, immunologic, or pharmacologic. Physical protection may range from the institution of certain infection control precautions through the use of fully encapsulated suits and self-contained breathing apparatuses. Issuance of complete physical protection to all inhabitants of a community is not feasible, although high-risk communities have considered issuance of protective hoods for temporary, partial protection. Expedient cloth masks may significantly reduce total inhaled inoculum in an overt attack. Intact skin provides an adequate barrier to all known bioagents with the exception of T2 mycotoxins. Although no consensus exists concerning physical protection, standard precautions with aerosol and droplet protection are adequate for most individuals in close contact with infected or contaminated victims [12,20]. Decontamination personnel should wear respiratory and splash protection, at a minimum (ie, Occupational Safety and Health Administration Level C). In the unlikely event that the time and location of the release is known, response personnel close to the scene should follow OSHA Level B guidelines, with closed system respiratory protection, because initially it may not be possible to differentiate between a biological and chemical release.

Immunologic protection involves the inducement of one's immune system to fight the pathogen. This is normally provided through prior exposure or active vaccination. Vaccination was key to the worldwide elimination of smallpox. Although intensive research continues, there are few vaccines for generally accepted potential bioagents, and widespread pre-exposure vaccination must be balanced against the risks, complications, and costs of such treatment.

Pharmacologic protection, the provision of specific chemoprophylaxis to susceptible or infected but asymptomatic individuals, may be administered before or after exposure. Pharmacologic protection may be accomplished through administration of antibiotics or immunoglobulins. Except in selected populations, similar risk and cost concerns preclude pre-exposure chemoprophylaxis. It may be determined ultimately that treated individuals were not at risk, but mortality of symptomatic victims is so high that delay is ill advised once release is known and the pathogen is presumptively identified. Loss of critical community personnel because of illness amongst themselves or their families will translate into overall degradation of response. Further discussion of mass post-exposure prophylaxis is covered later.

Psychologic protection (see chapter 7 in this issue for an in-depth discussion of the mental health aspects of bioterrorism) is crucial for responders, regardless of roles. Twenty percent of rescue personnel at the Oklahoma City bombing required mental health treatment. Prevention programs will better prepare them psychologically [21]. Post-event Critical Incident Stress Debriefing (CISD) and psychologic monitoring and support will be essential for the psychologic well being of healthcare workers and emergency personnel [4].

Management of the health consequences of the event. Mass healthcare management falls into four categories: victim decontamination, mass prophylaxis, mass patient care, and mass fatality management.

Decontamination. In contrast to chemical agent attacks, decontamination after a covert biological attack will probably not be required, owing to the delay between release and the development of symptoms [8]. In most cases patients will present days after exposure and already will have taken soap and water showers several times. Field decontamination may not be achievable with potential casualties in the tens of thousands, geographically separated over a wide area. Most organisms are fragile in the environment. Re-aerosolization is highly unlikely [20]. Decontamination with sodium hypochlorite solution has not been shown to have benefit for routine skin decontamination and is not recommended unless there appears to be grossly visible skin contact [20]. If necessary, removal of clothing and placement of it in a sealed plastic bag, and soap and water shower will suffice [22]. Effluent entrapment is not necessary, as noted in the chapter on federal response in this issue.

Mass prophylaxis. A plan for expeditious post-attack prophylaxis must be developed. Post-exposure prophylaxis serves to reduce individual morbidity and mortality and prevent secondary infections from transmissible diseases, thereby assisting in eradication of the epidemic. The prognosis in patients with active disease caused by many of the bioagents is uniformly poor, with mortality rates approaching 100% (inhalational anthrax, pneumonic plague) if treatment is delayed until patients are symptomatic [13]. For some, little treatment beyond supportive care is available. The Operation

TOPOFF exercise in May 2000 highlighted significant challenges in co-ordinating interaction between local and federal agencies [23].

Most hospitals and pharmacies have gone to "just in time" pharmaceutic procurement, and stockpiles to handle surge demand are meager at best. Strong consideration should be given to raising the par levels of antibiotics, antidotes, and antitoxins in the community. The federal government (primarily the CDC) has initiated programs to address this deficiency, and a community should anticipate the arrival of federal equipment and pharmaceutic stockpiles within 12 hours of a decision to release a stockpile.

Logistic problems of mass prophylaxis are magnified by difficulties in determining the population at risk. Initial estimates are likely to be high. Planners must have an accurate inventory of local pharmaceutic and medical supplies and detailed plans and procedures for safeguarding, distributing, and dispensing community stores, patient screening and tracking, and receiving, distributing, dispensing, and providing security for and traffic control at federal stockpile receiving locations and points of distribution (PODs). Few communities have implemented such plans. In the New York City model, PODs can process approximately 1000 patients per hour, and require 105 trained personnel each shift (James Alexander, University Medical Group, PC, New York, personal communication, September 2001). The American Red Cross (ARC) may play a key role in mobilizing volunteers to assist with dispensing the stockpile [24]. Ambulatory, home-ridden, and homeless patients require provisions. Sufficient numbers of PODs must exist to relieve hospitals of this burden and to ensure delivery of these medications in a timely fashion. Difficult ethical issues of prioritizing who receives medications if shortages are anticipated should be resolved before an event.

Mass patient care. Health care systems will have little time to prepare for a bioterrorism event after the fact, and may also suffer significant staff shortages because of absenteeism or illness among personnel, at the same time that they experience a surge in the demand. This surge will be composed of patients at risk, infected or affected, and many unaffected but susceptible and anxious individuals, frequently referred to as the "worried well" [12]. Indeed, this last category of individuals seeking healthcare may exceed those actually requiring services by a factor of 5–10:1. All healthcare systems will have to significantly modify operations to reduce routine demand for services while simultaneously taking actions to allow for graduated system expansion. A particularly vexing problem exists as a result of the free market approach to fixed site healthcare—whereas most public safety agencies, including EMS, serve a defined geographic area, multiple hospitals within that area may routinely function as independent, competing entities, rather than as an integrated, coordinated unit. Creative planning will be needed to overcome this. Ideally, fixed site operations would operate under the control of a predesignated control hospital.

Methods to reduce demand may include the following:

- Prospectively developed triage systems based on comparison of antici-pated victims and time-phased response capacity
- Diversion of certain patients to other sites of care that may entail estab-lishing health care centers physically separate from hospitals.
- Provision of enhanced telephonic advice obviates the necessity of seek-ing treatment at any facility. This may also reduce the likelihood of un-infected patients being exposed to those affected by the bioagent.
- Cancellation of elective appointments, procedures, and surgery to release space, supplies, and staff to augment other departments and services
- Institution of public information campaigns to reduce requests for am-bulance or other transportation services unless absolutely necessary

There are also methods to increase the capacity of healthcare services:

- Early discharge of unexposed patients home, to skilled nursing facilities, home health care, or remote health care facilities. Patient's families may be able to provide post-hospitalization care after brief education, or un-der the direction of visiting nurses or through telephonic instructions.
- Evacuation of exposed patients outside the affected area. The wisdom of evacuating patients who may transmit the disease to new communities must be balanced with the need to contain the spread of the disease and the desires of family members, and may ultimately have to be made by elected state or federal officials. Until outside resources are available, use of community patient transport systems for long distance transfer or transport will reduce the availability of these already overburdened re-sources.
- Doubling up single or even shared hospital rooms, and temporarily in-creasing lengths of healthcare personnel work shifts.
- Use of auditoriums or cafeterias within healthcare facilities or establish-ing expansion facilities may extend services to more patients than can be accomplished on wards with private rooms. Although patient privacy and comfort may be compromised, this method of expansion of facil-ities was used effectively during the influenza epidemic of 1918 [25]. One of many difficulties with this option is obtaining the necessary hu-man and material resources required to operate these facilities. Other than pre-established community or regional caches, possible procure-ment sites include local hospital supply distributors.
- Volunteers, retired health care workers, or medical, nursing, dental, and other allied healthcare students may expand the pool of available provi-ders, although their participation in a bioattack cannot be predicted. Orientation will be required, as will expeditious credentialing mechan-isms to prevent imposters from gaining access to the system.
- Many functions, such as epidemiologic data collection, do not require ad-vanced skills, and volunteers may free up these personnel. Augmentation

of EMS by commercial vehicle operators may release Emergency Medical Technicians for direct patient care with the ambulance service or at other locations. Alternate vehicles may also be used. In those communities that have already instituted Multi-Option Priority Dispatch (MOPD) procedures, enhanced protocols to select out those patients not requiring vehicular litter transport may be a viable option.

Mass fatality management. An event using a lethal pathogen will likely produce significant fatalities. Symptomatic patients misdiagnosed early in the epidemic have little chance for survival. Local morgues and funeral homes may not be able to absorb the surge and commercial establishments may be reluctant to accept infected remains for fear of contamination or disease transmission. Processes must be in place to establish temporary morgues [12]. These sites require environmental control, water, lighting, rest facilities, and viewing areas. These sites should have communications with patient tracking and emergency operations centers. Infection control procedures should parallel those at other healthcare sites during all phases of morgue operations, because survivability of potential pathogens in corpses has not been well studied. Security and pastoral care services should also be included. Legal, moral, ethical, psychologic, and religious reasons exist to identify the dead. Procedures must be in place to gather the information for positive identification. Similar issues are involved with decisions to release or cremate remains.

Management of response operations

Management of the diverse organizations and agencies involved with a bioterrorism response requires a clearly defined and well-coordinated structure that includes command, control, communications, and information management, and should optimally be organized under a Unified Command System (UCS). The UCS is an enhancement of the Incident Command System, developed as the result of problems identified in responses to wild land fires in the 1970s. UCS facilitates the coordination of multiple agencies, standardizes terminology, and provides a framework for communication [27–29]. The complexity of the incident also warrants an electronic database to document events or to assist in management decision-making [23,41]. There are several commercially available systems that link patient capacity data from local medical centers and EMS systems to an accessible database. A computerized Automated Decision Aid System for Hazardous Incidents (ADASHI), specifically designed to provide decision support in a chemical or biological incident, is currently under development [10].

Recovery

Following stabilization, recovery may be prolonged. Most disaster planning processes focus on disaster response to the exclusion of recovery. A biological event does not cause physical destruction, and physical infrastructure will remain intact. Issues facing communities and local healthcare systems are environmental surety, long-term community mental health, and rehabilitative services.

Environmental surety

Most bioagents have short life spans outside a host. Plague may become endemic among the rodent population of an area, posing a continued threat to the community. Anthrax spores have maintained viability under extreme environmental conditions for decades. Depending on the pathogen released, ensuring that areas of high concentration are safe for use is necessary. Schools, auditoriums, or other sites used as inpatient facilities may require confirmation of contamination removal, if for no other reason than legal liability and peace of mind for the community.

Long-term community mental health

In any disaster, the tendency is to underplay the importance of addressing the psychologic needs of the community—the victims and their families, survivors, and response personnel. The entire community may suffer short-term psychologic effects, and a significant percentage of the population may develop post-traumatic stress disorder. Failure to address this important aspect of recovery may have significant effects well after recovery operations have been completed. Short-term mass crisis counseling, beginning even during response operations, may mitigate these long-term effects [21,30,31].

Rehabilitative services

Most disasters in the United States have resulted in few casualties, and many of those injured do not even require hospitalization. Survivors of bioterrorist incidents may require prolonged inpatient and rehabilitative services and will usually want these services in their local communities. This potential burden on the healthcare industry should be addressed in recovery plans.

Forensic and legal issues

A myriad of diverse legal and forensic issues will be superimposed on a bioterrorist event disaster. Many of these have yet to be resolved at state or federal levels, and no standardized templates exist. Issues that may affect healthcare operations include:

- Pre- and trans-event communications and information sharing between the healthcare law enforcement communities
- Declaration and enforcement of quarantine
- Release of remains
- Legal requirements for community immunization or forced postexposure prophylaxis

- Security at healthcare facilities, temporary morgues, neighborhood treatment centers, and antibiotic dispensing stations
- Evidence collection
- Patient privacy
- Interstate licensing of providers and liability issues

Healthcare system biological terrorism response planning

Although no community will likely have sufficient resources and expertise to respond to a significant biological attack, inadequate preparation will magnify the consequences of this catastrophe. It should be clear from the earlier discussion that plans aimed at typical mass casualty situations will be inadequate in many aspects for managing the consequences of a terrorist attack involving biological agents and producing large numbers of casualties, and eventually will require outside assistance. Local planners should plan for self-sufficient operations for the first 12–48 hours. The following 10-step process is one method to approach community healthcare systems planning for response to a biological terrorism event.

1. Assemble planning committee. Preparedness requires a multidisciplinary approach. Many steps in response are concurrently or sequentially interdependent, often on the actions of organizations not directly affiliated with the healthcare system. In addition to members usually involved in disaster planning, laboratory officials, law enforcement agents, legal representatives, medical examiners, funeral home directors, and public health officials should be part of the process. The media should also be included to as great an extent as possible. A well-informed and educated media is more apt to work with emergency planners and response personnel to ensure that information of value is relayed to the community in a responsible fashion. There are benefits to including members of religious organizations and representatives of the community, including the business sector. Industries may have a greater appreciation for availability of certain resources, and may be a source of some funding for system enhancement. The local chapter of the American Red Cross may also be of great value because of its ability to mobilize volunteers from its nationwide network [24].

2. Review applicable documents. The optimal approach to system development is to build on existing "all-hazards" response plans, even though a bioattack would present differently. Many aspects of subsequent response do not fit into this traditional model, but this approach may prevent redundancy in systems or processes that are common to all events. Other documents for review would include state and federal response plans and concepts of operations, public health laws, and departmental or organizational standard operating procedures.

3. Perform vulnerability analysis. Emergency planners are familiar with threat and vulnerability analyses for traditional disasters. Geographic

areas prone to hurricanes, tornadoes, and floods can be identified. Local Emergency Planning Committees are well aware of the potential threat of significant hazardous materials. The difficulty with bioterrorism threat analysis is that any community could be a target. Vulnerabilities can be more easily identified. These might include weaknesses in public health, law enforcement, or overall disaster response systems capabilities, water purification systems, prevalent meteorologic conditions, or other specifics of the community (eg, age, special needs populations, population density) that would make it more vulnerable to either the attack itself or the consequences of such an attack. Review of these may facilitate mitigation actions to reduce the community's vulnerabilities.

4. Evaluate system capability and capacity. Capability refers to the qualitative ability to accomplish specific required response and recovery tasks, whereas capacity implies a quantitative measure of this ability. Capacity may be reflected in absolute units performed or by other measures of performance, such as units/time, depending on the task involved. Some tasks are absolute—they either can or cannot be accomplished.

5. Identify necessary tasks and determine requirements. A "mission essential task list" can be constructed of actions to be taken in the event of a bioterrorist incident. Required steps to accomplish the specific task should also be delineated. Requirements will fall into one or more of the following categories: (1) human resources—sufficient numbers of appropriately trained personnel, (2) material resources—facilities, vehicles, equipment, supplies (consumable and non-consumable), and (3) clear and concise, but flexible, guidance. Some tasks will be sequentially dependent on the success or failure of previous tasks and should be linked to these. It is also crucial to identify those tasks that are so critical that failure to accomplish them will have major ramifications on successful response. A prime example of this would be the failure to recognize early that an abnormal public health crisis was unfolding. A final factor in this equation is time—when the action is required, how long it may take, and when it is no longer required.

6. Match capability and capacity to requirements. By mapping existing human and material resources, techniques, tactics, and procedures to the identified tasks, planners may discern whether the response system has a capability to respond, and to what functional capacity. Most systems will have some capability. This approach will also lend itself to identifying those areas requiring the greatest improvement.

7. Enhance system capabilities and capacity. There are several methods to reduce weaknesses. Underused community resources may be adjusted to augment those functional areas that are overtaxed. Likewise, should resources not be needed during certain phases of response operations, these may be "re-used" at other times, to expand time-phased capacities. Review of certain processes may lead to improvements that require

less manpower or supplies, resulting in a "virtual" increase in capacity. Regional mutual assistance compacts may prevent redundancy across jurisdictional lines. Still likely, some new procurement will be required. Many states offer grants as part of overall EMS programs. Grants are also available to those communities that qualify under a number of different federal programs. For example, the Office of Domestic Preparedness/Department of Justice "Fiscal Year 1999 State Domestic Preparedness Equipment Program" provides guidance to states and local jurisdictions in risk assessments and strategies for training, technical assistance, and equipment identification [32]. Ultimately, however, emergency preparedness is a community responsibility; regardless of the size of the disaster, the community will bear the brunt.

8. Develop plans, techniques, tactics, and procedures. A standard disaster plan usually is composed of a "basic" plan with a series of appendices for the major functional areas (eg, fire services, EMS, law enforcement), and annexes that each provides specific variations for individual threats, such as hazardous materials, hurricanes, or earthquakes. An "allhazard" disaster plan should have a health and medical services appendix that may or may not include public health/preventive medicine. A bioterrorism annex should be developed that outlines deviations from the base plan and appendices. Plans should be of sufficient detail that all parties could understand the concepts of operations, but not so all-inclusive that they are cumbersome to use in actual events. Plans should also describe the process for incorporating state or federal resources as they become available. Detailed guidance more appropriately should be placed in organizational standard operating procedures, such as Federal Bureau of Investigation (FBI) notification procedures by public health departments in the event of suspected attacks [12]. Further detail may require individual departmental techniques, tactics, and procedural manuals. Examples of these latter documents include forensics, evidence collection, and chain-of-custody procedures [33]. There are a number of national consensus guides that have been developed that are adaptable for local use. For example, the CDC has developed guidelines for treatment and prophylaxis, and information sheets for clinicians, laboratories, and patients, on many biological agents [12].

9. Educate, train, and exercise. Virtually all participants in response management and operations will require some additional education. First responders must be able to quickly recognize clinical syndromes and event characteristics unique to bioterrorist attacks. Training should include safety, self-protection, personal protection equipment, patient care, decontamination, triage and mass casualty management, and incident command operations, commensurate with assigned roles [34]. Healthcare providers, especially primary care and emergency nurses and physicians, should receive education to promote awareness and

facilitate diagnosis, initial treatment, enhanced infection control, and reporting procedures [11]. Others such as radiologists and pathologists may also benefit from awareness programs. Targeting providers-in-training seems optimal. Education must include interventional techniques to mitigate psychologic sequelae, including community anxiety [12,30,35]. Laboratory professionals require training in the recognition of the critical biological agents most likely to be used in a bioterrorism attack. Trained epidemiologists are needed to identify critical parameters of ensuing epidemics [25]. All healthcare personnel must be totally familiar with the unified command structure, the overall general concepts of operations and their roles in response, vertical and horizontal communications, and the specifics of techniques, tactics, and procedures unique to their roles. Public awareness and response education must also be provided, because the average citizen will be the true first responder [26].

Detailed and realistic exercises should be conducted. Exercises may be tabletop, functional component, or full scale. Plans should be tested under a variety of scenarios involving agents of different characteristics, and should be of various magnitudes, because response procedures may vary with differing conditions. An important scenario that may be overlooked involves a bioagent-release hoax. Addressing hoaxes is important for two reasons—they are historically more likely to occur than actual releases, and even hoaxes can significantly tax community resources. Drills should be conducted on a periodic basis to identify potential problems, to understand the characteristics of command and control and incident response involving mass-casualties, and to evaluate the communications infrastructure [36]. Success requires an interdisciplinary approach (eg, EMS, fire, law enforcement, hospitals, HAZMAT units), and must include hands-on experience. Multi-jurisdictional exercises are a critical part of the community preparedness program. They should also test integration and coordination with state and federal agencies [34]. Exercises and exercise programs should be externally reviewed.

10. Establish a continuous disaster preparedness improvement program. There is no "perfect" disaster plan. Consumable materials expire, education and training is extinguishable if not used, and new technologies may be developed that are more affordable. Reviews, tabletops, or functional exercises will most likely uncover deficiencies or identify unexpected problems. These should lead to "Issues for action" that require resolution. A continuous disaster preparedness improvement program should ensure overall system sustainment that includes initial and ongoing training, replacement or replenishment of material resources, technologic upgrades as available, and process modifications as necessary based on lessons learned, statutory requirements, or as the result of innovative thinking.

Summary

Disaster planning is an arduous task. Perhaps no form of disaster is more difficult to prepare for than one resulting from the intentional, covert release of a biological pathogen or toxin. The complexities of response operations and the perils of inadequate preparation cannot be overemphasized. Even with detailed planning, deviations from anticipated emergency operations plans are likely to occur. Several federal programs have been initiated to assist communities in enhancing their preparedness for events involving biological and other agents of mass destruction. Many of these, such as the Metropolitan Medical Response Systems (MMRS) Program [37,38], will be discussed elsewhere. Community preparedness will be enhanced by:

1. Implementing a real-time public health disease surveillance program linking local healthcare, emergency care, EMS, the CDC, local law enforcement, and the FBI
2. Improved real-time regional patient and healthcare capacity status management
3. Development of affordable, accurate biological agent detection systems
4. Incorporation of standardized education and training curricula (appropriate for audience) on terrorism and biological agents into healthcare training programs
5. Expansion of federal and state programs to assist communities in system development
6. Increased public awareness and education programs

References

[1] Federal Emergency Management Agency. Guide for all-hazards emergency operations planning. State and local guide (SLG 101). Emmitsburg, PA; 1996.
[2] Fine A, Layton M. Lessons from the West Nile viral encephalitis outbreak in New York City, 1999: implications for bioterrorism preparedness. Clin Infect Dis 2001;32:277–82.
[3] Henderson DA, Inglesby TV, O'Toole T. Implications of pandemic influenza for bioterrorism response. Clin Infect Dis 2000;31:1409–13.
[4] Simon JD. Biological terrorism: preparing to meet the threat. JAMA 1997;278(5):428–30.
[5] Kuhr S, Hauer JM. The threat of biological terrorism in the new millennium. Am Behav Sci 2001;44(6):1032–41.
[6] Khan AS, Morse S, Lillibridge S. Public-health preparedness for biological terrorism in the USA. Lancet 2000;356:1179–82.
[7] Franz DR, Jahrling PB, Friedlander AM. Clinical recognition and management of patients exposed to biological warfare agents. JAMA 1997;278(5):399–411.
[8] Kortepeter MG, Cieslak TJ, Eitzen EM. Bioterrorism. Environ Health 2001;Jan/Feb:21–4.
[9] US Army Soldier and Biological Chemical Command (SBCCOM). Biological Integrated Detection System (BIDS). Available at: http://www.sbccom.apgea.army.mil/products/bids.htm Accessed July 1, 2001.
[10] US Army Soldier and Biological Chemical Command (SBCCOM). ADASHI—a training tool for CB defense. Available at: http://www.sbccom.apgea.army.mil/RDA/hld/adashi.htm. Accessed July 1, 2001.
[11] Pavlin J. Epidemiology of bioterrorism. Emerg Infect Dis 1999;5(4):528–30.

[12] English JF, Cundiff MY, Malone JD, et al. Bioterrorism readiness plan: a template for healthcare facilities. Atlanta, GA: Centers for Disease Control and Prevention; 1999.

[13] Kaufmann AF, Meltzer MI, Schmid GP. The economic impact of a bioterrorist attack: are the prevention and postattack intervention programs justifiable? Emerg Infect Dis 1997;3(2): 83–94.

[14] Inglesby TV, Henderson DA, Bartlett JG, et al. Anthrax as a biological weapon: medical and public health management. JAMA 1999;281(18):1735–45.

[15] Waeckerle JF, Seamans S, Whiteside M, et al. Executive summary: developing objectives, content, and competencies for the training of emergency medical technicians, emergency physicians, and emergency nurses to care for casualties resulting from nuclear, biological, or chemical (NBC) incidents. Ann Emerg Med 2001;37(6):587–601.

[16] Pesik N, Keim M, Sampson TR. Do US emergency medicine residence programs provide adequate training for bioterrorism? Ann Emerg Med 1999;34(2):173–4.

[17] Bradley R. Health care facility preparation for weapons of mass destruction. Prehosp Emerg Care 2000;4(3):261–9.

[18] Moran GJ. Bioterrorism alleging use of anthrax and interim guidelines for manage-ment—United States, 1998. Ann Emerg Med 1999;34(2):229–31.

[19] Meltzer MI, et al. Modeling potential responses to smallpox as a bioterrorist weapon. Emerg Inf Dis 2001;7(6):959–69.

[20] Keim M, Kaufmann AF. Principles for emergency response to bioterrorism. Ann Emerg Med 1999;34(2):177–82.

[21] Institute of Medicine, National Research Council. Chemical and biological terrorism: re-search and development to improve civilian response. Washington, DC: National Academy Press; 1999.

[22] Macintyre AG, Christopher GW, Eitzen E, et al. Weapons of mass destruction events with contaminated casualties: effective planning for health care facilities. JAMA 2000; 283(2):242–9.

[23] Hoffman R, Norton J. Lessons learned from a full-scale bioterrorism exercise. Emerg Infect Dis 2000;6:652–3.

[24] Healy B. Hearing on terrorism and US government capabilities [written statement]. Senate Appropriations Committee, May 10, 2001. Available at: http://www.senate.gov/~appro-priations/commerce/testimony/terrheal.htm. Accessed July 15, 2001.

[25] Henderson DA. The looming threat of bioterrorism. Science 1999;283:1279–82.

[26] Taylor ER. Are we prepared for terrorism using weapons of mass destruction? Govern-ment's half measures. Policy Anal 2000;387:1–19.

[27] Brennan RJ, Waeckerle JF, Sharp TW, et al. Chemical warfare agents: emergency medical and emergency public health issues. Ann Emerg Med 1999;34:191–204.

[28] Irwin RL. The incident command system (ICS). In: Auf der Heide E, editor. Disaster response: principles of preparation and coordination [online edition]. Atlanta, GA: Erik Auf der Heide; 1989. Available at: http://coe-dmha.org/dr/index.htm. Accessed 30 July 2001.

[29] US Government. CONPLAN United States Government Interagency Domestic Terrorism Concept of Operations Plan, January 2001. Available at: http://www.Fema.gov./R-N-R/ Conplan/. Accessed 30 July 2001.

[30] Dembert ML, Simmer ED. When trauma affects a community: group interventions and support after a disaster. In: Klein R, Shermer V, editors. Group psychiatric treatment for psychological trauma. New York: Guilford Press; 2000. p. 239–64.

[31] North CS, Nixon SJ, Shariat S, et al. Psychiatric disorders among survivors of the Oklahoma City bombing. JAMA 1999;282:755–62.

[32] Office for State and Local Domestic Preparedness Support. Assessments. Available at: http://www.ojp.usdoj.gov/osldps/assessments.htm. Accessed July 1, 2001.

[33] Yeskey KS, Llewellyn CH, Vayer JS. Operational medicine in disasters. Emerg Med Clin N Am 1996;14:429–38.

[34] Department of Defense. Domestic preparedness program in the defense against weapons of mass destruction. Report to Congress. Washington, DC; May 1, 1997. Available at: http://www.defenselink.mil/pubs/domestic/toc.html. Accessed 30 July 2001.

[35] DiGiovanni C. Domestic terrorism with chemical or biological agents: psychiatric aspects. Am J Psychiatry 1999;156:1500–5.

[36] Richards CF, Burstein JL, Waeckerle JF, et al. Emergency physicians and biological terrorism. Ann Emerg Med 1999;34:183–90.

[37] US Department of Health and Human Services, Office of Emergency Preparedness. Origin of the MMRS. Available at: http://www.mmrs.hhs.gov/About/Origin.cfm. Accessed July 15, 2001.

[38] US Department of Health and Human Services, Office of Emergency Preparedness. National Disaster Medical System (NDMS): about teams. Available at: http://www.oep-ndms.dhhs.gov/NDMS/About_Teams/about_teams.html#dmat. Accessed July 15, 2001.

[39] Centers for Disease Control and Prevention. Epidemiological Surveillance. Available at: http://www.bt.cdc.gov/EpiSurv/ Accessed June 1, 2001.

[40] Centers for Disease Control and Prevention. Health Alert Network. Available at: http://www.phppo.cdc.gov/han/ Accessed June 1, 2001.

[41] Effler P, Ching-Lee M, Bogard A. Statewide system of electronic notifiable disease reporting from clinical laboratories: comparing automated reporting with conventional methods. JAMA 1999;282:1845–50.

[42] The Defence Research Establishment Suffield. The Canadian Integrated Biochemical Agent Detection System (CIBADS). Available at: http://www.dres.dnd.ca/Products/RD98002/index.html Accessed June 1, 2001.

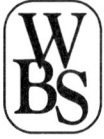

EMERGENCY
MEDICINE
CLINICS OF
NORTH AMERICA

Emerg Med Clin N Am
20 (2002) 477–500

Bioterrorism preparedness III:
state and federal programs and response

Jerry L. Mothershead, MD, FACEP,[a],*
Kevin Tonat, DrPH, MPH,[b]
Kristi L. Koenig, MD, FACEP[c]

[a]Navy Environmental Health Center, 620 John Paul Jones Circle,
Suite 1100, Portsmouth, VA 23708, USA
[b]Office of Emergency Preparedness, Department of Health and Human Services,
Twinbrook Metro Plaza, 12300 Twinbrook Pkwy, Rockville, MD 20857, USA
[c]Emergency Management Strategic Healthcare Group, Veterans Health Administration,
Department of Veterans Affairs, Washington, DC 20001, USA

The initial response to any type of disaster, whether bioterrorism or not, is local. With the current lack of healthcare surge capacity in the United States, however, a bioterrorism attack of any significant magnitude would likely rapidly overwhelm the resources and capabilities of even the best regional healthcare systems. A framework exists by which state and federal agencies may respond with assistance to such an event. Indeed, any bioterrorism event would prompt a federal response because of the criminal nature of the act.

This article discusses the evolution of federal efforts to respond to disasters and epidemics, applicable to bioterrorism incidents, and focuses on three broad categories of initiatives and response to bioterrorism: executive and legislative branch actions, federal agency counterterrorism programs, and bioterrorism emergency operations, with a primary focus on health and medical operations. Because state governments exercise important legal oversight within their borders, are benefactors of federal programs, and will be intimately involved with operations in the event of such an attack, a discussion of a typical state's laws and operations related to epidemic and disaster response are described also. Recent legislation facilitating interstate assistance is also reviewed. Federal actions taken after the terrorist attacks

---

* Corresponding author.
E-mail address: usna1974@cox.net (J.L. Mothershead).
The views expressed in this article are not official government statements, are the authors' views, and do not necessarily represent the views of the Departments of Defense, Health and Human Services, or Veterans Affairs, or of the United States Government.

against the World Trade Center and the Pentagon and the ensuing anthrax mailings are also addressed. However, counterterrorism and consequence management programs continue to evolve at an accelerated pace as the result of those events, and certain information accurate at the time of the writing of this article might not be so by date of publication.

Initiatives and response as used in this article refer to preparedness programs and response operations. It must be kept in mind, however, that the precepts of an all-hazards approach to disasters—mitigation, preparedness, response, and recovery—are important; the basic tenets of this approach to disaster planning and response are equally as applicable to a disaster resulting from an act of bioterrorism as they are to any disaster, whether caused by natural or technologic causes. The specific application of these principles, however, may differ significantly, as is true in the case of a bioterrorism attack.

Historical perspective

Major disasters, epidemics, and terrorism in American history

The United States has been fortunate—only a few disasters have resulted in great loss of life. There have been only seven disasters in American history, barring combat, with greater than 1000 fatalities [1]. Some international disasters by comparison have produced death counts in the hundreds of thousands. The United States event with the largest loss of life is believed to be the Battle of Antietam in 1862. An estimated 7000 Americans died, more than 3200 in the first day [2]. Disasters before the twentieth century were primarily caused by natural causes. Technologic catastrophes have increased over the last century, and urbanization of America over the last 100 years has increased the cost of all disasters [3].

In contrast, the effects of epidemics have been greatly reduced, in large part because of public health and preventive medicine initiatives and better overall health and hygiene among the US population. The most significant epidemic in US history was the Spanish influenza epidemic of 1918. More than 20 million persons lost their lives worldwide, and in the United States an estimated 650,000 people died over a four-month period, at a time when the US population was approximately 76 million [4]. In Philadelphia, more than 3000 victims died and another 12,000 became acutely ill in one week during the peak of the epidemic. This probably represents the last time in modern history that the US health care system was overwhelmed to any significant extent. The last plague epidemic occurred in Los Angeles in 1924 [5]. Approximately 20,000 deaths occur annually from influenza. Vaccination of the populations at risk, however, has significantly reduced morbidity and mortality from prior times.

Terrorism has increased in lethality, although absolute numbers of terrorist events have declined since peaking in 1979 [6]. Weapons of choice for terrorists remain guns, pipe bombs, and explosives. Over the past decade, there has been concern that rogue states or terrorist organizations domestic or foreign may use chemical, biological, or radiologic weapons. The attacks in the last quarter of 2001 using anthrax-laced letters that, at the time of this publication, infected 22 individuals (11 cutaneous and 11 inhalational), caused 5 deaths, and resulted in nearly 40,000 people requiring prophylactic antibiotics, may be a harbinger of the future, should the international community not be able to curb worldwide terrorism and eliminate the potential for future use of such weapons [7].

Evolution of federal response to disasters and epidemics

Disaster response

Federal response to disasters can be traced to a Congressional Act of 1803 that provided assistance to a New Hampshire town following an extensive fire [8]. In the ensuing century, ad hoc legislation was passed more than 100 times in response to hurricanes, earthquakes, and other natural disasters. In the 1930s, the Reconstruction Finance Corporation made loans to repair certain public facilities following disasters. By 1934, the Bureau of Public Roads was providing funds for damaged highways and bridges. The Flood Control Act gave the US Army Corps of Engineers authority to implement flood control projects. This fragmented approach to disaster assistance was problematic, and prompted legislation requiring greater cooperation among federal agencies. In 1974 the Robert T. Stafford Disaster Relief and Emergency Assistance Act firmly established the process of Presidential disaster declarations [9]. Federal disaster response remained fragmented, however—disasters associated with nuclear power plants and other hazardous substances required cooperation among more than 100 federal agencies. In 1979, an Executive Order transferred many disaster-related responsibilities, including civil defense, to the newly established Federal Emergency Management Agency (FEMA) [10]. Today FEMA is the Lead Federal Agency (LFA) for the coordination of all federal assistance in managing the consequences of disasters within the United States.

Public health emergency response

Responsibility for the control of infectious diseases and epidemics resides with the Department of Health and Human Services (DHHS), the core of which is the Public Health Service (PHS). PHS traces its beginning to the passage of a 1798 act that provided for the care of sick and injured seamen [11]. Reorganization in 1870 resulted in a centrally controlled Marine Hospital Service (MHS). The National Quarantine Act of 1878 conferred quarantine authority, initially the responsibility of the states, on the MHS. Quarantine was primarily enforced at seaports. The MHS uniformed services component was formalized as the Commissioned Corps in 1889. As the federal government took over immigration processing in 1891, MHS became responsible for medical inspection of arriving immigrants, and played a major role in preventing disease from entering the country. Renamed the Public Health Service in 1912, its uniformed personnel became crucial in controlling the spread of contagious diseases such as smallpox and yellow fever, conducting important biomedical research, regulating the food and drug supply, providing healthcare to underserved groups, and supplying medical assistance in the aftermath of disasters.

Between 1862 and the present, federal offices were created with various roles in public health and prevention. The Communicable Disease Center, forerunner of the Centers for Disease Control and Prevention (CDC) was established in 1946 [12]. The Department of Health, Education and Welfare (HEW) was established in 1953. In 1979, the Department of Education Organization Act provided for a separate Department of Education. HEW became the Department of Health and Human Services (DHHS). Currently DHHS primarily consists of five staff offices, ten Regional Health Administrators, eight public health operating divisions, and three human services operating divisions. A new Office of Public Health Preparedness has also been established as a result of events in the fall of 2001 [13].

Federal response to terrorism

Executive and legislative branch actions and issuances

Laws concerning terrorism have existed for many years, but were primarily passed to combat bombings during the civil unrest of the 1960s and the rash of airplane hijackings of the 1970s. Even at the time of the poisoning of salad bars in The Dalles, Oregon, there were no federal laws that dealt with terrorist use of unconventional weapons of mass destruction (WMD) [14]. A review of legislation and resolutions introduced in Congress indicates that the total number of such introductions gradually increased from 11 in 1973 to 176 in the 106th Congressional session (2000). Peaks in legislative activities usually occurred immediately following specific terrorist events, such as the hijackings of TWA Flight 847 and the cruise ship *Achille Lauro* in 1985, or the terrorist bombing of Pan Am Flight 103 over Lockerbie, Scotland in 1988. Still, Public Law enactment remained low, averaging less than ten laws each year, and many bills languished and eventually died [15]. Events in the mid-1990s focused major attention on terrorism and the use of unconventional, highly lethal devices and agents selected to cause significant death, injury, societal disruption, and public panic. These events included the first World Trade Center bombing, the highly publicized release of sarin nerve agent into a Tokyo subway system by the Aum Shinrikyo religious cult in 1995 (the second of such releases by that religious sect), the destruction of the Murrah Federal Building in Oklahoma City by an improvised bomb, and several hoaxes involving chemical or biological agents. These and other events led to legislation targeting terrorism and use of WMD.

The Antiterrorism and Effective Death Penalty Act of 1996 [16] made terrorism a federal crime punishable by death, and provided legislation to improve investigation, capture, and prosecution of terrorists in the United States. It further allowed the government to institute deportation proceedings without divulging classified information, disallowed fundraising that supports terrorist organizations, and barred terrorists from entering the United States. It also provided the initial definitions for what were to become "Weapons of Mass Destruction," and established legislation to safeguard the illicit procurement of certain biological pathogens or precursors of highly lethal chemical compounds.

In 1997, Congress enacted the Defense Against Weapons of Mass Destruction Act [17] (commonly referred to as the Nunn-Lugar-Domenici Act). This broad-sweeping legislation was designed to improve overall national preparedness for large-scale terrorist attacks using chemical, biological, radiologic, nuclear, or high-yield explosives (CBRNE). Among its provisions, it provided civilian response personnel with CBRNE detection and monitoring equipment, and provided educational and other assistance to state and local providers through the Domestic Preparedness Program. It also authorized use of the National Guard (state asset unless federalized) and other military reserve components in responding to WMD, and established a domestic terrorism rapid response team within the Department of Defense, the Chemical and Biological Rapid Response Team (CB-RRT) [18]. DHHS was directed to establish civilian health and medical response teams/systems (originally designated Metropolitan Medical Response Teams, or MMST) in the largest metropolitan areas of the country [19], and FEMA was directed to incorporate guidance into the Federal Response Plan (FRP) for responding to WMD events and to develop a rapid response information system for use by response organizations [20,21].

Significant legislative action to improve the nation's public health posture to defend against and respond to threats from biological weapons, however, would have to wait until 2000, with the enactment of the Public Health Improvement Act, intended to improve a broad array of federal and state public health programs [22]. Several sections applied specifically to programs targeting bioterrorism. These included funding to states and localities to improve public health structures and capabilities, educational programs for hospitals, institutions, clinical, and public health professions, and a variety of grants for demonstration projects or improvements in surveillance systems.

Several Executive Orders and Presidential Decision Directives were also enacted in the 1980s and 1990s to combat terrorism and protect American citizens. An Executive Order established the National Communications System, a federal interagency group assigned the responsibility of ensuring the survivability of national security and emergency preparedness telecommunications in all circumstances, including conditions of crisis or emergency [23]. Executive Order 12656 assigned security emergency preparedness responsibilities to federal departments and agencies, based on, but separate from, their regular missions [24]. Although this document did not address WMD, it did discuss measures to protect American citizens from hazards associated with these agents, and further assigned counterterrorism responsibilities to the Department of Justice. An Executive Order issued in 1994 addressed the proliferation of such agents by foreign states, and outlined measures to re-duce this threat but did not specifically target terrorists' use of these weapons [25]. It was not until Presidential Decision Directive (PDD) 39 [26] was issued in 1995 that terrorism and the use of WMD were linked. PDD 39 detailed national policy to deter, defeat, and respond vigorously to all terrorist attacks, including those involving such weapons. Two other PDDs, issued over the next four years, further refined this policy and addressed protection of public and private sector operations deemed critical to the continuity of government of the United States [27,28]. PDD 62 specifically tasked DHHS to work with the Veterans Administration (VA) to ensure adequate stock-piles of antidotes and other necessary pharmaceuticals nationwide and the training of medical personnel in National Disaster Medical System (NDMS) hospitals.

Federal antiterrorism and weapons
of mass destruction preparedness programs

As a result of these legislative and executive actions, a series of antiterror-ism initiatives have been instituted, and have resulted in a complex web of programs to improve local, state and federal preparedness and response ca-pabilities by providing equipment, training, and planning assistance. Feder-al funding for these programs was in excess of $1.4 billion in 2000 [29], and virtually all federal agencies have such programs. Of the 40 federal agencies involved with combating terrorism, several have significant preparedness programs [30]. These include the Departments of Justice, Health and Human Services, and Defense, and FEMA and the Federal Bureau of Investigation (FBI). The following examples are by no means a complete listing, but rather those of the greatest importance to the health and medical communities.

The Domestic Preparedness Program, originally assigned to the Depart-ment of Defense (DoD) under the Nunn-Lugar-Domenici Act, was insti-tuted to provide training, expertise, and equipment grants to the 120 largest US cities. This program was transferred in 2000 to the Department of Justice (DoJ), Office of Justice Programs, under the Office for State and Local Domestic Preparedness Support, recently renamed the Office of Domestic Preparedness [31]. DoJ also oversees the National Domestic Preparedness Consortium and the Metropolitan Fire and Emergency Medical Services Training Program. The consortium has several testing and training centers in New Mexico, Texas, Alabama, Louisiana, and Nevada.

The FBI operates two programs supporting state and local preparedness, the National Domestic Preparedness Office (NDPO) and the Bomb Data Cen-ter (BDC). NDPO is an information clearinghouse on all aspects of domestic preparedness and coordinates federal policy regarding this assistance to state and local jurisdictions [32]. BDC develops bomb disposal techniques, technology, and equipment, administers the Hazardous Devices School (HDS) that trains public safety personnel in explosive device render-safe technology, and manages the State and Local Bomb Technician Equipment Program [32].

The National Institute of Justice (NIJ) is the DoJ research and development agency. Its Office of Law Enforcement Standards (OLES), as the agent for the Interagency Board of Equipment Standardization and Interoperability (IAB) [73], published the Guide for the Selection of Chemical Agent and Toxic Industrial Material Detection Equipment for Emergency First Responders [33]. At the time of this writing, four additional guides are in draft [34].

FEMA has been assisting states with disaster planning, training, and exercising for years. It provides grants to state emergency management agencies to fund terrorism consequence management and preparedness. The National Emergency Training Center (NETC) develops courses, offers on-site training, and distributes training material to state and local jurisdictions. FEMA also supports training activities by the 50 state fire-training centers, and maintains the Rapid Response Information System (RRIS), an on-line database of training and planning resources related to WMD terrorism [20]. In May of 2001, at the direction of the President, the Vice President was tasked to develop an overarching national strategy to address WMD terrorism, and FEMA established the Office of National Preparedness to coordinate all federal programs dealing with WMD consequence management [35].

Since 1995, DHHS has administered two programs to improve preparedness for bioterrorism events: the Nunn-Lugar-Domenici-mandated MMRS that evolved from the MMST concept, and the Bioterrorism Preparedness and Response Program (BPRP). The MMRS program, administered by the Office of Emergency Preparedness (OEP), is designed to enhance a community's overall health and medical capabilities to respond to WMD events. Under this program, a community must develop programs that comply with OEP guidelines and performance standards to receive federal grants. MMRS programs have been instituted in 97 cities to date, and the ultimate goal of OEP is to continue this program until the 200 largest communities have received this assistance [36]. The BPRP, established by CDC in 1998, targets five initiatives: (1) Preparedness Planning and Readiness; (2) Epidemiology and Surveillance Capacity; (3) Biological Laboratory Capacity; (4) Chemical Laboratory Capacity; and (5) State/Local Public Health Communication through the Health Alert Network (HAN). CDC has also established the Laboratory Response Network (LRN) to link public health departments at all levels to advanced diagnostic capabilities. The program is designed to increase the number of laboratories capable of detecting critical biological agents, reduce the time needed to confirm the presence of a critical agent in a clinical or environmental sample, and improve communication of testing results within the public health community. DHHS has also sponsored several other bioterrorism preparedness initiatives through OEP, CDC, the Agency for Healthcare Research and Quality (AHRQ), the Food And Drug Administration (FDA), and the National Institutes of Health (NIH) [30]. These initiatives focus on such issues as healthcare provider education and methods of early detection and diagnosis of diseases caused by potential bioterrorism pathogens and toxins. In fiscal year 2002, it is anticipated that other public health service agencies such as Health Resources and Services Administration (HRSA) and the Substance Abuse and Mental Health Services Administration (SAMHSA) will also be funded for specific bioterrorism preparedness initiatives.

As the largest national integrated healthcare system with facilities and personnel across the country, VA plays an important role in supporting federal and local counterterrorism efforts. The executive agent for Veterans Health Administration (VHA)'s Fourth Mission (emergency management) is the Emergency Management Strategic Healthcare Group (EMSHG). EMSHG coordinates emergency management programs that ensure health care for eligible veterans, military personnel, and the public during DoD contingencies and natural, manmade, and technologic emergencies. EMSHG plans and coordinates VA's role as the primary backup to DoD during war or national emergencies under the Federal Response Plan and Federal Radiological Emergency Response Plan (discussed later). EMSHG also supports continuity of operations plans through maintenance of relocation sites, and operates a remote site VA Emergency Operations Center. EMSHG's Area Emergency Managers provide support for VA healthcare facilities designated as Federal Coordinating Hospitals for the NDMS.

DoD was initially responsible for the Domestic Preparedness Program. Administered by the Soldier's Biological and Chemical Command (SBCCOM), most functions of that program were transferred to the DoJ. SBCCOM does maintain its many WMD equipment test programs and technical advisory capability, and continues to develop and exercise its Biological and Chemical Weapons Improved Response Programs [37]. These programs model incidents involving pathogens and agents and develop templates and guidelines to assist communities in improving their overall preparedness for such events. The Joint Task Force for Civil Support (JTF-CS) plans and, when directed, controls DoD's WMD and high-yield explosive consequence management capabilities in providing support during a domestic terrorism incident. JTF-CS and its parent command, US Joint Forces Command (USJFCOM), work in support of FEMA and DHHS OEP to plan Force Packages, which are groupings of military units designated to respond to an incident [38]. Under the Nunn-Lugar-Domenici Act, DoD also administers the Weapons of Mass Destruction Civil Support Team (WMD-CST) Program, providing equipment and training to these 22-person National Guard teams. WMD-CSTs, which are rapidly responsive diagnostics and communications units, remain state assets, but could be federalized if necessary. Thirty-two teams have been established, and as of this writing, twenty-six have been certified as ready for operations.

DoD has several other programs involving simulation, research and development, and equipment testing and evaluation. These focus primarily on the wartime requirement, but many of their accomplishments have application in the civilian sector. Most of these offices coordinate through the Joint Program Office for Biological Defense (JPOBD), the Defense Advanced Research Projects Agency (DARPA), or the Defense Threat Reduction Agency (DTRA). The US Army Medical Research Institute of Infectious Diseases (USAMRIID) continues its work in countermeasures against biologic warfare agents, and the Navy Medical Research Center investigates technologies such as highly accurate immune-absorbent assays.

Virtually all other federal agencies, including the Environmental Protection Agency (EPA) and Departments of Commerce, Transportation, Treasury, and Agriculture, have research or preparedness programs related to disaster preparedness, terrorism, or WMD. The Department of Energy national laboratories (Oak Ridge, Argonne, Los Alamos, Pacific Northwest, and Sandia) also perform applied and pure scientific research in biodefense. The burgeoning of such programs led the government's General Accounting Office (GAO) to conclude in the fall of 2001 that, although these departments and agencies have engaged in many efforts to coordinate these activities, collaboration between departments and agencies remains fragmented [33].

Federal response to bioterrorism: emergency operations

The Stafford Act provides the infrastructure for assistance to state and local governments by the federal government during Presidential declared disasters [39]. Federal emergency operations in response to a bioterrorism event follow these procedures, with the exception that, under PDD 39 and the Terrorist Incident Annex to the FRP, a bioterrorism incident automatically triggers a presidential declaration, and because of the criminal nature of the event, there will be superimposed federal law enforcement activities that would usually not occur as the result of natural or unintentional disasters.

Expected local response

Before or concurrent with federal actions, local community authorities are expected to take certain steps. These would include providing initial response, establishing an incident command system, and centralizing local coordination. Simultaneously with community warning and potential enactment of evacuation procedures, local emergency managers should be assessing the situation, matching requirements with capabilities, identifying further requirements, and requesting assistance through mutual aid agreements from neighboring jurisdictions and the state. If it were known at the time of discovery that a terrorism event is the cause of the disaster, local law enforcement and FBI officials would be drawn in.

Expected state response

Once a request has been received, the state is expected to respond and match needs with state capabilities. Under a State of Emergency declaration, the governor may, subject to state constitutional limitations, exercise his unique authority to suspend existing statutes and regulations and mobilize National Guard, including the WMD-CSTs and other state resources. It is believed that most states' laws concerning public health, especially as they pertain to epidemic and bioterrorism control, need updating in light of current threats. As a result, an initiative to improve this aspect of state capabilities has been undertaken, and CDC, in conjunction with the George Washington University Center for Law and Public Health and Johns Hopkins University, developed model legislation to assist the states in upgrading their statutes on this important function [40]. Although a bioterrorism event would automatically trigger involvement of the FBI, a request for outside assistance—personnel, equipment and supplies, and funding—in managing the consequences of the event would still have to be made, if deemed necessary. Such requests can go to the federal government, other state governments, or both. Section 319 of the Public Health Service Act provides specific authority for the Secretary of Health and Human Services (in consultation with the Public Health Service agency heads such as NIH, CDC, and FDA) to declare a public health emergency and take appropriate actions to prevent or respond to such emergencies.

Emergency Management Assistance Compact

Few states possess all necessary resources to respond to catastrophic disasters. Realizing that there may be emergencies requiring immediate access to outside resources to make a prompt and effective response to such emergencies, in 1996 Congress enacted the Emergency Management Assistance Compact (EMAC) [41], a mutual aid agreement that allows states to assist one another in responding to governor-declared state disasters of all types. Assistance, including personnel, material resources, or the use of the states' National Guard forces, may be provided regardless of whether a national emergency has been declared. EMAC also allows for the use of resources of signatory states during disaster training and exercises. Although originally developed for 13 states, as of April 2002, 45 states and 2 territories have signed this agreement and 2 states have legislation pending.

Any Compact state requested to render assistance to a declaration of a state of emergency or disaster or to conduct mutual aid training agrees to provide available resources. Responding personnel are afforded the same duties, rights, powers, and protections as those of the requesting state. The only exception to this is detention and arrest authority unless specifically authorized. Signatory states will also provide aid and comfort to evacuees from other Compact states. Requesting states are responsible for reimbursing all out-of-state costs and for providing death or injury benefits to responders, and are legally liable for out-of-state personnel. Any person holding a license, certificate, or other permit issued by a Compact state is deemed to be licensed, certified, or permitted by the requesting state, and state employees are considered agents of the requesting state for tort liability and immunity purposes. Allowable supplementary agreements may include provisions for evacuation and reception of injured and other persons and the exchange of medical, fire, police, public utility, reconnaissance, welfare, transportation and communications personnel, and equipment and supplies. Responding medical personnel, under the Compact supplementary umbrella, fall into the same category as responding state employees [42]. Without such supplemental agreements, however, specific authorities for such actions as quarantine might not be clear or enforceable.

Federal response

A bioterrorism event will produce little if any physical destruction, and therefore federal response will focus primarily on medical and public health operations and logistics to contain the epidemic and assist state and local agencies in providing healthcare services, including mass prophylaxis, mass patient care, and mass fatality management. The exception to this would be a combined event (ie, conventional explosion coupled with a bioterrorism agent release). Response to the consequences of a bioterrorism attack will occur simultaneously with federal criminal investigation and evidence collection. A bioterrorism event of any significant magnitude would be a national disaster, and as such, the federal government would respond to mitigate the consequences within the context of existing response plans and using existing structures, but only at the request of state and local officials. Some understanding of these plans and structures is therefore necessary to fully appreciate the complexities involved.

Several plans have been developed over the past half century, usually in response to one or more significant disasters. These plans, which cover a range of hazards and responses, are often referred to as the federal "Family of Plans." The National Oil and Hazardous Substances Pollution Contingency Plan, more commonly called the National Contingency Plan or NCP, is the federal government's blueprint for responding to oil spills and hazardous substance releases [43]. First published in 1968, it provides a comprehensive system of reporting, containment, and cleanup, and establishes a response headquarters, and national and regional reaction teams. The NCP was initially revised in 1973 [44], was broadened in 1980 [45], and further updated in 1994 [46]. Another program, the Chemical Stockpile Emergency Preparedness Plan (CSEPP), was devised to protect the public from an accident involving storage or incineration of chemical weapons at eight Army installations within the continental United States, scheduled for decommissioning over the next several years, as directed by Congress [47]. The Federal Radiological Emergency Response

Plan (FRERP) [48] sets out federal agency roles and assigns tasks regarding federal assistance to state and local governments in their radiologic emergency planning and preparedness activities. Officials are currently attempting to fold the FRERP into the Federal Response Plan as an annex. Because of its unique expertise in dealing with nuclear weapons, the DoD promulgated a separate Nuclear Accident/Incident Response Plan (NARP) [49]. Of these plans, the one most applicable to a bioterrorism event would be the NCP. Several federal agencies are also included in government plans to pre-position resources and personnel in preparation for designated high-risk events such as the Olympic Games, Presidential Inauguration, or certain international functions.

Many of these plans (NCP is a notable exception) are subsumed under the Federal Response Plan or FRP, developed under the authorization of the Stafford Act [39]. The FRP, an agreement between 27 federal agencies and one volunteer agency, the American Red Cross, is the template for overall federal assistance to state and local authorities in responding to presidentially declared disasters. Unfortunately, at present there are no clear criteria for what "qualifies" for such requests and affirmative response. The FRP was first promulgated by FEMA in 1992 and then updated in 1999. Portions of it have been revised several times, most recently in 2000 with the incorporation of the Terrorist Incident Annex, which modifies the FRP to conform with the requirements as set down by the previously discussed executive orders and public laws. In conjunction with the United States Government Interagency Domestic Terrorism Concept Of Operations Plan (CONPLAN) [50] and other agency-specific plans, the FRP provides guidance to federal, state and local agencies concerning how the federal government would respond to a potential or actual terrorist threat or incident that occurs in the United States, particularly one involving WMD.

The complete organizational structure and inter-relationships of the FRP are complex and beyond the scope of this article. As previously stated, disaster response and mitigation are deemed responsibilities of state and local governments. If the President declares a national disaster, the entire resources of the federal government may be brought to bear to stabilize the consequences of the disaster and assist in recovery operations. The FRP identifies 12 Emergency Support Functions (ESFs), each with a Primary Federal Agency (PFA) (Table 1).

According to guidance of PDD 39 as incorporated into the Terrorist Incident Annex of the FRP, the federal response to a terrorist incident involving use of WMD is divided into two phases:

- "Crisis management" includes "measures to identify, acquire, and plan the use of resources needed to anticipate, prevent, and/or to resolve a threat or act of terrorism." Primary authority for crisis management has been assigned to the federal government; state and local governments provide assistance as required. Crisis management is predomi-

Table 1
Federal response plan emergency support functions

Emergency support function and primary federal agencies	
Emergency support function	Responsible agency
1 Transportation	Department of Transportation
2 Communications	National Communications System
3 Public works and engineering	US Army Corps of Engineers
4 Firefighting	Department of Agriculture
5 Information and planning	Federal Emergency Management Agency
6 Mass care	American Red Cross
7 Resource support	Government Services Administration
8 Health and medical services	Department of Health and Human Services
9 Urban search and rescue	Federal Emergency Management Agency
10 Hazardous materials	Environmental Protection Agency
11 Food	Department of Agriculture
12 Energy	Department of Energy

nantly a law enforcement response. The FBI is the designated LFA for crisis management in the United States.

- "Consequence management" includes "measures to protect public health and safety, restore essential government services, and provide emergency relief to governments, business, and individuals effected by the consequences of terrorism." Primary authority for consequence management remains with the state and local authorities, with the federal government providing assistance if required. FEMA remains the LFA for consequence management.

The CONPLAN Biological Terrorism Incident Annex outlines initial actions and responsibilities required to respond to a biological weapon attack to protect the public's health and well being, including federal interagency actions and responsibilities in support of crisis management and consequence management operations.

In the event of an actual bioterrorism attack, the FBI will activate multiagency crisis management structures at FBI Headquarters, the responsible FBI Field Office, and the incident scene. Federal agencies requested by the FBI, including FEMA, will deploy representatives to the FBI Headquarters Strategic Information and Operations Center (SIOC). The FBI Field Office responsible for the incident site modifies its Command Post to function as a Joint Operations Center. Although the FBI On-Scene Commander retains authority over crisis management decisions, operational decisions are made cooperatively, or by higher authority, to resolve conflicts.

The Director of FEMA will consult immediately with the White House to determine if FEMA is permitted to act under the Stafford Act. If so, identified PFAs will support FEMA in overall federal response. FEMA will provide centralized consequence management coordinating all federal response assets. Because the effects of a bio-terrorism event may be manifested at multiple sites, coordinated response management on a large scale may be required. Although all PFAs will probably play some role, the principal agencies involved with health and medical consequence management operations will be DHHS, VHA, and DoD. The American Red Cross (ARC) and the EPA will also have a significant contribution.

HHS has the lead federal responsibility for the health and medical service requirements (ESF #8) resulting from biological terrorism (or all disasters, for that matter) in the United States. Categories of this functional support are listed in Table 2. The broad health objectives of the US government consequence management response to a bioterrorism event are to detect a biological release and identify the pathogen or toxin, control the epidemic, and augment patient services. These actions will require a coordinated bioresponse and close cooperation among all supporting departments and federal agencies. HHS has a primary responsibly to support state and local authorities in these objectives, with detection and agent identification capabilities, mass casualty management, protection of the "at-risk" population through immunization/prophylaxis, and direct patient care. The OEP is delegated responsibility for national implementation and coordination of this function. OEP also directs and manages the NDMS, discussed later. OEP will, after conducting a needs assessment, coordinate the mobilization and deployment of resources.

The unique attributes of a biological terrorism incident will require response elements tailored to specific health concerns and effects of each class of biological agent (eg, bacteria, viruses, toxins). A biological agent release into the population either by natural or deliberate forces may occur silently and be detected only by increased demand on the health delivery system. The route of transmission can occur by way of aerosol, person-to-person spread, or intentionally contaminated food and water. An effective detection, epidemiologic and surveillance system, and laboratory support network are therefore required. In all instances, local communities will first experience and respond to the effects of a biological release. In keeping with the template of the FRP, local response will initially be assisted by state resources and subsequently by federal ones.

CDC, which is an agency under DHHS, can provide epidemiologic and laboratory expertise to help determine the causative agent, the affected and

Table 2
Functional federal health and medical support categories (ESF #8)

Health needs assessment	In-hospital care
Health surveillance	Food/drug/medical device safety
Medical care personnel	Worker health and safety
Medical equipment and supplies	Potable water
Patient evacuation	Mental health care
Public health information	Victim identification/mortuary services
Vector control	Veterinary services
Wastewater and solid waste disposal	Radiologic/chemical/biologic hazard consultation

at-risk population, and recommended control measures, including isolation/ quarantine, and treatment and prophylactic regimens, the rapid implementation of which may be key in mitigating the consequences of the attack. HHS is also responsible for determining the need for increased surveillance in states or localities not initially involved in the outbreak, and provide recommendations to state and local health officials, to notify international health authorities, and to assist local and state authorities in establishing appropriate isolation and quarantine measures.

Beyond detection and identification, the primary HHS roles will be in coordinating control mechanisms of mass immunization/prophylaxis of the population at risk, direct patient care, and fatality management. If the biological agent involved is communicable, or if multiple geographic areas are affected, OEP will coordinate a plan for protecting public health on the national level.

Based on the size of the population at risk and availability of local resources, CDC and OEP will determine the amount and distribution of stockpiled pharmaceuticals, vaccines (if available), and supplies needed. OEP or CDC can make recommendations to the Secretary, HHS who has the final authority to mobilize the National Pharmaceutical Stockpiles (NPS). NPS consists of eight "push packs" that are supposed to be delivered to the scene within 12 hours of mobilization. Each of these weighs nearly 50 tons, occupies 124 cargo containers, and requires more than 5000 square feet of warehouse storage space [51]. Contents include antibiotics for prophylaxis or treatment, other medicines, and medical equipment and supplies. Before deployment, local officials, who are responsible for distribution of the stockpile materials, must have a plan in place to receive, store, protect, distribute, and dispense these supplies and medications. Push packs may be followed by tailored packages referred to as Vendor Managed Inventory (VMI), procured under prearranged contracts with pharmaceutical and medical supply companies. OEP will also mobilize and deploy other supplies under their control, such as those of the National Medical Response Teams (see later discussion), and may direct release of supplies from undisclosed VA locations.

If quarantine measures become necessary, CDC can provide specific recommendations regarding persons who require it and methods and time periods of such actions. The Surgeon General is empowered to enforce quarantine measures to restrict spread of disease across state lines, or into or out of the country, but it is a state responsibility to enact those measures within its boundaries, as discussed previously [52]. The quarantine authorities have not been used since the 1918 influenza pandemic and would likely be problem atic to enforce. Public education and isolation would be key measures for effective containment of a contagious biological agent. Indeed, a recent article critically examines the potential use of mass quarantine measures following a bioterrorism attack, and concludes that this method of disease containment is fraught with problems and should only be used as a last resort [53]. The CDC has also recently published interim guidance concerning a response to an outbreak of smallpox. In this document are specific guidelines concerning individual and cohort isolation. Mass quarantine is discussed, but again, this document recommends other actions, such as infected and close contact surveillance and isolation, concentric "ring" quarantine, and aggressive vaccination programs as first-line methods for disease containment [54].

If local hospital capacity is exceeded, several approaches may be used, including activating the patient evacuation and definitive care elements of the NDMS, mobilizing local auxiliary care resources, or deploying mobile treatment resources to the affected areas.

NDMS was developed in 1981 to improve response to large-scale disasters, by supplementing state and local capabilities. The four federal partners that comprise NDMS are DHHS, DoD, VA, and FEMA. Currently operating under a Memorandum of Understanding, legislation was introduced in 2001 to codify the NDMS [55]. NDMS components include medical response, patient evacuation, and definitive medical care.

Medical response is provided primarily through deployment of Disaster Medical Assistance Teams (DMATs). DMATs are locally operated and supported voluntary teams of approximately 100 people with varying medical skills. A deploying team consists of 35 people. There are currently more than 60 DMATs, of which 27 are fully capable of deploying within six hours of notification, can provide medical care for approximately 250 patients per day, and are self-sustaining for 72 hours without replenishment [56]. In addition to primary DMATs, there are several specialty teams (eg, burn, pediatrics, crush injury, veterinary medicine) [57]. There are also four National Medical Response Teams (NMRTs), located in California, Colorado, North Carolina, and Washington, DC. These teams are equipped and trained to manage casualties from chemical, biological, radiologic, or nuclear incidents. All are deployable within four hours, except the Washington, DC team, which is held in reserve [58]. DMATs provide triage and treatment of casualties in the disaster area, and can prepare patients for evacuation to other cities if necessary. Medical evacuation is coordinated by the DoD. The Aeromedical Evacuation System (AES), US Transportation Command (USTRANSCOM), has aeromedical evacuation capabilities used daily for transportation of DoD patients and in military and NDMS patient movement exercises. Though never fully tested in a real-life scenario, these resources can be re-tasked for this mission [59].

DoD, VHA, or NDMS hospitals from the private sector comprise the sites of definitive medical care for casualties resulting from an overseas war (VA-DoD Contingency Hospital System) or national disaster (NDMS). More than 2000 civilian hospitals have pledged the availability of staffed beds (total estimated at 100,000) in the event of a national disaster or major theater war. Regionally, VA or DoD Federal Coordinating Centers recruit and provide oversight in enrolling civilian hospitals that would accept civilian casualties from overwhelmed local communities. Military casualties would be placed in DoD and then VA medical centers. Patient movement to distant geographic regions through the NDMS might not be possible with a contagious biological agent, however. Hence, plans to augment local resources at the scene are required.

Fatality management is a local Medical Examiner responsibility. If local capability is overwhelmed, DHHS can offer support by activating Disaster Mortuary Operational Response Teams (DMORTs), a component of the NDMS. One of these teams is trained and equipped to process the remains of individuals that may be contaminated with an infectious agent.

DoD also has significant resources that could be used in response to disasters. The limits of such support are outlined in departmental directives that state that the military services shall plan for and respond to requests from civil government agencies for military support in dealing with the actual or anticipated consequences of civil or national security emergencies or attacks requiring federal response [60], but may not participate in law enforcement activities except under extraordinary circumstances, commonly referred to as the *Posse Comitatus* Act [61]. In general, the military may not respond to civilian requests for assistance without a Presidential declaration of an emergency. Any military commander may however provide local humanitarian assistance without higher authority to prevent significant property damage or loss of life, commonly referred to as the "Immediate Response Clause."

A complex chain of events must occur before DoD resources may deploy. First, regardless of resources required, FEMA must receive a Request for Assistance (RFA) from the affected PFA. This request must be for actual resources needed, and not for a particular military unit. If these resources are requested as a result of a disaster not related to terrorism or WMD releases, the US Army Director of Military Support (DOMS), as the operational arm of the DoD executive agent for military support to civil authorities, coordinates identification of military services' resources that can match the requirements. If, however, a bioterrorism event were to occur, approvals for these resources must be given first by the Secretary of Defense and then the Chairman of the Joint Chiefs of Staff. Validated requests are then passed to JFCOM, who, in conjunction with DOMS, tasks the services to provide appropriate units. Even JTF-CS cannot deploy without approval from the Secretary of Defense. Once deployed, however, JTF-CS assumes on-scene command of all military forces deployed for response to the event, and coordinates those forces' involvement with consequence management operations.

DoD has three categories of resources to contribute to consequence management from a bioterrorism event. expertise, medical personnel, and transportation assets. Although a part of NDMS, total fixed-site hospital capacity within DoD is less than 6000 beds, most of which are occupied. There are, however, more than 12,000 physicians and 125,000 other medical personnel on active duty, and approximately that same number in the reserve forces. There are also a significant number of deployable medical platforms (hospitals or the equivalent), ranging from the 25-bed US Air

Force Air Transportable Hospitals to the two 1000-bed hospital ships. All three services have several mobile hospitals with bed capacities in the 500-bed range. The major difficulties in using these deployable platforms are that, for the most part, they were designed for combat-related trauma casualties and they are large, requiring significant transportation assets to move, needing at least one week to be fully operational, and requiring more than 20 acres of land. The platforms also do not have significant capabilities to isolate patients with highly contagious diseases (eg, negative pressure room). Theoretically, personnel assigned to these deployable platforms could be mobilized without equipment, to augment existing healthcare facilities to staff expansion facilities, assuming equipment, most likely through the Government Services Administration (GSA), were available. With recent guidance from the Quadrennial Defense Review, which is the DoD blueprint for the future, some retooling of these assets to provide greater mobility and flexibility may occur, but that will likely take a few years [62]. DoD also has smaller, more responsive medical teams, such as the Army SMART teams, the Navy SPRINT teams, and the Air Force SPEARR teams that could be deployed more rapidly.

VA has several resources that may be used in the event of a large bioterrorism event. VHA has several emergency management functions, including participation in the NDMS and provision of support to several other agencies in their PFA roles. VHA has 163 hospitals, 130 nursing homes, and many more ambulatory care clinics and domiciliaries that could be pressed into service. It also operates more than 200 counseling centers that may be required in the aftermath of a bioterrorism event. As mentioned earlier, selected sites are repositories of additional pharmaceutical stockpiles that could be mobilized. More than 15,000 physicians and 200,000 staff are part of the VHA system. The Disaster Emergency Medical Personnel System is a database of fulltime VA employee volunteers who could be deployed to assist with disaster response and recovery. Members of VHA regional Emergency Medical Response Teams, similar but larger than DMATs, could also augment federal response under ESF #8.

The ARC, which is the PFA for ESF #6 "Mass Care," can provide vital support for massive events that includes expertise, facilities, and personnel needed to care for many casualties. The ARC can mobilize volunteers from a nationwide network to provide assistance in sheltering, feeding, emergency first aid services, and disaster welfare services. Currently, 75 chapters of the ARC are working with Metropolitan Medical Response Systems throughout the country [63].

The number of other specialty teams is staggering. In addition to those previously mentioned, DoD has explosive ordnance teams, the Chemical and Biological Immediate Response Force (CBIRF), several Technical Escort Units (with specialized chemical and biological detection equipment), and deployable public health laboratories, to name a few. Emergency Response Teams from the EPA and Strike Teams from the US Coast Guard might also be of assistance in a bioterrorism event. A GAO report concluded that, although these teams usually have unique functions, better coordination and collaboration would improve capabilities [64].

Actions since 9-11-2001

Even before September 11, 2001, several reports critical of the federal government's approach to combating terrorism and the use of WMD had been issued. These reports called for strengthening antiterrorism programs, improving overall public health infrastructure, consolidating programs, and providing greater oversight to those programs [33,65]. Weakness in response capabilities were also identified in the Operation TOPOFF exercise in May of 2000, in which a simulated bioterrorism-induced pneumonic plague epidemic occurred in Denver, Colorado, simultaneously with a chemical agent release in Portsmouth, New York and a radiologic dispersal device explosion near Washington, DC [65], and in a senior leadership tabletop exercise involving a multiple site release of smallpox, called "Dark Winter," in 2001 [66].

The events of September 11 and the subsequent anthrax-laden mailings to news media figures and government offices have prompted immediate attribution of responsibility and retaliatory actions by the federal government. In addition to the more obvious military actions undertaken against the Taliban government and Al Qaeda network in Afghanistan, evidence of the strong governmental reaction to these attacks can be seen in further executive and legislative actions. Of the 402 bills and resolutions regarding terrorism submitted during the current 107th Congress, 333 were submitted after the World Trade Center and Pentagon attacks, including the Presidential request for $40 billion in emergency funding that was approved. Twelve of the 17 Public Laws enacted were signed into law after September 11, the most significant of which is the so-called "Patriot Act," designed to strengthen intelligence gathering, border protection, and criminal prosecution of terrorists [67]. At the time of this writing, two Homeland Security Presidential Directives, four Executive Orders, and one Military Order [68] (authorizing military tribunals in lieu of criminal court actions against foreign terrorists) have also been signed.

In an attempt to provide better coordination in antiterrorism programs and terrorism response operations, the President established the Office of Homeland Security to develop and coordinate the implementation of a comprehensive national strategy to secure the United States from terrorist threats or attacks, and a Homeland Security Council to advise and assist in coordination of homeland security-related activities of executive departments and agencies and to begin effective development and implementation of homeland security policies [69]. The effectiveness of this Office and Council remain to be seen, but certain members of Congress have already opined that a cabinet-level position would work more effectively, as was recommended by at least one previous report [70].

Summary

Management of a bioterrorism event will begin with early detection and intervention at the local level. Any large-scale event will require rapid state and federal assistance. Federal initiatives targeting bioterrorism have increasingly become a complex web of executive and legislative actions, frequently initiated in reaction to specific events, and often unrelated to this threat. Multiple executive and legislative branch actions have resulted in a proliferation of federal programs, and coordination of these efforts remains a significant challenge. Still, great strides have been taken to improve our defensive posture against this emerging threat, and, at all levels, governmental authorities and agencies are much better prepared to respond to such events than they were a decade ago.

The events of September 11, 2001 and subsequent events are clear indicators that the timeline for preparedness has been significantly compressed. Federal emergency operations, historically designed more for recovery than response, seemed up to the task in the wake of the World Trade Center and Pentagon attacks, although there was criticism of federal responsiveness to the subsequent anthrax incidents [71,72], and the timeliness of federal resources in the event of a large-scale outbreak resulting from a bioterrorism attack has yet to be truly tested. The recent establishment of the Office of Homeland Security and the Homeland Security Council holds promise that some of these inefficiencies may be rectified and overall coordination of programs will improve.

Continued improvements in the effectiveness of the federal government in meeting the challenges of this and other emerging threats to homeland security will require:

- Establishment of consensus standards, metrics, and measures of effectiveness for all aspects of disaster, epidemic, and terrorism management at the local, regional, state, and federal levels
- Delineation of expected, quantifiable state and local capabilities to mitigate, prepare, respond, and recover from all disasters, including those caused by terrorist actions
- Development of predefined or clear and rapidly discernible criteria for deployment of state and federal emergency resources
- Full accountability of program costs and expenditures
- Continued consolidation or coordination of the many overlapping and at times redundant federal programs

References

[1] Auf der Heide E. Disaster response: principles of preparation and coordination. St. Louis: Mosby; 1989. p. 20.
[2] Antietam, Battle of. Microsoft® Encarta® Online Encyclopedia 2000. [at http://encarta.msn.com©1997–2000 Microsoft corporation.] Accessed: 04-14-2002.

[3] Federal Emergency Management Agency. Disaster costs: 1990–1999. April19, 2000. Available at: http://www.fema.gov/library/df_7.htm. Accessed: 04-14-2002.

[4] Kolata GB. Flu: the story of the great influenza pandemic of 1918 and the search for the virus that caused it. New York: Simon & Schuster; 2001.

[5] Viseltear AJ. The pneumonic plague epidemic of 1924 in Los Angeles. Yale J Biol Med. 1974;47(1):40–54.

[6] Department of State. Office of the Coordinator for Counterterrorism. Patterns of global terrorism—2000. April 2001 Available at: http://www.state.gov/s/ct/rls/pgtrpt/2000/. Accessed: 04-14-2002.

[7] Centers for Disease Control and Prevention. Update: investigation of bioterrorism-related anthrax—Connecticut. Morb Mortal Wkly Rep 2001;50(48):1077. pp. 1077–9.

[8] Federal Emergency Management Agency. History of the Federal Emergency Management Agency. May 28, 1999. Available at: http://www.fema.gov/about/history.htm. [Accessed: 04-14-2002.

[9] United States Code 5121, et seq. Cornell Legal Information Institute at http://www4.law.cornell.edu/uscode/. Accessed: 04-14-2002.

[10] Executive Order 12127. Federal Emergency Management Agency. March 31, 1979. National Archives and Records Administration. Available at: http://www.nara.gov/fedreg/eo1979.html. Accessed: 04-14-2002.

[11] Department of Health and Human Services. Office of the Public Health Historian. The History of the Commissioned Corps. Available at Thomas Legislative Information on the Internet. http://thomas.loc.gov/. Accessed: 04-14-2002.

[12] Department of Health and Human Services. HHS: historical highlights. November 15, 2001. Available at: http://www.hhs.gov/about/hhshist.html. Available at Thomas Legislative Information on the Internet. http://thomas.loc.gov/. Accessed: 04-14-2002.

[13] Department of Health and Human Services. Factsheet: What we do. November 15, 2001. Available at http://www.hhs.gov/news/press/2001pres/01fsprofile.html. Accessed: 04-14-2002.

[14] Miller J, Broad S, Engelberg S. Germs: biological weapons and America's secret war. New York: Simon & Schuster; 2001.

[15] Review of Congressional Sessions 1973-present by author, at Thomas Legislative Information on the Internet. http://thomas.loc.gov/. Accessed: 04-14-2002.

[16] Public Law 104–132. Antiterrorism and Effective Death Penalty Act of 1996. Available at Thomas Legislative Information on the Internet. http://thomas.loc.gov/. Accessed: 04-14-2002.

[17] Public Law 104–201. Defense Against Weapons of Mass Destruction Act of 1997. Available at Thomas Legislative Information on the Internet. http://thomas.loc.gov/. Accessed: 04-14-2002.

[18] Soldiers' Biological and Chemical Command. Chemical and Biological Rapid Response Team Concept of Operations. Aberdeen Proving Grounds. September 23, 1999.

[19] Henderson DA DHHS FY2000 Anti-terrorism funding: $277,553,000. In: Biodefense Quarterly 2000;1(4) Baltimore, MD: Center for Civilian Biodefense Studies, Johns Hopkins University.

[20] Federal Emergency Management Agency. Rapid response information system internet homepage. [at http://www.rris.fema.gov/]. Accessed: 04-14-2002.

[21] Federal Emergency Management Agency. Terrorist incident annex to the federal response plan. June 3, 1999. Available at: http://www.fema.gov/r-n-r/frp/frpterr.htm. Accessed: 04-14-2002.

[22] Public Law 106–505. Public Health Improvement Act of 2000. Available at Thomas Legislative Information on the Internet. http://thomas.loc.gov/. Accessed: 04-14-2002.

[23] Executive Order 12472. Assignment of national security and emergency preparedness telecommunications functions. April 3, 1984. Available at: http://www.fas.org/irp/offdocs/eo/eo-12472.htm. Accessed: 04–14-2002.

[24] Executive Order 12656. Assignment of emergency preparedness responsibilities. Federal Register Vol. 53. No. 228, November 23, 1988.

[25] Executive Order 12938. Proliferation of weapons of mass destruction. White House Fact Sheet. November 14, 1994. Available at: http://www.fas.org/irp/offdocs/eo12938.htm. Accessed: 04-14-2002.

[26] Presidential Decision Directive 39. US Policy on Counterterrorism. June 21, 1995. Available at: http://www.fas.org/irp/offdocs/pdd39.htm. Accessed: 04-14-2002.

[27] Presidential Decision Directive 62. Combating Terrorism. May 22, 1998. Available at: http://www.fas.org/irp/offdocs/pdd-62.htm. Accessed: 04-14-2002.

[28] Presidential Decision Directive 63. Critical Infrastructure Protection. May 22, 1998. Available at: http://www.fas.org/irp/offdocs/paper598.htm. Accessed: 04-14-2002.

[29] Department of Defense. Annual report to congress on combating terrorism, including defense against weapons of mass destruction/domestic preparedness and critical infrastructure protection. Government Printing Office, Washington; DC; May 18, 2000. p. 45.

[30] General Accounting Office. Bioterrorism: federal research and preparedness activities. GAO-01-915. Washington, DC: Government Printing Office; September 2001.

[31] Clinton WJ. Designation of the Attorney General as the Lead Official for the Emergency Response Assistance Program Under Sections 1412 and 1415 of the National Defense Authorization Act for Fiscal Year 1997 (Public Law 104-201). Memorandum 2000; April:6.

[32] National Domestic Preparedness Office. Blueprint for the National Domestic Preparedness Office, undated, p. 5–7. [at http://www.ndpo.gov/blueprint.pdf.] Accessed: 04-14-2002.

[33] Heinrich J. Bioterrorism: coordination and preparedness. Statement of the Director, Health Care–Public Health Issues, General Accounting Office, before the Subcommittee on Government Efficiency, Financial Management, and Intergovernmental Relations, Committee on Government Reform, House of Representatives, October 5, 2001.

[34] National Institute of Justice, Federal Bureau of Investigation website. http://www.ojp.usdoj.gov/nij/new.htm#pubs Accessed 04-14-2002.

[35] Federal Emergency Management Agency News on the Internet. FEMA announces organizational and functional changes. Washington, DC. June:18, 2001. Available at: http://www.fema.gov/nwz01/nwz01_60.htm. Accessed: 04-14-2002.

[36] Office of Emergency Preparedness. Department of Health and Human Services. Metropolitan Medical Response System program. [at http://www.mmrs.hhs.gov/About/ProDesc.cfm]. Accessed: 04-14-2002.

[37] Soldiers' Biological and Chemical Command. Homeland Defense Website. [http://www.sbccom.army.mil/]. Accessed: 04-14-2002.

[38] Lawlor B. Military capabilities and domestic terrorism: perspectives on preparedness. Cambridge, MA: John F. Kennedy School of Government, Harvard University publication No. 2; August 2001.

[39] Public Law 93-288. Disaster Relief Act Amendments of 1974. May 22, 1974. Available at Thomas Legislative Information on the Internet. http://thomas.loc.gov/. Accessed: 04-14-2002.

[40] Gostin LO, Terret SP, Burris S, Vernick JS. Model State Emergency Health Powers Act. Center for Law and the Public's Health, Johns Hopkins and George Washington Universities. October 23, 2001. Available at: http://www.publichealthlaw.net. Accessed: 04-4-2002].

[41] Public Law 104-321. Granting the Consent of Congress to the Emergency Management Assistance Compact. Available at Thomas Legislative Information on the Internet. http://thomas.loc.gov/. Accessed: 04-14-2002.

[42] Emergency Management Assistance Compact available at National Emergency Management association webiste. [at http://www.nemaweb.org]. Accessed: 04-14-2002.

[43] Public Law 101-380. Oil Pollution Act of 1990. August 18, 1990. Available at Thomas Legislative Information on the Internet. http://thomas.loc.gov/. Accessed: 04-14-2002.

[44] Public Law 93–207. A bill to amend the Federal Water Pollution Control Act, as amended. December 28, 1973. Cornell Legal Information Institute at http://www4.law.cornell.edu/uscode/. Accessed: 04-14-2002.

[45] Public Law 96–510. Comprehensive Environmental Response, Compensation, and Liability Act of 1980. December 11, 1980. Available at Thomas Legislative Information on the Internet. http://thomas.loc.gov/. Accessed: 04-14-2002.

[46] Public Law 103–311. Hazardous Materials Transportation Act Amendment. August 26, 1994. Available at Thomas Legislative Information on the Internet. http://thomas.loc.gov/. Accessed: 04-14-2002.

[47] Public Law 99–145, Title 14, Part B, Section 1412. Department of Defense Authorization Act of 1985. November 8, 1985. Cornell Legal Information Institute at http://www4.law.cornell.edu/uscode/. Accessed: 04-14-2002.

[48] Public Law 96–295, Section 304. A bill to authorize appropriations to the Nuclear Regulatory Commission.; June 30,1980.

[49] Department of Defense Directive 3150.8 DoD Response to Radiological Accidents. Government Printing Office, Washington; DC.

[50] Federal Emergency Management Agency. United States Government Interagency Domestic Terrorism Concept Of Operations Plan. Cornell Legal Information Institute at http://www4.law.cornell.edu/uscode/. Accessed: 04-14-2002.

[51] National Pharmaceutical Stockpile 2001. Presentation by Centers for Disease Control and Prevention, National Center for Environmental Health, Division of Emergency and Environmental Health Services. Washington, DC, May 13, 2001.

[52] United States Code. Sections 264 and 271. Public Health Service Act. Cornell Legal Information Institute at http://www4.law.cornell.edu/uscode/. Accessed: 04-14-2002.

[53] Barbera J, MacIntyre A, et al. Large-scale quarantine following biological terrorism in the United States: scientific examination, logistic and legal limits, and possible consequences. JAMA 2000;286(21):2711–7.

[54] Centers for Disease Control and Prevention. Interim smallpox response plan and guidelines (draft 2.0). Available at: http://www.bt.cdc.gov/DocumentsApp/Smallpox/RPG/index.asp. Accessed November 21, 2001.

[55] House Resolution 2333. National Disaster Medical System Act. July 16, 2001.

[56] Committee on research and development needs for improving civilian medical response to chemical and biological terrorism incidents. Institute of Medicine. Chemical and Biological Terrorism: Research and Development to Improve Civilian Medical Response. National Academy Press; 1999.

[57] Office of Emergency Preparedness. Department of Health and Human Services. Disaster Medical Assistance Teams Factsheet. [at http://ndms.dhhs.gov/NDMS/About_Teams/about_teams.html]. 04-14-2002.

[58] Office of Emergency Preparedness. Department of Health and Human Services. National Medical Response Team Factsheet. [at http://ndms.dhhs.gov/CT_Program/NMRTs/nmrts.html]. Accessed: 04-14-2002.

[59] US Transportation Command Pamphlet 35–1. September 1, 1997. Available at: http://www.transcom.mil. Accessed: 04-14-2002.

[60] Department of Defense Directive 3025.1 Military Support to Civil Authorities. Government Printing Office, Washington; DC.

[61] 18 United States Code Section 1385, PL86–70, Section 17[d] Use of Army and Air Force as posse comitatus. Cornell Legal Information Institute [at http://www4.law.cornell.edu/uscode/]. Accessed: 04-14-2002.

[62] Department of Defense. Quadrennial Defense Review 2001. Government Printing Office; September 30, 2001. pp. 3–6.

[63] Healy B. Hearing on terrorism and US government capabilities [written statement]. Senate Appropriations Committee. May 10, 2001. Available at: http://www.senate.gov/~appropriations/commerce/testimony/terrheal.htm. Accessed: 04-14-2002.

[64] General Accounting Office. Combating terrorism: federal response teams provide varied capabilities; opportunities remain to improve coordination. GAO-01-14. Washington, DC: Government Printing Office.; November 30, 2000.

[65] Inglesby TV, Grossman R, O'Toole T. A plague on your city: observations from TOPOFF. Clin Infect Dis 2001;32:436–45.

[66] Inglesby TV, O'Toole T. Shining light on Dark Winter. Baltimore, MD: Center for Civilian Biodefense Studies, Johns Hopkins University. Available at: http://www.hopkins-biodefense.org. Accessed: 04-14-2002.

[67] Public Law 107–56. Uniting and strengthening America by providing appropriate tools required to intercept and obstruct terrorism (USA Patriot Act) Act of 2001. October 26, 2001. Cornell Legal Information Institute at http://www4.law.cornell.edu/uscode/. Accessed: 04-14-2002.

[68] Military Order of November 13, 2001. Detention, treatment, and trial of certain noncitizens in the war against terrorism. Federal Register: Presidential Documents. November 16, 2001;66(222)57831–6.

[69] Executive Order 13228. Establishing the Office of Homeland Security and the Homeland Security Council. October 8, 2000. [http://www.fas.org/irp/offdocs/eo/eo-13228.htm]. Accessed: 04-14-2002.

[70] US Commission On National Security In The 21st Century: seeking a national strategy. A concert for preserving security and promoting freedom. Washington, DC; 2001. [http://www.nssg.gov/Reports/reports.htm]. Accessed: 04-14-2002.

[71] McClam E. CDC under fire for failure to test. Chicago, IL: Southtown Daily News (Associated Press) October 24, 2001.

[72] Waeckerle JF. Testimony before the House Committee on Government Reform, Subcommittee on National Security, Veterans Affairs, and International Relations. November 29, 2001.

[73] National Law Enforcement and Corrections Technology Center Internet site. [at http://www.nlectc.org/techproj/nij_p52.html]. Accessed: 04-14-2002.

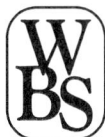

EMERGENCY
MEDICINE
CLINICS OF
NORTH AMERICA

Emerg Med Clin N Am
20 (2002) 501–524

Future challenges in preparing for and responding to bioterrorism events

Jessica Jones, MD[a,*], Thomas E. Terndrup, MD, FACEP[b],
David R. Franz, DVM, PhD[c],
Edward M. Eitzen, Jr., MD, MPH, FACEP[d]

[a]*Department of General Internal Medicine, University of Alabama at Birmingham,
619 South 19th Street, MEB 608, Birmingham, AL 35249, USA*
[b]*Department of Emergency Medicine, University of Alabama at Birmingham,
619 South 19th Street, JTN 266, Birmingham, AL 35249, USA*
[c]*Chemical and Biological Defense Division, Southern Research Institute,
365 West Patrick Street, Suite 223, Frederick, MD 21701, USA*
[d]*US Army Medical Research Institute of Infectious Diseases,
1425 Porter Street, Fort Detrick, MD 21702, USA*

Before 1990 and the Gulf War, the possibility of biological warfare or a biological terrorist attack against the United States seemed remote. At the time of the Gulf War and afterwards, we learned that Iraq had attempted to weaponize the etiologic agents of anthrax and botulism. The United States and some coalition forces were immunized and diagnostic tools were quickly developed. Fortunately the primitive Iraqi biological weapons were never used. Shortly thereafter, Colonel Kanatjan Alibekov (now known as Dr. Ken Alibek), Deputy Director of Biopreparate, the civilian research and production arm of the Soviet biological weapons program, defected to the United States with stories that made the Iraqi program look like a shoe-string terrorist effort. During the cold war, Russia, the United States, and other nations developed biological agents for use on the battlefield against military forces, or for strategic use against their wartime enemies. They learned that only 10 or 20 agents of the thousands in nature had the pathogenic characteristics, growth characteristics, and stability to survive long enough in the environment to be inhaled by their unsuspecting victims. Thousands of scientists and engineers were employed in these programs.

This work was supported by The Agency for HealthCare Research and Quality (contract #290-00-0022).

* Corresponding author.
E-mail address: jesjones@rocketmail.com (J.W. Jones).

The most virulent strains of agents like *Bacillus anthracis* were painstakingly selected before the four to six year process of weaponization began. This culminated in an efficient weapon of war that could kill or incapacitate humans inhabiting thousands of square kilometers. With the apparent demise of the Russian bioweapons (BW) program, the perceived threat has diminished in size—and possibly lethality—but is much broader in scope. Subsequently, the economy of the former Soviet Union imploded under the pressures of western free enterprise and many of the highly skilled and experienced Russian weaponeers were suddenly without paid employment. The concern in this country was "brain-drain" to states that might employ these weaponeers to develop their own bioweapon programs. At the same time several conventional terrorist attacks against American assets, the Aum Shinrikyo chemical attack in the Tokyo subway, and a surge of hoaxes and media attention gave the American public a growing realization that the next terrorist attack might be with a disease-causing agent. Tragically, the events of September 11, 2001 and those in the weeks following have demonstrated that the perceived threat is indeed a real one.

The current threat: terrorism versus warfare

The spectrum of the bioterrorist threat has broadened in the last few decades. Today we are concerned about an attack by an individual or small group on one of our cities, a large sporting event, or a unit of our military forces deploying from one of our bases to stabilize a situation in a developing country. The new bioweaponeer may be state-sponsored or simply a disgruntled employee. In the case of a state-sponsored terrorist group, the weapon might be a pound of talcum powder-like bacteria, genetically engineered for vaccine and antibiotic resistance and professionally stabilized for easy dissemination, or in the latter case, it might be human body fluids sprayed on a cafeteria serving line. In the future, it could be a microorganism genetically engineered or stabilized using the latest pharmaceutic technologies.

Future bioterrorist attacks are likely to be smaller in scale than were planned during the period of the United States and Soviet programs. Certainly, states with bioweapon stocks may resort to their use as an act of desperation. This type of "asymmetric" warfare is a viable alternative for a nation that cannot match the arsenal of the United States. Although a large-scale state-sponsored attack is believed to be unlikely, the aftermath would be disastrous not only in lives lost, but also in the potential for significant social, psychologic, and economic destruction.

Attackers may more likely be small, non-government–sponsored splinter groups isolated from the mainstream, paranoid, grandiose, and who see terrorist actions as defensive. They may use fairly low-tech and often inexpensive, available devices. Many experts believe that aerosolization of microorganisms into a building HVAC system or sprayed on food are likely mechanisms for organism dissemination. There seems to be a trend among conventional terrorists to choose either a single symbolic building such as a government or financial building, or to try to affect as many innocent civilians as possible. This was the case in the Aum Shinrikyo sarin nerve gas attack on a Tokyo subway. Common motivations of terrorist groups now tend to be either apocalyptic or anti-government, although a variety of anarchist groups such as the anti-globalization, eco-environmental, and others may resort to using biological weapons as a means of advancing their agendas. As evidenced by the recent incidents of bioterrorism dispersed through the mail, whatever the dispersion method or the target, the resultant disruption to our infrastructure and societal confidence is severe.

A hoax can be nearly as disruptive as an actual attack. The frequency of hoaxes and attacks continues to increase. According to a 1999 analysis by Tucker et al, there have been 415 total chemical, biological, radiologic, or nuclear purported terrorist attacks worldwide since 1900, with 74 in 1997, and 181 in 1998. Thirty-three of these attacks were biological in nature, and 80% were hoaxes. In addition to hoaxes, there have been many copycat incidents, particularly after widely publicized attacks such as Aum Shinrikyo [1,99]. In the past, intense and sometimes exaggerated media attention has stimulated copycat hoaxes [98]. Appropriate media coverage puts these disruptions into proper community perspective.

Potential impact of biotechnology

We know that scientists in the former Soviet Union experimented with modifying many agents such as smallpox, tularemia, and the plague bacillus, attempting to make them more virulent or resistant to available vaccines or antibiotics. The Soviets may have developed a vaccine-resistant strain of *Bacillus anthracis*. It has been alleged that the Soviet program may have the capability to create a recombinant Ebola-smallpox weapon, or a tularemia weapon encoding genes for the production of a myelin-toxin, causing the victim to display symptoms of multiple sclerosis after recovering from tularemia [2]. Genetically altered mousepox has been created in a laboratory in Australia that expresses interleukin 4. Not only does this dramatically increase virulence but it kills previously immunized mice [3]. Although the completion of the sequencing of the human genome represents a great medical advance, this data may be used by scientists and others for less than beneficial reasons. Sophisticated bioengineers may be able to design biological weapons that attack our immune system in ways that make us less capable of responding in the event of infection.

The notion of genetically enhanced virulence factors in viruses causing human infection is conceivable, but remains enormously difficult without significant resources and futuristic technical developments. Future bioterrorist attacks would likely resemble natural outbreaks initially. Clinicians must keep in mind, however, that although bioterrorist-induced illness may resemble natural outbreaks, the microorganisms may have been modified for increased virulence, may have resistance to antibiotics or vaccines, or may have had recombinant genes inserted in them to resemble multiple, simultaneous infections, so-called binary agents.

Prevention

The complete prevention of biological warfare or biological terrorism, however desirable, may not be feasible. Treaties have not been followed in the past, and may not be followed in the future [2]. There is also an ongoing effort to develop international law that would hold leaders of proliferating states or organizations responsible for the illegal use of biological agents as weapons. Some scientists and ethicists believe that international non-governmental collaboration between scientists may be the best hope for limiting possible threats from government-sponsored terrorism [4]. For instance, a microbiologist with strong research ties to many other international scientists might have greater reservations about participating in weapons research. Broad preparation is a deterrent: a terrorist may be less likely to attack given the knowledge that we are prepared to minimize the consequences. An effective forensic capability to characterize a bioagent, making attribution and response possible, may also be a deterrent for state-sponsored terrorism. Biologic weapons in the future, however, also may be used by terrorists with either minimal or no ties to any government, which would make attribution more difficult.

Early detection and early response are critical in defense against bioterrorist attacks. The importance of appropriate surveillance systems cannot be overemphasized. Ideally, the public health system should lead preparation efforts. Augmenting public health services not only helps detect and defend against bioterrorism, but also helps protect our increasingly urban and mobile population from the growing threat of emerging infectious diseases. Sufficient preparation to detect and rapidly respond to bioterrorism may be the best deterrent to an attack.

Clearly emergency medicine plays a leading role in disaster preparedness and response, especially to a bioweapons incident, but also in a natural epidemic. The most recent data on Emergency Department (ED) visits indicates continued escalation in the number of encounters in the United States, including a significant concentration of patients with infectious disorders. Bioterrorism preparedness has the additional benefit of augmenting the ED's ability to recognize and treat emerging infections. It is likely that victims will first be encountered in the ED. This article lays out what the authors believe are important future challenges for the health care community in becoming better prepared for biological terrorism.

Identification of a biological attack

Biologic attacks may be either overt (announced) or covert (unannounced). In either case, awareness or recognition of the event is the first step in response management. Overt attacks require rapid assessment of the veracity of the incident, then an appropriate response as indicated. A covert attack will be obvious only after victims present for medical care, after the incubation period has passed and clinical signs begin to manifest. Overt and covert attacks may require different types of biodetection technology. Environmental detection may, in the future, be useful in determining the necessary level of response. Early diagnostic evaluation and assessment of host responses will play a role in both types of attacks. Surveillance systems remain the most important means for early detection of a covert event and management of an overt attack.

Surveillance system issues

Increasing the timeliness and accuracy of public health surveillance can promote early identification of an outbreak. A nationally computerized database of unusual or prevalent medical conditions will promote earlier recognition of bioterrorist events, emerging infections, and outbreaks or epidemics. Victims of a covert bioterrorist attack are unlikely to present to the same hospital or clinic. Given the delayed onset and insidious nature of most diseases caused by likely bioterrorism agents, victims may present in a delayed and geographically diverse fashion, even after traveling to other cities and states. Because an epidemic may arise on many fronts, computerized, real-time surveillance may be indispensable in promoting early detection of an attack.

Current routine surveillance did not detect the West Nile Virus outbreak in New York City in 1999. The system in place at that time, despite detecting nine reports of encephalitis and 172 reports of aseptic meningitis, did not sound the alarm. An alert clinician noticed the unusual pattern first. In addition, there was ineffective recognition of the importance of veterinary reports of avian encephalitis cases. Animal outbreaks may be the first manifestation of a bioterrorist or agricultural attack against humans or animals. Involvement of veterinarians in disease surveillance and bioterrorism planning is needed. Improved surveillance might have detected West Nile Virus earlier, preventing morbidity and mortality [5]. In the future, bioterrorists may in fact seek to use animal diseases to cripple the United States economically. The implications of the recent "mad cow" and "foot and mouth" disease outbreaks serve as important indicators of the impact of animal disease on society.

One model that may be appropriate is increased local surveillance, like that which took place during the 1996 Atlanta Olympic Games. In addition to having onsite biodetection systems, vaccine and antibiotic stockpiles, and staff trained in recognition of agent-related illnesses, there was also active surveillance of local disease incidence. Physicians were not only instructed to report any unusual symptoms, but standardized patient data were transmitted and collated daily [6]. Geographic Information Systems (GIS) software has also been shown to be useful in tracking infectious disease outbreaks [7].

A recent promising development is syndromic surveillance. Several "applications" have been piloted with encouraging results. One such system, LEADERS (Lightweight Epidemiological Advanced Detection Emergency Response System), works by collecting data by way of the internet or a faxed sheet listing the types of syndromes seen in the ED. Results are compiled every 12 hours and distributed to ED workers and public health authorities. When unusual patterns appear, alerts are generated and an investigation is initiated. A similar system, ENCOMPASS (Enhanced Consequence Management Planning And Support System), was used in Washington, DC during the inauguration and was the first local system to detect an outbreak of influenza [8]. Other similar systems have been developed to collect data from alternate sources, for example, the ESSENCE system used to monitor disease trends at military hospitals in the Washington, DC area. Computer-assisted syndromic recognition also may be useful for healthcare professionals. Some experts recommend routine surveillance for disease syndromes such as "fever and rash," "acute hepatitis," "rapidly progressive pneumonia," and "influenza-like illness," among others. Education of clinicians is required to consider a syndromic approach to diagnosis. Computerized reporting of such syndromes, whether through LEADERS or other similar systems, can provide early warning of suspicious patterns, and earlier recognition than might be provided by even well prepared clinicians [9]. A potential benefit of such surveillance could be to trigger the targeted use of other, more expensive technical diagnostic measures. For instance, it may not be feasible to routinely use high-technology diagnostics on every patient who presents with flu-like symptoms in the ED, but in the event of a suspicious pattern, high-level identification and diagnostic tools could be applied to assess for the confirmation of a threat agent.

Future surveillance challenges will include the creation of the technical infrastructure to survey as many computerized data entry points as possible, to allow the earliest possible warning of bioterrorism attacks and emerging infections. For example, computerized surveillance of the numbers of ED encounters for specific complaints or syndromes, the total number of ambulance calls, total ED visits, school or work absenteeism, microbiology laboratory data, over-the-counter drug purchases and pharmacy prescriptions, and other medical data, with evaluation of suspicious patterns, may assist in early detection [10]. One promising approach would be to monitor real-time prescription drug use by national pharmacy benefits management companies. These organizations provide electronic data collection and feedback to pharmacies on drug coverage by insurance companies. Rapid upsurges in certain filled drug prescriptions may indicate the beginnings of an infectious disease outbreak. If privacy and proprietary concerns can be overcome, this data may serve as an important aspect of surveillance.

Public health "infrastructure" has been defined as "a system of well trained persons who have the right tools and equipment to prevent disease and protect the public's health" [11]. Public health infrastructure not only includes improved surveillance and improved computer technology and well-trained individuals, but established communication pathways. The importance of communication cannot be overemphasized. Better communication with not just the medical community but also law enforcement, intelligence communities, first responders, and environmental authorities such as municipal water quality managers is also needed [12,13].

In the future there will be greater need for more public health officials with specialized epidemiology training to better determine the source of a covert attack or natural outbreak, and to trace individuals who may have been exposed. The epidemiology of a bioterrorism attack is likely to be consistent with classic infectious disease epidemiology. There are however some potential differences. There may be a shorter incubation period secondary to higher exposure doses, better delivery systems, different routes of exposure, or alterations in the bioagents themselves. Other clues might include a compressed epidemic curve in a focal population, unusually severe disease, an outbreak unusual for the geographic area or season, multiple outbreaks of different diseases, unusual strains, or atypical exposure patterns such as an outbreak only in personnel from a single office building [14]. Thus, there will be a need for personnel with epidemiologic and surveillance training in public health and other medical professions [11]. It is hoped that the public health system of the new century will play a much more vital role in medical care than it has for the last several decades. We are beginning to understand the importance of preventive medicine, not just acute care, and we are thinking of the health of populations rather than isolated individuals.

Environmental detection

Most of the work on environmental biodetection devices has been in a military context. Current detection devices are slow, lack sensitivity for some agents, and are plagued by false positive results. Early warning in a civilian context might involve either assessment of the threat of covert attack or surveillance in a high-risk area. Biodetectors could be calibrated to the calculated risk assessment in appropriate locations to tune the surveillance system to risk. Although current technology is not sufficiently developed to have a system of sensors work as "bio-alarms," in the future it may be feasible to have biosensors placed in high-risk areas to provide immediate detection and warning of an attack.

Two types of biosensors have been developed for use in a military or field setting: immunoassay-based sensors and instruments based on spectral analysis. For example, the Portal Shield is a 120-pound immunochromatographic sensor that can detect eight different agents in 20 minutes. The RAPTOR, at 12 pounds, is another field detector that uses an immunoassay-based fiberoptics biosensor [15,16,100]. There are several genetically based agent identification devices in development that use nucleic acid analysis. Handheld, lightweight, fully automated PCR-based agent identification devices that provide results in less than half an hour are now in the final stages of development [17]. Researchers also are working on sensors based on biological systems such as cellular response and cell membrane response [18,19]. All of the above methods are limited in the sense that one must be looking for a specific pathogen to create the appropriate antibody or gene probe to find it. A completely different approach based on time-of-flight mass spectrometry can overcome this difficulty, but presently this technology has limitations regarding specificity [20–23].

Sensitivity and specificity are important issues to consider in designing and using an environmental biosensor. The appropriate level of sensitivity will vary based on the situation and the agent. Increasing the level of sensitivity may result in decreased specificity and an increased false positive rate. This may be appropriate in certain settings where there is an increased risk and adequate preparations for a possible attack have been made. False positive results from biodetectors may lead to panic, (especially in untrained populations), and could lead to unnecessary closings of major institutions, airports, and subways. One way to increase the accuracy of sensors in the environment is to integrate multiple sensors of the same type or perhaps to use a quick antibody-based test to screen and a nucleic acid-based test to confirm a positive result (much as HIV testing is routinely confirmed). Another approach to area coverage is to integrate input from an array of environmental sensors to reduce the likelihood of false positive results. An array of confirmatory (ie, not screening) identification tools is used in certain high-risk situations so that immediate field decisions can be made [19].

Antibody-based chromatographic field assays have been fielded for six to eight of the key threat agents. Although considered by many to be diagnostic tools, the CDC has recommended that they be used only for screening of environmental samples. The sensitivity and specificity of these portable assays is better for some agents than others. Unfortunately the assays for *Bacillus anthracis* have suffered from a high rate of false positive results. The state-of-the-art diagnostics include traditional clinical laboratory microscopic staining, antigen and antibody ELISA, and for some agents, specific or other metabolic assays. Definitive laboratory identification is currently by nucleic acid-based assays. Several forms of PCR can be used for quick and definitive screens. Restriction fragment length polymorphism (RFLP) and amplified fragment length polymorphism (AMFLP) are used for quick strain identification, and targeted sequencing is used for definitive strain identification. These nucleic acid-based assays are generally more specific and sensitive than antibody-based assays. We have just begun moving the nucleic acid-based assays out of the laboratory and into the field. In the future the equipment will become smaller and hand-held, and sample preparation will be automated. Finally, the real breakthrough in diagnostics for triage will come when we can identify exposed individuals before the onset of clinical signs.

Because of the technical difficulty of environmental detection of biological agents, outbreak identification through early clinical recognition will remain the most feasible and effective means of detection in the foreseeable future. Environmental detection technology will be most useful in a supportive role, after surveillance methods have noted an unusual number of cases or atypical syndromes. Currently, the Agency for Healthcare Research and Quality (AHRQ) is sponsoring research into the sensitivity, specificity, and delay of "alarms" from environmental detection and various surveillance systems.

Laboratory diagnostics and identification issues

Currently many hospital laboratories must send out suspicious specimens to reference laboratories, delaying diagnostic confirmation. Furthermore, laboratory staff may not be suspicious of exotic agents. In a recent example, four out of four labs in New Mexico did not evaluate *B. anthracis* specimens further than "bacillus species, probable contaminant" [24]. Other laboratories at highly respected institutes such as Johns Hopkins have also failed similar tests [25]. Some microbiology laboratories have been underfunded, have undergone consolidation, and may have lost adequate clinical contact with physicians [26]. Education of hospital laboratory employees is needed in the recognition of potential implications of anthrax bacillus and its characteristic morphology under suspicious circumstances. A national Laboratory Response Network (LRN) is being developed by the Centers for Disease Control to provide reagents and training, along with a system of rapid regional laboratory referral. The system consists of Levels A through D laboratories, with Level A laboratories having basic rule-out capability, then progressively more capability up to the two Biosafety Level (BSL)-4-capable Level D laboratories, one at the CDC's National Center for Infectious Diseases and the other at USAMRIID [27]. Future plans include increasing the number of laboratories involved in this system, improving regional forensic identification capabilities, furthering the education of laboratory technicians, and pushing nucleic acid-based diagnostic technologies to the state laboratory level.

Future laboratory needs include the further development of nucleic acid technology for increased diagnostic ability and increased forensic capability. A diagnostic computerized "zebra chip" would use nucleic acid technology to quickly screen a sample from an ill patient, potentially providing an immediate diagnosis and identifying an unusual or man-made agent from a natural infection. Although this technology will probably take years to develop and implement, increased forensic capability may not be as far off. A database of all known threat agents and their genomic signature would be useful for attribution. A bioagent once identified could be compared with the database, and its source might be identified.

Pre-clinical diagnostics

It is likely even in the event of a small-scale attack that many individuals will present for medical care out of concern that they may have been exposed. Even patients who have not been exposed may present with symptoms suggesting exposure [28]. Mass hysteria will make it extremely difficult to sort out individuals who truly have been exposed and would benefit from prophylactic therapy, from worried well and patients with other illnesses or psychogenic symptoms. A simple, rapid means of detecting early or asymptomatic infection would be especially useful in such circumstances. High sensitivity would be required, even at the expense of specificity. There are several cytokines that are elevated early in some infections. A sensitive assay for one of these cytokines, or the gene expression that precedes their presence, could be helpful in determining who had been exposed to an infectious agent and who may benefit from post-exposure antibiotic prophylaxis, vaccination, or quarantine.

Prophylaxis, post-exposure measures, and treatments

Vaccines

Vaccination is an effective means of prophylaxis, and for a few infectious diseases it is a useful means of helping to prevent disease in exposed individuals or terminating outbreaks. Vaccines are unlikely to be useful in protecting the general population from all agents used by bioterrorists. In addition to lack of public acceptance of additional vaccination and its attendant risks, attempting to immunize the entire population would be too expensive and would result in too little potential benefit. Vaccines will likely be of greater use for military personnel, and possibly emergency medical technicians (EMTs), law enforcement personnel, laboratory workers, and frontline healthcare providers. For certain agents such as anthrax and smallpox, however, it is essential to have a supply of vaccine for post-exposure prophylaxis, and in the case of smallpox, for contacts of ill patients and healthcare providers [29,30].

The current US anthrax vaccine is a cell-free filtrate of a protein antigen (protective antigen) that is also produced by *B. anthracis* during infection; it requires a six-dose series over 18 months, with annual boosters thereafter [30,31]. A similar vaccine was tested in at-risk woolen mill workers in the late 1950s. Available for military use and other high-risk professions, the vaccine has been shown to be nearly 100% effective in preventing anthrax in aerosol challenges of non-human primates, and has few side effects, mainly mild local reactions [32]. Currently, research is underway to reassess the anthrax vaccination schedule to determine if a less onerous schedule is equally efficacious in producing an antibody response, and if intramuscular rather than subcutaneous delivery will result in a lower incidence of local reaction without decreasing the immune response.

In 1999, $51 million was appropriated to the Department of Health and Human Services (DHHS) by Congress for development of vaccine and drug stockpiles [33]. For smallpox, there are 15.4 million doses of vaccine available, but fewer than 7 million may remain effective after years of storage. There is enough vaccinia immune globulin to treat serious vaccinia reactions in less than 1000 people. Before the recent bioterrorist attacks on the United States, Acambis had been funded by DHHS to produce 40 million doses of a cell culture-derived vaccinia vaccine [10]. More recently, 155 million doses of smallpox vaccine, enough for every US citizen if needed, has been ordered through Acambis and Baxter International (Cambridge, Massachusetts). Delivery is expected in the fall of 2002. The CDC has also recently updated the smallpox containment strategy, basing the planned response on the smallpox eradication campaign.

Future challenges include not only the development of better vaccines but also better maintenance of adequate supplies and rapid, effective distribution systems. With vaccines there is broad overlap between current public health issues and bioterrorism defense. The public health community has traditionally been heavily involved in vaccine efforts and has a great deal of experience to share in this field. Targeted pre-attack vaccination of first-responder and emergency personnel, combined with a coordinated distribution plan post-exposure, may prove valuable for selected high-risk biological agents once new, rapid genetic production methods become accepted [34].

Decontamination

Decontamination is unlikely to be of any significant value with any of the probable bioterrorism agents. For additional information on decontamination issues, see chapter by Drs. Fred Henretig, Cieslak, Kortepeter, and Fleisher in this issue. Anthrax is probably only infectious during primary aerosolization; secondary aerosolization may not occur to any significant degree. An analysis of the Sverdlosk epidemic curve does not suggest cases resulting from secondary aerosolization. Exposed persons should wash their skin and clothes with soap and warm water [35]. Anthrax spores, however, may survive in the environment for some time. Bioengineered microbial methods of decontaminating the environment are in development [36]. Other developments include novasomes (microscopic liposomes) to dissolve pathogens that may be used topically or may be inhaled or ingested (as protection for soldiers or first responders to a domestic attack), or possibly to decontaminate food and water. These agents appear to be safe and effective topically [37].

Environmental decontamination is also problematic for some bioterrorist agents. Although agents such as smallpox, plague, and botulinum toxin have a short half-life in the environment, other agents can remain stable in the environment for long periods of time. In the case of anthrax, the spores may remain stable for many years. Decontaminating the environment must proceed with forethought and care; tragically, using air pressure to clean postal offices may have re-aerosolized anthrax spores. Finally, as seen with the Hart building, decontamination procedures must take valuable art and other objects into consideration.

Better personal protection devices are also needed, as current devices are cumbersome and fatiguing [38]. Examples of attempts to develop new approaches are a helmet that uses a photo-electrochemical reactor, and an advanced toxic environment combat helmet that also incorporates improved communication measures [39]. Another proposal is for the use of a simple biological facemask, possibly even for civilian use, especially in high-risk areas [40].

Antimicrobial agents

Historically, biowarfare agents have been modified to be resistant to multiple antibiotics. In addition, multi-resistant nosocomial infections are a major emerging public health threat. The Defense Advanced Research Projects Agency (DARPA), in its Unconventional Pathogen Countermeasures program, and USAMRIID, are sponsoring several projects that not only have great potential in combating bioterrorism but also in making advances in public health and medical science. Several researchers are looking for new bacterial targets found across a broad range of pathogens that would not only provide defense against a biowarfare agent but would represent new classes of broad spectrum antibiotics. Development of new antiviral drugs may progress much more rapidly in the future in part through Department of Defense (DOD) activities supporting current HIV and hepatitis research.

Given the urgency of producing new vaccines and medications to combat bioterrorism, the Food and Drug Administration (FDA) is assisting research by participating in an interagency bioterrorism preparation group. This group includes other members such as the Veterans Administration, DOD, DHHS, CDC, National Institutes of Health, and the Office of Emergency Preparedness. The Federal Drug Administration is also doing research in many relevant areas, including how to facilitate review of new vaccines and immunoglobulins, for example, and when it is reasonable to accept animal data instead of human data in the case of countermeasures for which efficacy cannot be tested in humans [41].

Healthcare professionals' education and system preparedness issues

A domestic bioterrorist attack is unprecedented in differing from conventional military or terrorist actions, because the first responders are likely to be physicians and not law enforcement personnel [33]. Thus, education of civilians in the medical and public health field is essential for an appropriate response. Although federal programs have focused heavily on first-responder communities in weapons of mass destruction (WMD) training (eg, Metropolitan Medical Response Teams and the National Institute of Justice Domestic Training Program in Anniston, Alabama), hospital-based and primary care medical personnel have received little preparedness training.

Hospital-based personnel are important, because acutely ill patients representing the earliest cases after a covert attack will likely seek care in EDs. Less ill patients at the onset of an illness may also seek care in primary care facilities. Physicians, nurses, and physician extenders must therefore be trained in recognition and early treatment of biological casualties, and must understand and be able to carry out their roles and responsibilities in the event of a terrorist attack [42]. An optimally prepared medical community will have addressed the educational needs of all these groups, including the important interaction between public health and healthcare providers.

There is a general absence of disaster and biological casualty management in medical school curricula, and few (if any) American Board of Medical Specialty examinations include certification questions in this field. The American Medical Association's Council on Scientific Affairs has been charged with getting physicians more involved in community-wide planning before a bioterrorism crisis occurs. Clearly, if we are to directly improve the education of physicians and hospital-based personnel, appropriate continuing education programs must be developed and implemented [43]. Coroners, pathologists, and medical examiners also need to be educated on the pathologic features of the most likely bioterrorist agents because they may be the first to recognize an outbreak. Radiologists and infection control practitioners should become more aware of agents of biological terrorism and their clinical presentations. Anthrax, for instance, has characteristic pathology such as hemorrhagic mediastinitis and meningitis that may be the first clues to add it to the differential diagnosis. Coroners and medical examiners also need to know how to handle deaths and resources following an attack and must have access to appropriate diagnostic tools [44].

The American College of Emergency Physicians has recently completed a WMD curriculum design under contract with DHHS that includes objectives, content, and competencies for EMTs and ED personnel for situations involving nuclear, biological, or chemical incidents [45]. The Agency for Health Care Research and Quality is providing support for several prominent academic and commercial contractors who are developing innovative educational strategies for training clinicians to respond to a bioterrorism attack. USAMRIID and USMRICD have produced live, interactive satellite distance learning programs that have reached out to military and civilian healthcare providers. USAMRIID's medical response to biological warfare and terrorism program has trained nearly 55,000 healthcare workers.

Hospital and system preparedness

State public health systems continue to be underfunded. Public health systems will benefit in other ways from preparations for bioterrorism [46]. In a recent survey of hospitals in four states by Wetter et al, overall preparedness was shown to be inadequate; specifically, less than 20% had plans for a chemical or biological attack, and only 64% had enough antibiotics on hand to treat 50 cases of anthrax [100]. Although all US hospitals are required to have a disaster plan, the extent of planning is variable. Traditional disaster management involves augmenting resources. Excessive resources can complicate a disaster response. Area hospitals tend not to communicate well with each other in their response plans. A community-wide disaster plan involving the area hospitals and other emergency community agencies improves disaster operational knowledge. Another suggested approach is to plan for likely events and to anticipate "planned improvisation" for events that are unlikely [48]. Frequent drills for chemical events have helped revise and improve disaster plans, and have reduced staff anxiety regarding the outcome of a chemical event [49]. Drills for biological events are far more complicated, but developing them is indispensable in developing response plans, improving communication, and improving staff role acceptance. Many experts in the natural disaster field are moving toward mitigation in addition to incident response. Mitigation involves minimizing the effects of a disaster before, during, and after, whereas response is merely minimizing the suffering post-consequence [50].

Many hospitals operate near capacity on a daily basis and had little flexibility even to accommodate the increased burden of the 1999–2000 flu season [51]. During a bioterrorism outbreak with a significant number of casualties, additional hospital capacity will likely be required, and planning efforts defining operating procedures during this period are needed.

There may be lessons we can learn from other types of disasters. For instance, in the Oklahoma bombing, many victims, rather than panicking, assisted search and rescue teams. The overloaded telephone lines impeded communication and thus runners were used to help facilitate transfer and discharge decisions within the hospital. Less seriously injured victims were often brought to the closest hospital in private cars, and critically injured patients were moved by way of ambulance to more distant hospitals to balance patient load. Volunteer physicians and nurses recruited to new facilities needed assistance in areas such as finding supplies. Thus, stationing a person who was familiar with the supply area was helpful. Other lessons learned included the need to plan ahead for staffing, addressing stress early, and the need for a patient tracking system [52]. In staged exercises, computerized patient identification band bar coding to facilitate registration and diagnosis has been studied. Patient identification information, diagnostic information, and location and time of presentation were entered. Tests during exercises showed improved quantity and accuracy of information from these resources [53].

The sarin attack in Tokyo also produced some useful lessons, such as pointing out the need for disaster drills for relevant organizations, regional mediators, and a real-time multi-directional communication system. Multiple means of communication are necessary, such as television, radio, personal pagers, satellites, and other means. EMTs in Tokyo had to use public phones to coordinate patient movement. Appropriate protective wear must be available for in-hospital and out-of-hospital providers; in Tokyo, staff suffered secondary contamination from off-gassing of sarin [54,55]. Hospital staff may be subject to infection with some bioterrorist agents. Fortunately anthrax is not communicable, but smallpox, the worst-case scenario from a communicable disease standpoint, is highly contagious. How will hospital staff react to possible exposure? Will they be less likely to come to work? Should there be a prophylactically vaccinated group of volunteer healthcare workers to respond to a crisis?

Future challenges include involving more physicians and other medical staff in preparations for bioterrorism and continuing to move from a HAZ-MAT/first responder model to an ED/hospital provider model with less emphasis on decontamination and more emphasis on diagnosis [56]. Other aspects of preparedness include logistic concerns such as infrastructure, including hospital beds, quarantine facilities, and stockpiling of pharmaceuticals and supplies. Finally, the unresolved challenge still exists of how to prepare the community. When should quarantine be implemented? Should there be a single designated hospital per community for victims of a bioterrorist attack? How should we protect providers? Physicians and other healthcare providers will be the first responders in a biological attack and must be aware of the possibility of bioterrorism and become involved in preparations and policy.

Media and public education and preparedness

The media must be educated on how to support the response to an attack rather than providing sensationalist coverage that can promote panic. In a smallpox attack, for instance, without adequate vaccine, quarantine may be our best defense. The media could be extremely useful in educating civilians on the need for this, or extremely harmful in promoting panic and rioting over the limited supply of vaccine. Sensationalist coverage has also been associated with an increased incidence of copycat hoaxes, for example, after the Aum Shinrikyo sarin attack in Tokyo [1]. In the event of an attack, some experts recommend a centralized joint information and operations center to supply the media with consistent and credible information [57]. Public health, medical, and law enforcement agencies should form relationships with the media that facilitate constructive information to educate but not frighten citizens.

The public must understand the risk and response balance to properly prepare for correct actions during a bioterrorist attack. Increased public awareness currently is due in large part to the recent anthrax incidents and in small part to popular movies and novels, the latter of which take certain factual liberties, often resulting in non-scientifically based responses [51]. The better the public understands the threat and response before an attack, the more rational will be their response after an attack. Prior data on public preparedness for bioterrorism is limited. We must carefully examine the usefulness of preparedness efforts that are not strongly linked to long lasting and parallel improvements in public health and protection from naturally occurring disease outbreaks. Improved biological preparedness, especially among hospital-based personnel and public health authorities, will improve our ability to recognize natural and man-made infectious outbreaks earlier, lessening casualties and improving chances for preventing further spread.

Communication

There is a need to include the healthcare community as part of the medical intelligence network, and to alert the medical community of any threatened bioterrorist attacks. The importance of a good, pre-existing communication plan with a clear, widely understood and practiced chain of authority cannot be overemphasized. In analyses of the Tokyo sarin subway disaster and simulations of possible attacks in the United States, the lack of clear communication, unclear legal issues, and an uncertain chain of authority stand out as key factors in promoting confusion and hampering rapid and efficient patient care [58–60]. In the future, satellite-based handheld terminals for phone, fax, and internet access will provide additional technologies to facilitate communication [61].

Legislative activity

The steps in jurisdiction and prosecution following an attack are being clarified. Until recently, deliberate infection of another person with a biological agent or intentional contamination of food and water was not even illegal. The legal authority of public health officials and the CDC is unclear. Public health authority varies by state and most power rests with states and localities. A significant lesson learned from the Operation TOPOFF exercise of May 2000 was that leadership and decision-makers were hindered by a lack of understanding between agencies regarding operating procedures and lack of an ability to rapidly identify key contacts. Clarification of roles and responsibilities in surveillance, biodetection, communication, consequence management, and other operational aspects is needed, especially at the local level. Other legal issues raised by TOPOFF include quarantine, forced treatment, vaccination, and travel limitations [58]. A thorough discussion of the legal issues is beyond the scope of this article.

Future research

Not only can bioterrorism defense research borrow from advances in better understanding and treatment of HIV, hepatitis, and cancer, but the converse is also true. Many of the future biotechnologic innovations and developments may benefit other current medical and public health problems. Research to facilitate preclinical diagnosis of infection with a biowarfare agent through early human or microbial gene products, or early cytokine production, is of use for a variety of important microbes. Antimicrobial resistance is of growing worldwide significance in hospitals and long-term care facilities, and development of new antimicrobials is of great importance. Furthermore, some biodefense researchers are investigating entirely new concepts regarding ways of combating infection through immune system augmentation and genetic microbial targets. The knowledge gained can contribute to the development of therapies for emerging infections such as HIV and prion diseases, to prolonging the survival of organs after transplantation, and to discovering more effective cancer chemotherapies. Much of the basic science research into bioterrorism defense is potentially of extremely broad use throughout medicine.

Cytokines and pre-clinical diagnostics

One study noted increased serum levels of tumor necrosis factor (TNF) alpha, interleukin (IL)-6, and nitric oxide (NO) among emergency room patients with sepsis who were admitted, compared with septic patients who were discharged. Levels of these cytokines were also elevated in patients with sepsis compared with patients with non-infectious systemic inflammatory immune response (SIRS) [62]. Other proinflammatory and anti-inflammatory mediators or markers involved in sepsis include prostaglandins, leukotrienes, cytokines, especially IL-6, -8, and -18, procalcitonin, type I phospholipase A2 propeptide, endorphins, histamine, serotonins, platelets, neutrophils, macrophages, monocytes, complement, protein kinase, tyrosine kinase, toxic oxygen metabolites, endotoxin, neopterin, plasminogen activator inhibitor-1 CD 14, vasoactive neuropeptides, monocyte chemoattractant protein, IL-1 receptor antagonist, type 2 IL-1 receptor, IL-4, -10, and -13, transforming growth factor beta, NO, soluble TNF receptor, soluble CD 14, lipopolysaccharide binding protein, and defensins [63–66]. The role of these factors in pathogenesis of disease is being studied. Much of this research involves searching for ways to mediate the severity of the inflammatory response. The unraveling of the cytokine story may be applicable to bioterrorism defense research in two ways. There are suggestions that qualitative patterns of elevation or the gene expression that precedes it may provide early signatures for specific disease agents. Simultaneous testing of multiple factors may improve sensitivity and specificity. Furthermore, immunomodulation of the body's response to sepsis may prove to be of use in treating victims of a biological attack.

Other means of preclinical diagnosis currently being researched are immunoassays, advanced PCR techniques, evaluation of host response, and time-of-flight mass spectrometry. Immunoassays are quick and simple to perform; however, searching for the host immune response may be of limited usefulness in early diagnosis because the immune response does not develop for days to more than a week in most infections. Of more use may be immunologic techniques to look for pathogenic antigens, perhaps through using samples obtained by swabbing nasal mucosa [67]. PCR has undergone immense development in the past 10 years. Other research is attempting to identify common microbial gene products expressed early in infection to treat preclinical infections [68]. Gene "chips" are being developed that might make possible a broad range of diagnostic tests from a single blood sample. A chip might eventually allow for the simultaneous assessment of genetic material from, or stimulated by, multiple pathogens in the ED or critical care unit in less than 30 minutes [47]. Data suggest that different pathogens induce different host genes. Thus, the immediate specific identification of the pathogen may not be necessary to begin treatment, but rapid PCR to determine the host response may allow for determination of the type of infection even before changes in cytokine levels are observed [69,70]. These methods are limited in the sense that one must be looking for a specific pathogen to find it. Mass spectrometry for preclinical diagnosis may overcome this difficulty but is early in research and development for these biological pathogen-screening purposes [71].

Continued research in the area of rapid preclinical diagnosis is important for several reasons. Some diseases caused by biological agents are treatable if diagnosed early. Some, such as anthrax, are probably only treatable before the development of signs and symptoms. The worried well can be safely triaged if it can be confirmed that they were not exposed. If the disease is preventable with post-exposure vaccine but not treatable with anti-microbial agents (eg, smallpox), then limited vaccine supplies may need to be distributed to have the greatest benefit, and individuals not exposed can be spared unnecessary quarantine. Without a way to identify who has been infected, all who have been possibly exposed may be subjected to quarantine. Limited supplies of drugs or vaccines can be used most effectively if the diagnosis can be made before clinical onset or early in the disease.

Antimicrobials

Under sponsorship by DARPA, researchers are investigating the potential of developmental proteins in limiting the cellular damage of viral infection. In vitro studies have demonstrated not only a broad spectrum of antiviral effects, but also inhibition of breast cancer and lung cancer cell growth [72]. The antiviral effect of pokeweed antiviral protein to combat bioterrorist viral agents, HIV and CMV is under scrutiny [73]. Research is being done to develop intracellular antibodies to treat CMV and potentially threat viruses [74]. Other investigators are targeting a viral RNA polymerase in efforts to find a new antiviral agent [75]. Many other groups, also sponsored by DARPA, are investigating antiviral compounds [76,77]. The dual purpose of bioterrorism funding is thus demonstrated again. Not only will this research help in limiting the effects of bioterrorism agents, but it will also contribute to treatment of HIV and CMV and provide insight into cancer research.

High throughput screening is being researched to find a way to inhibit FtsZ, a tubulin-like GTPase important in bacterial cell division [78]. Other investigators are also using molecular libraries and computerized software to locate microbial-specific essential RNA sequences and to design targeted drugs [79,80]. Another project to target a newly discovered DNA-methylating enzyme common to *B. abortus* and several other pathogens is underway [81].

Recently isolated is a dominant negative mutant protective antigen, a component of anthrax toxin. The mutant subunit assembles with wild-type subunits and blocks a necessary conformation of the toxin. Results in vivo with rats are encouraging, and suggest that this mutant subunit may be a possible therapy for anthrax. Furthermore, as the mutant subunit is similar to the current vaccine, it may also induce immunity [82]. Other current research concepts include the use of large random peptide libraries to screen for possible antitoxins to superantigens such as Staph enterotoxin B [82], to block the induction of cytokines [83], or to elicit protective immunity [84].

The CDC now has contracted with pharmaceutic providers and has stockpiles of drugs and antidotes, and agreements with the industry for rapid production. The current plans are to stock enough antibiotics to treat 10 million humans for six weeks, to pretreat after anthrax exposure [9]. Shelf-life issues make stockpiling expensive, however. Research is being done in stockpiling subunits of DNA- and RNA-binding antimicrobials for rapid assembly and synergy [85].

Immunomodulators

Conversely, another concept is to use immunomodulators to stimulate the body's own immune system. There may be synergies with ongoing clinical research with HIV-infected patients. Patients with HIV are deficient in CD4 cells that regulate cell-mediated immunity (CMI) and humoral immunity. HIV patients are thus more susceptible to viral, bacterial, and fungal disease. Several agents have been shown to successfully treat cutaneous viral infections in HIV patients. For example, Imiquimod for genital warts (HSV2) and aliretinoin gel for Kaposi's sarcoma (HHV8) work through immunostimulation [86]. Imiquimod has no antiviral effects in vitro but induces cytokines, including interferon alpha, tumor necrosis factor-alpha, G-CSF, GM-CSF, interferon gamma, IL12, and Langerhan's cells [87].

A potential approach to treating infections is to focus not on killing the microorganism, but on limiting the cellular and organic damage they cause. For instance, most of the pathologic changes from tuberculosis are caused not by the bacteria but by the immune system's response to it. Alpha-melanocyte–stimulating hormone peptides, which are neuroimmunumodulators, not only help modulate inflammation but also slow viral and bacterial growth; these peptides are under investigation [88]. Nitric oxide can mediate cellular injury in infection; research is being conducted in inhibiting the production of nitric oxide and scavenger peroxynitrite, a related mediator of cellular injury [89].

Several other compounds are potentially of interest in the event of biological warfare with an agent for which there is no specific therapy. GCSF (granulocyte-colony stimulating factor), which is a factor produced by many cell types, works by augmenting the differentiation of neutrophils, recruiting neutrophils, and by stimulating the function of neutrophils. It is used in patients with granulocytopenia, such as after myelosuppressive chemotherapy, to hasten recovery, and may also be of benefit in non-neutropenic patients [90]. GCSF seems to be safe in patients with pneumonia and severe sepsis or septic shock. [91] GCSF may potentially be of use in treating other severe infections. Finally, ways to use CpG motifs (a DNA molecular pattern specific to microbes) to activate the innate immune system rapidly and non-specifically to a wide variety of microorganisms are being investigated [92]. Other researchers are also investigating ways to augment the immune system's ability to fight viral infection while limiting physiologic damage [93].

Old concepts for treating bacterial disease are being rediscovered. An effort is underway to investigate the potential uses of bacteriophage (viruses that infect bacteria) as therapeutic agents or in vaccine production [94]. Finally, new technologies are being developed to treat old bacterial infections. Research is ongoing into inhibiting the expression of pathogenic virulent genes in infected host cells with DNA nanobinders, compounds that bind to specific DNA sequences [95,96,97].

Summary

The future success of our preparations for bioterrorism depends on many issues as presented in this article. If these issues are properly addressed, the resulting improvements in bioterrorism preparations will allow us to better deter and mitigate a bioterrorism incident and will also provide us with the added benefit of improvements in early detection, diagnosis, and treatment of natural disease outbreaks. Emergency physicians must take an active leading role in working with the various disciplines to produce a better-prepared community.

References

[1] Tucker J. Historical trends related to bioterrorism: an empirical analysis. Emerg Infect Dis 1999;4:498–504.

[2] Alibek K. Biohazard. New York: Dell Publishing; 1999.

[3] Jackson R, Ramsay A, Christensen C, et al. Expression of mouse interleukin 4 by a recombinant ectromelia virus suppresses cytolytic lymphocytic responses and overcomes genetic resistance to mousepox. J Virol 2001;75:1205.

[4] Zilinskas R. Bioethics and biologic weapons. Science 1998;279:635.

[5] Fine A, Layton M. Lessons from the West Nile Viral encephalitis outbreak in New York City, 1999: implications for bioterrorism preparedness. Clin Infect Dis 2001;32:277.

[6] Sharp T, Brennan R, Keim M, et al. Medical preparedness for a terrorist incident involving chemical and biological agents during the 1996 Atlanta Olympic games. Ann Emerg Med 1998;32:214.

[7] Mckee K, Shields T, Jenkins P, et al. Application of a geographical information system to the tracking and control of an outbreak of shigellosis. Clin Infect Dis 2000;31:728.

[8] DARPA epidemiology software used during presidential inauguration. DARPA news release.

[9] Khan A, Morse S, Lillibridg S. Public health preparedness for biological terrorism in the USA. Lancet 2000;356:1179.

[10] Pavlin J. Epidemiology of bioterrorism. Emerg Infect Dis 1999;5:528.

[11] Bryan J, Fields H. An ounce of prevention is worth a pound of cure—shoring up the public health infrastructure to respond to bioterrorist attacks. AJIC 1999;27:465.

[12] Hamburg M. Addressing bioterrorist threats: where do we go from here? Emerg Infect Dis 1999;5:564.

[13] Macintyre A, Christopher G, Eitzen E, et al. Weapons of mass destruction events with contaminated casualties: effective planning for health care facilities. JAMA 2000;283:242.

[14] Torok T, Tauxe R, Wise R, et al. A large community outbreak of salmonellosis caused by intentional contamination of restaurant salad bars. JAMA 1997;278(5):389–95.

[15] Anderson G, King K, Gaffney K, et al. Multi-analyte interrogation using the fiber optic biosensor. Biosens Bioelectron 2000;14:771.

[16] Rowe C, Scruggs S, Feldstein M, et al. An array immunosensor for simultaneous detection of clinical analytes. Anal Chem 1999;71:433.

[17] Pourahmadi F, Taylor M, Kovacs G, et al. Toward a rapid, integrated, and fully auto-mated DNA diagnostic assay for *Chlamydia trachomatis* and *Neisseria gonorrhoeae*. Clin Chem 2000;46:1511.

[18] Guiliano K. Fluorotox system: rapid toxicological assessment of biological threats.

[19] Bayne P, Zdanovsky A. Rapid sensitive universal detection system for biological agents of mass-destruction. Accessed July 11, 2001.

[20] Demirev P, Ho Y, Ryzhov V, et al. Microorganism identification by mass spectrometry and protein database searches. Anal Chem 1999;71:2732.

[21] Hill S, Pinnick R, Niles S, et al. Real-time measurement of fluorescence spectra from single airborne biological particles. Field Analytical Chem Technol 1999;3:221.

[22] Hart K, Wise M, Griess W. Design development and performance of a fieldable chemical and biological agent detector. Field Analytical Chem Technol 2000;2:93.

[23] Iqbal S, Mayo M, Bruno J. A review of molecular recognition technologies for detection of biological threat agents. Biosensors and Bioelectronics 2000;15:549.

[24] State labs flunk tests on spotting anthrax.

[25] Bartlett J. Applying lessons learned from anthrax case history to other scenarios. Emerg Infect Dis 1999;5:561.

[26] Peterson L, Hamilton J, Baron E, et al. Role of clinical microbiology laboratories in the management and control of infectious diseases and the delivery of health care. Clin Infect Dis 2001;32:605.

[27] Gilchrist M. A national laboratory network for bioterrorism: evolution from a prototype network of laboratories performing routine surveillance. Mil Med 2000;165:28.

[28] Jones T, Craig A, Hoy D, et al. Mass psychogenic illness attributed to toxic exposure at a high school. N Engl J Med 2000;342:96.

[29] Russell P. Vaccines in civilian defense against bioterrorism. Emerg Infect Dis 5:531.

[30] Cieslak J, Christopher G, Kortepeter M, et al. Immunization against potential biological warfare agents. Clin Infect Dis 2000;30:843.

[31] Shafazand S, Doyle R, Ruoss S, et al. Inhalational anthrax: epidemiology, diagnosis and management. Chest 1999;116:1369.

[32] Friedlander A, Pittman P, Parker G. Anthrax vaccine: evidence for safety and efficacy against inhalational anthrax. JAMA 1999;282:2104.

[33] Henderson D. The looming threat of bioterrorism. Science 1999;283:1279.

[34] McDade J. Addressing the potential threat of bioterrorism: value added to an improved public health infrastructure. Emerg Infect Dis 1999;5:591.

[35] Inglesby T, Henderson D, JG B, et al. Anthrax as a biological weapon: medical and public health management. JAMA 1999;281:1735.

[36] Stemmer W, Longchamp P, Giver L, et al. Decontamination methods based on industrial enzymes optimized for killing of biological warfare spores.

[37] Baker J, Kukowska-Latallo J, Hayes M, et al. Molecular decoys to soak up pathogens.

[38] McClellan T. Work performance at 40 degrees C with Canadian Forces biological and chemical protective clothing. Aviation Space Environ Med 1993;64:1094.

[39] Pirich R, Hoffman M, Hofacre K, et al. Personal environmental protection system.

[40] Lowe K, Pearson G, Utgoff V. Potential values of a simple biological warfare protective mask. In: XXX, editors. Biological weapons: limiting the threat. Cambridge, MA: MIT press; 1999.

[41] Zoon K. Vaccines, pharmaceutical products and bioterrorism: challenges for the US Food and Drug Administration. Emerg Infect Dis 1999;5:534.

[42] Rega P. Disaster medical education for all physicians and physician extenders. Ann Emerg Med 2000;35:314.

[43] Cole T. When a bioweapon strikes who will be in charge? JAMA 2000;284:944.

[44] Nolte K, Yoon S, Pertowski C. Medical examiners, coroners, and bioterrorism. Emerg Infect Dis 2000;6:559.

[45] Waeckerle J, Seamans S, Whiteside M, et al. Developing objectives, content, and competencies for the training of emergency medical technicians, emergency physicians, and emergency nurses to care for casualties resulting from nuclear, biological or chemical (NBC) incidents [executive summary]. Ann Emerg Med 2001;37:587.

[46] Rosen P. Coping with bioterrorism is difficult but may help us respond to new epidemics. BMJ 2000;320:71.

[47] Wang J. Survey and summary: from DNA biosensor to gene chips. Nucl Acids Res 2000; 28:3011–6.

[48] Auf der Heide E. Disaster planning part II: disaster problems, issues and challenges identified in the research literature. Emerg Med Clin N Am 1996;14:453.

[49] Tur-Kaspa I, Lev E, Hendler I, et al. Preparing hospitals for toxicological mass casualties events. Crit Care Med 1999;27:1004.

[50] Mitigation emerges as major strategy for reducing losses caused by natural disasters. Board on Natural Disasters, 1943–1947; 1999.

[51] Schoch-Spana M. Implications of pandemic influenza for bioterrorism response. Clin Infect Dis 2000;31:1409.

[52] Anteau C, Williams L. The Oklahoma bombing: lessons learned. Crit Care Nurs Clin N Am 1997;9:231.

[53] Noondergraff G, Bouman J, Van Den Brink E, et al. Development of computer-assisted patient control for use in the hospital setting during mass casualty incident. Am J Emerg Med 1996;14:257.

[54] Okumura T, Kouichiro S, Atsauhiro F, et al. The Tokyo subway sarin attack: disaster management, part 3: national and international responses. Acad Emerg Med 1998; 5:625.

[55] Okumura T, Kouichiro S, A A, et al. The Tokyo subway sarin attack: disaster management, part 2: hospital response. Acad Emerg Med 1998;5:618.

[56] Waeckerle J. Domestic preparedness for events involving weapons of mass destruction. JAMA 2000;283:252.

[57] Bardi J. Aftermath of a hypothetical smallpox disaster. Emerg Infect Dis 1999;5:547.

[58] Inglesby T, Grossman R, O'Toole T. A plague on your city: observations from TOPOFF. Clin Infect Dis 2001;32:436–45.

[59] Okumura T, Suzuki K, Fukuda A, et al. The Tokyo subway sarin attack: disaster management, part 1: community emergency response. Acad Emerg Med 1998;5:613.

[60] O'Toole T. Smallpox: an attack scenario. Emerg Infect Dis 1999;5:540–6.

[61] Garshnek V, Burkle F. Telecommunications systems in support of disaster medicine: applications of basic information pathways. Ann Emerg Med 1999;34:212.

[62] Terregino C, Lopez B, Karras D, et al. Endogenous mediators in emergency department patients with presumed sepsis: are levels associated with progression to severe sepsis and death? Ann Emerg Med 2000;35:26.

[63] Symeonides S, Balk R. Bacterial sepsis and septic shock: nitric oxide in the pathogenesis of sepsis. Infect Dis Clin N Am 1999;13:449.

[64] Opal S, Cross A. Bacterial sepsis and septic shock: clinical trials for severe sepsis. Past failures and future hopes. Infect Dis Clin N Am 1999;13:285.

[65] Opal A, DePal V. Anti-inflammatory cytokines. Chest 2000;117:1162.

[66] Casey L. Immunologic response to infection and its role in septic shock. Crit Care Clin 2000;16:193.

[67] Hail A, Rossi C, Ludwig G, et al. Comparison of noninvasive sampling sites for early detection of *Bacillus anthracis* spores from rhesus monkeys after aerosol exposure. Mil Med 1999;164:833.

[68] Rosenberg M. Novel broad spectrum antimicrobial agents—gene expression.

[69] Cummings C, Relman D. Using DNA microarrays to study host-microbe interactions. Emerg Infect Dis 6:13.

[70] Diehn M, Relman DA. Comparing functional genomic datasets: lessons from DNA microarray analyses of host-pathogen interactions. Curr Opin Microbiol 2001;4:95.

[71] Nelson R, Nedelkoy D, Tubbs K. Biosensor chip mass spectrometry: a chip-based proteomics approach. Electrophoresis 2000;6:1155.

[72] Barnea E, Leavis P, Choi Y, et al. Developmental proteins to prevent human injury from pathogens.

[73] Uckun F. Pokeweed antiviral protein as a universal virus neutralizer.

[74] Ghazal P, Burton D. Invasive (intracellular) antibodies.

[75] Kirkegaard K, Richmond K, Kim C, et al. A common target for positive-strand RNA viruses.

[76] Shope R. Structure-based design of acute countermeasures to viruses.

[77] Kornguth S, Niber M, Dahlberg J, et al. Non peptide antiviral agents that interdict host cell transport.

[78] Kirschner K, Evans L, Chaudhuri D. To exploit the essential cell division protein FtsZ as a broad spectrum anti-bacterial target.

[79] Griffey R, Ecker D. Universal pathogen countermeasures.

[80] Ecker D. Drugs to protect against engineered biological warfare bacteria.

[81] Shapiro L. Novel targets of pathogen vulnerability.

[82] Sellman B, Mourez M, Collier R. Dominant-negative mutants of a toxin subunit: an approach to therapy of anthrax. Science 2001;292:695.

[83] Kaempfer R. Superantigen toxin antagonist and vaccine.

[84] Cohen S, Leppla S. Creating cellular resistance to toxins in mammals.

[85] Bruice T. Stockpiling drug subunits for rapid response to biological warfare.

[86] Conant M. Immunomodulatory therapy in the management of viral infections in patients with HIV infection. J Am Acad Dermatol 2000;43:S27–30.

[87] Sauder D. Immunomodulatory and pharmacologic properties of imiquimod. J Am Acad Dermatol 2000;43:S6–11.

[88] Lipton J, Lipton M. Neuroimmunomodulatory alpha-MSH peptides.

[89] Southan G, Salzmann A. Mercaotiethylguanide: a revolutionary generic immunomodulatory countermeasure for biological warfare defense.

[90] Van der Poll T. The use of granulocyte colony-stimulating factor in critically ill patients. Crit Care Med 2000;28:3758.

[91] Wunderink R, Leeper K, Schein R, et al. Filgrastim in patients with pneumonia and severe sepsis or septic shock. Chest 2001;119:523.

[92] Krieg A. Activation of innate immunity by CpG DNA for broad spectrum protection against pathogens.

[93] Scadden D, Seed B, Walker B. Super immune cells.

[94] Mekalanos J, Tobias J, Lin W, et al. Novel bacteriophage therapies for Vibrio cholerae infection.

[95] Tanaka R. Genetic countermeasures: regulation of pathogen gene expression by DNA-binding polyamides.

[96] Centers for Disease Control and Prevention. Bioterrorism alleging use of anthrax and interim guidelines for management—United States, 1998. JAMA 1999;281:787.

[97] Gupta G. Structural biology of bacterial toxins.

[98] Osterholm M. Bioterrorism: media hype or real potential nightmare? AJIC 1999;27:461.

[99] Stern J. The prospect of domestic bioterrorism. Emerg Infect Dis 1999;5:517.

[100] Wetter D, Daneill W, Treser C-S. Hospital preparedness for victims of chemical or biological terrorism. Am J Public Health 91:710.

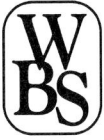

EMERGENCY
MEDICINE
CLINICS OF
NORTH AMERICA

Emerg Med Clin N Am
20 (2002) 525–535

Index

Note: Page numbers of article titles are in **bold face** type.

A

Advanced Trauma Life Support, for diagnosis of multiple trauma victims, 353
    secondary survey, expansion of, 356–362
    traditional survey, expansion of, 356

Alphaviruses, clinical presentation of, 317–318
    diagnostic testing in, 318
    treatment of, 318

Anthrax, bioterrorism-related inhalational, 280, 281
    clinical presentation of, 278
    cutaneous, 278–279
    diagnosis of, 280–282
    endemic inhalational, 279–280
    gastrointestinal, 279
    history and significance of, 274–278
    in children, diagnosis and treatment of, 379–380
    in pregnancy, treatment of, 372
    infection control precautions and, 282–283
    terrorism involving, 332
    treatment and prophylaxis of, 283–284

Anthrax Vaccine Adsorbed, 283–284

Antibiotic therapy, for children, in bacterial agents of bioterrorism, 386
    in bacterial agents of terrorism in pregnancy, 371–372, 373–374

Antimicrobials, bioterrorism defense research and, 518–519
    biowarfare agents and, 512
    in pregnancy, risk categories of, 369

Antiterrorism, federal programs and, 482–485

Arena viruses, 376–377

Aum Shinrikyo, contamination of Tokyo subway system by, 262

B

Bacillus anthracis. See *Anthrax.*

Biologic agent(s), critical, Centers for Disease Control and Prevention 1997 study
    and, 265
    identification of, in biologic agent-caused syndromes, 331

Changing Your Address?

Make sure your subscription changes too! When you notify us of your new address, you can help make our job easier by including an exact copy of your Clinics label number with your old address (see illustration below.) This number identifies you to our computer system and will speed the processing of your address change. Please be sure this label number accompanies your old address and your corrected address—you can send an old Clinics label with your number on it or just copy it exactly and send it to the address listed below.

We appreciate your help in our attempt to give you continuous coverage. Thank you.

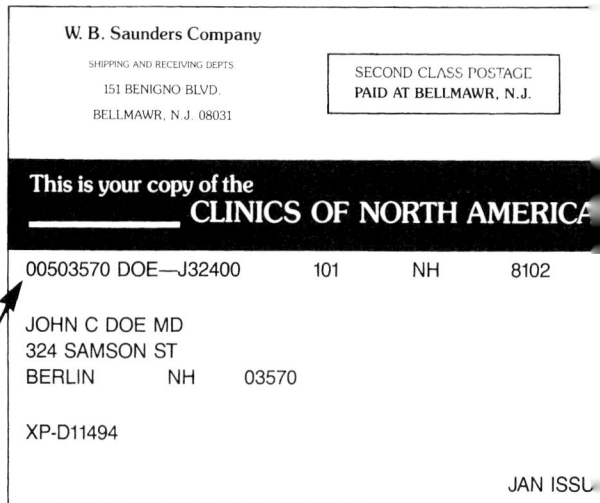

W. B. Saunders Company

SHIPPING AND RECEIVING DEPTS.
151 BENIGNO BLVD.
BELLMAWR, N.J. 08031

| SECOND CLASS POSTAGE |
| PAID AT BELLMAWR, N.J. |

This is your copy of the
_____ CLINICS OF NORTH AMERICA

| 00503570 DOE—J32400 | 101 | NH | 8102 |

JOHN C DOE MD
324 SAMSON ST
BERLIN   NH   03570

XP-D11494

JAN ISSU

Your Clinics Label Number
Copy it exactly or send your label
along with your address to:
W.B. Saunders Company, Customer Service
Orlando, FL 32887-4800
Call Toll Free 1-800-654-2452

Please allow four to six weeks for delivery of new subscriptions and for processing address changes.